Chapman & Hall/CRC Biostatistics Series

Elementary Bayesian Biostatistics

T0248583

Chapman & Hall/CRC Biostatistics Series

Editor-in-Chief

Shein-Chung Chow, Ph.D.
Professor
Department of Biostatistics and Bioinformatics
Duke University School of Medicine
Durham, North Carolina, U.S.A.

Series Editors

Byron Jones
Senior Director
Statistical Research and Consulting Centre
(IPC 193)
Pfizer Global Research and Development
Sandwich, Kent, UK

Jen-pei Liu
Professor
Division of Biometry
Department of Agronomy
National Taiwan University
Taipei, Taiwan

Karl E. Peace
Director, Karl E. Peace Center for Biostatistics
Professor of Biostatistics
Georgia Cancer Coalition Distinguished Cancer Scholar
Georgia Southern University, Statesboro, GA

Chapman & Hall/CRC Biostatistics Series

Published Titles

1. *Design and Analysis of Animal Studies in Pharmaceutical Development,* Shein-Chung Chow and Jen-pei Liu
2. *Basic Statistics and Pharmaceutical Statistical Applications,* James E. De Muth
3. *Design and Analysis of Bioavailability and Bioequivalence Studies, Second Edition, Revised and Expanded,* Shein-Chung Chow and Jen-pei Liu
4. *Meta-Analysis in Medicine and Health Policy,* Dalene K. Stangl and Donald A. Berry
5. *Generalized Linear Models: A Bayesian Perspective,* Dipak K. Dey, Sujit K. Ghosh, and Bani K. Mallick
6. *Difference Equations with Public Health Applications,* Lemuel A. Moyé and Asha Seth Kapadia
7. *Medical Biostatistics,* Abhaya Indrayan and Sanjeev B. Sarmukaddam
8. *Statistical Methods for Clinical Trials,* Mark X. Norleans
9. *Causal Analysis in Biomedicine and Epidemiology: Based on Minimal Sufficient Causation,* Mikel Aickin
10. *Statistics in Drug Research: Methodologies and Recent Developments,* Shein-Chung Chow and Jun Shao
11. *Sample Size Calculations in Clinical Research,* Shein-Chung Chow, Jun Shao, and Hansheng Wang
12. *Applied Statistical Design for the Researcher,* Daryl S. Paulson
13. *Advances in Clinical Trial Biostatistics,* Nancy L. Geller
14. *Statistics in the Pharmaceutical Industry, Third Edition,* Ralph Buncher and Jia-Yeong Tsay
15. *DNA Microarrays and Related Genomics Techniques: Design, Analysis, and Interpretation of Experiments,* David B. Allsion, Grier P. Page, T. Mark Beasley, and Jode W. Edwards
16. *Basic Statistics and Pharmaceutical Statistical Applications, Second Edition,* James E. De Muth
17. *Adaptive Design Methods in Clinical Trials,* Shein-Chung Chow and Mark Chang
18. *Handbook of Regression and Modeling: Applications for the Clinical and Pharmaceutical Industries,* Daryl S. Paulson
19. *Statistical Design and Analysis of Stability Studies,* Shein-Chung Chow
20. *Sample Size Calculations in Clinical Research, Second Edition,* Shein-Chung Chow, Jun Shao, and Hansheng Wang
21. *Elementary Bayesian Biostatistics,* Lemuel A. Moyé
22. *Adaptive Design Theory and Implementation Using SAS and R,* Mark Chang

Other books by Lemuel A. Moyé

- *Statistical Reasoning in Medicine: The Intuitive P–Value Primer.*
- *Difference Equations with Public Health Applications* (with Asha S. Kapadia).
- *Multiple Analyses in Clinical Trials: Fundamentals for Investigators*
- *Finding Your Way in Science: How You Can Combine Character, Compassion, and Productivity in Your Research Career*
- *Probability and Statistical Inference: Applications, Computations, and Solutions* (with Asha S. Kapadia and Wen Chan)
- *Statistical Monitoring of Clinical Research: Fundamentals for Investigators*
- *Statistical Reasoning in Medicine: The Intuitive P–Value Primer. 2nd Edition*
- *Face to Face with Katrina Survivors: A First Responder's Tribute*

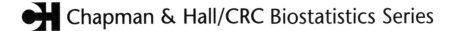

Chapman & Hall/CRC Biostatistics Series

Elementary Bayesian Biostatistics

Lemuel A. Moyé
University of Texas
Houston, U.S.A.

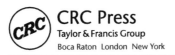

CRC Press
Taylor & Francis Group
Boca Raton London New York

CRC Press is an imprint of the
Taylor & Francis Group, an **informa** business

A CHAPMAN & HALL BOOK

CRC Press
Taylor & Francis Group
6000 Broken Sound Parkway NW, Suite 300
Boca Raton, FL 33487-2742

First issued in paperback 2019

ISBN-13: 978-1-58488-724-9 (hbk)
ISBN-13: 978-0-367-38879-9 (pbk)

Visit the Taylor & Francis Web site at
http://www.taylorandfrancis.com

and the CRC Press Web site at
http://www.crcpress.com

To Dixie and the DELTS

Contents

Preface

My fascination with the flexibility that Bayesian approaches offer the practicing biostatistician is one motivation for this book. If you have a moment, I'll share another.

The Bayes perspective carries a new and refreshing point of view about the field of biostatistics. Like a fresh spring breeze blowing through a room closed off all winter, inhaling its new, warm currents can be dizzying. Allowing scientists to focus on the hypothesis that they believe (rather than being forced to disprove what they don't believe) is a powerful attractor. Incorporating relevant prior information about the parameter of interest adds to the appeal. In fact, the common reaction of both physician-researchers and uninitiated biostatisticians to the Bayes approach is a sense of relief. Here, at last, is a collection of processes that fits their intuition and appreciation of the scientific method.

However, great hazard commonly accompanies great benefit; we must carefully examine the pitfalls of this alternative philosophy before falling into its embrace. The Bayes thought process is order shattering, overturning a paradigm that successfully dominated biostatistics throughout the twentieth century — that researchers in health care must separate belief from knowledge. This philosophical challenge to the frequentists' entrenched belief-set must be critically examined before abandoning ourselves to Bayes procedures in biology and medicine.

Whether you believe in the alternative Bayes perspective or not, the truth is that it's here. Bayesians are no longer banging at the door of accepted biostatistics, demanding to be let in; they are sitting across the table from us. Adaptive randomization and predictive power are each Bayesian procedures that have fought their way into the mainstream of clinical trial methodology. We, as health care scientists, must understand their interesting, sometimes natural, sometimes alien assumptions if we are to use them wisely in our work. Yet, unfortunately, there are no introductory textbooks on the modern Bayes perspective written for health care providers and researchers who themselves have a limited mathematics background.

Of course, elegant textbooks abound in this field. J.O. Berger's *Statistical Decision Theory* is a classic text. In fact, it was my textbook when I was a graduate student at Purdue University. However, its fine treatment requires a grasp of mathematics that many physicians lack. Other textbooks either do not focus on biostatistics, or delve into the material at a deeper mathematical level than most physicians and health care workers can stand. The writings of Dani Ganerman, Chen Ming-Hue Chen et al., Richardson Gilks et al., James H. Albert, B.P. Carlin et al., Gelman et al., each expertly focus on the computational procedures underpinning Bayes analyses. However, this important, technical topic is not the direct interest of the audience of this book.

My purpose was to write a treatment of Bayesian biostatistics that someone in health care without a strong calculus background could appreciate. This is a daunting task since at one point or another biostatistics involves calculations. Accepting this challenge required me to keep the mathematical computations in the background, or when appropriate, to embed them within a clear explanation. The product, I hope, resembles more of a conversation than a sequence of dry derivations.

Unique in its invented dialogue, Chapter Five requires a special explanation. The Bayesian-frequentist relationship has been a fractious one, with the history of debate going back to the eighteenth century. These vitriolic discussions sixty years ago sadly produced more heat than light. Yet, sharp debate can produce a clear view of a philosophy's jagged edges. Chapter Five portrays a fictitious debate between a cardiologist, and two statisticians; one Bayes, the other frequentist. The fictitious characters convey the intense feelings and beliefs that many contemporary workers in both fields experience, as well as conveying the merits and disadvantages of each approach in an educational but inoffensive manner.

Lemuel A. Moyé
University of Texas
School of Public Health
June 2007

Acknowledgments

My grandmother descended from one of the few North Carolina Cherokee who did not take the *Nunadautsun't* to the western reservations in Oklahoma. An important lesson she taught her grandchildren was never to begin the day until you have given thanks to God for the people He has placed in your life to guide you.

Kevin Sepulvida and several reviewers provided important advice and corrections for me. Dr. Claudia Pedroza, a Bayesian biostatistician and colleague, was frequently kind enough to take time from her busy schedule to discuss and debate my understanding of the modern Bayesian approach, sharpening my writing.

In addition, Kai Sun, Dawen Sui, and Charles Baimbridge provided important and careful edits of the chapters. More important, with the good impudence of graduate students, they challenged my approaches and discussions, leading to important changes in the manuscript as it evolved.

Finally, Dr. Stephen Stigler, the eminent historian of statistical sciences, kindly gave me permission along with the Bayes to use the only known picture of (someone reputed to be) Thomas Bayes. Ms. Prudence Board was particularly helpful with the final preparations for this book.

Finally, my dearest thanks go to Dixie, my wife, on whose personality, character, love, and common sense I have come to rely, and to my daughter Flora and her sister Bella, whose continued emotional and spiritual growth reveals anew to me each day that, through God, all things are possible.

Introd ction

Bayesian analyses have come of age in 21st century clinical investigation. Already well established in astrophysics, computer science, and business, Bayes procedures have blazed important inroads into modern health care research methods. Tools such as adaptive randomization and predictive power, both rooted in the Bayesian philosophy, have developed into useful statistical implements in modern clinical trials.

Recently, application of the Bayes approach to pharmaceutical and device development has attracted attention from regulatory agencies such as the U.S. Food and Drug Administration (FDA). This analytic philosophy is now accepted as a standard approach for the development of medical devices by the Center for Devices and Radiological Health (CDRH) of the FDA. Approximately 10% of FDA approvals for medical and radiological devices are based on Bayesian analysis, including spinal implants and cardiovascular stents.

The explosion of Bayes procedures in health care has compelled investigators to learn how to use them. However, many health care researchers struggle with the Bayesian approach. While the concept of prior information and loss functions is straightforward, how one combines them to generate insightful, defensible results is not. The absence of the typical hypothesis testing paradigm further disorients the researcher with only a short exposure to biostatistics.

Elementary Bayesian Biostatistics is an introduction to the modern world of Bayes procedures for the clinical scientist with a minimal background in biostatistics. This book offers the practicing biostatistician with no formal training in Bayes procedures a clear, uncomplicated overture to the topic and its application to health care research. Through its nonmathematical explanations of the basic concepts, it illustrates the use of the Bayesian thought process at an introductory level. This easy-to-read book brings the essentials of Bayesian statistics to those investigators who have the desire but not the background to understand the commonly available but more advanced treatments of Bayesian statistics.

The thesis of *Elementary Bayesian Biostatistics* is that clinical scientists with only a modicum of training in biostatistics and a limited exposure to calculus can understand Bayesian principles. Upon finishing the book, the investigator will be able to recognize if a health care research issue fits the Bayesian framework. If so, they can develop a prior distribution based on both the available medical literature and the experience of practitioners. In addition, the investigator will understand the role of the conditional and posterior distribution, and draw the most useful conclusions from their posterior distribution based on the intelligent choice of a loss function. This training will be provided building on only the basics of classic biostatistics and algebra. Derivations that require calculus are relegated to the appendix.

The Prologue, a must read for any scientist new to the Bayesian concept, reviews the interesting and controversial history of Bayes procedures. Describing the mysterious paper authored by the reverend who never intimated his work should be published, this prolusion depicts the controversies and obstacles that have obstructed the field's advance. In addition, the prologue delineates the fractious intellectual conflicts between the Bayesians of the 20th century and the "frequentists," who supported the hypothesis testing paradigm of Ronald Fisher.

Chapter One provides a review of probability, contrasting subjective and objective probability while motivating their use in both clinical investigation and practice. It also develops Bayes theorem from first principles, and provides several useful illustrations of its use.

Chapters Two and Three review the basic probability distributions commonly used in biostatistics. However, the cynosure of this work is the Law of Total Probability. The use of this tool serves not just as a stepping stone to the development of the posterior distribution; its application produces interesting probability distributions itself.

Chapter Four, entitled "Completing Your First Bayesian Computation" introduces the Bayes paradigm. It defines 1) the prior distribution, 2) the conditional distribution, and 3) the posterior distribution. Using elementary health care examples, the reader has the opportunity to examine the role of each of these three concepts in formulating the final Bayes solution. Since this is the natural point to introduce the influential effect of the prior distribution on the posterior distribution, examples allow the reader to observe how changes in the prior distribution influence the location and shape of the posterior distribution. These examples spark the development of intuition about Bayes procedures.

Chapter Five describes the differences between the frequentist and Bayes approach. With Chapter One's review of basic probability and statistics, and Chapter Four's Bayesian perspective as background, the reader is now in a position to compare the perspectives offered by each of these philosophies, and gauge which is most useful in a given circumstance. This chapter illuminates in a fair and balanced fashion the different emphases of the frequentist versus the Bayesian perspective. These are important messages that can be absorbed without a heavy mathematical preamble, and are necessary for the reader to internally integrate if they are to gain the skill to determine if a problem in health care research is a Bayesian problem or not (the topic of Chapter Eleven).

Chapter Six focuses on the generation of prior distributions. Discussion begins with three useful and ubiquitous prior distributions: uniform, beta, and normal. The use of mixture distributions, first introduced in Part I, is more completely developed here. Probability mixtures are a valuable resource to health care researchers who commonly feel that they must "make up their minds" about a single prior distribution (e.g., normal with $\mu = 13$ and $\sigma^2 = 5$). In addition, this chapter sharply differentiates between information available before a research effort begins from an investigator's beliefs and biases.

The concept of the loss function and Bayes risk is developed from an elementary level in Chapter Seven. While the examination begins with standard loss functions (e.g., linear loss and squared error loss), other functions more directly related to clinical interest will be provided. Chapter Eight offers several contemporaneous examples of the use of posterior distribution. Taking a step-by-step approach, this chapter converts the prior and conditional distributions into a posterior distribution, then uses the loss function to create the Bayes estimator δ_B. Sensitivity analysis, first discussed in Chapter Six, is developed here to demonstrate the relationship between choice of prior distributions and the selection of posterior distributions. The illustrations demonstrate how to select realistic choices for prior distributions.

Chapters Nine and Ten discuss two important implementations of Bayes procedures in clinical trials. Chapter Nine focuses on Bayesian sample size computations. Chapter Ten focuses on adaptive randomization and Bayes monitoring procedures for clinical trials. Each of these topics has surpassed the threshold of acceptance in the clinical research communities, and requires special treatment. In addition, a detailed reference list is provided that will ease the transition of the reader to the more advanced literature in the field.

Chapter Eleven is perhaps the most innovative chapter of the book. Entitled "Is My Problem a Bayes Problem?" it illustrates for the reader how to appraise a research scenario in health care to determine whether the frequentist or Bayesian perspective is most appropriate. This chapter recommends that the investigator consider whether the incorporation of available prior information and or a loss function will provide an appreciable update to the traditional frequentist solution. The book ends with a conclusion and commentary on the current implementation of Bayes procedures in health care.

Elementary Bayesian Biostatistics is the only book that the investigator will need for an understandable and balanced introduction to Bayes procedures in health care research.

Opening Salvos

Old Conflicts, New Wars

Open warfare swept across the great European landmass in ghastly waves that consumed entire cities. Hungry English citizens hunkered down on long stretches of frigid beaches awaiting invasion. Hundreds of miles to the east, Germans soldiers courageously battled hand-to-hand against Swedish and Russian troops for control of Berlin. War catapulted through the southern India territories to the rich eastern province of Bengal where British regulars engaged French corsairs in fierce, determined fighting. On the high seas, opposing fleets fought to the death for control of vital sea routes. In America, a British expeditionary army braved subzero weather in a daring invasion of Canada, while determined French guerrilla brigades along with skilled Native American forces picked off starving English loyalists in their isolated Ohio river outposts. Each belligerent nation had the same goal — total war for empire!

In Europe, the years of destruction were called The Seven Years War. In Asia, the conflict was known as The Great Carnatic War. In America, its name was The French and Indian War. It is only tradition that denies this conflagration the name it deserves — World War I [1]. And, in 1763, it was finally over.

Jubilation filled the streets of London as citizens and soldiers alike celebrated Britain's victory. The Treaty of Paris signified not just the end of the war; it announced Great Britain's insurmountable control of the seas, her undisputed control of India, and her dominance in Canada and the American colonies.

No celebrant in this season of victory noted the quiet, opening salvo of a different war. Its initiation heralded a mathematical and philosophical clash that would cycle through ever-growing intellectual explosions for over two hundred and forty years.

The first shots were not hot lead and buckshot — only wet ink and parchment. But, as in so many wars, confusion reigns over who actually fired the first shot.

Bayes' Quiet Bombshell

In 1763, a paper entitled, "An Essay Towards Solving a Problem in the Doctrine of Chances" appeared in the *Philosophical Transaction of the Royal Society of London* [2]. Few paid attention to the contents of this confusing paper. However, if a dogged reader persisted, they would have learned two remarkable things. First, its author was a reverend. Second, he was dead [3]! The Reverend Thomas Bayes, having published only three manuscripts during his entire life, died two years before the appearance of his final manuscript (Figure 1).

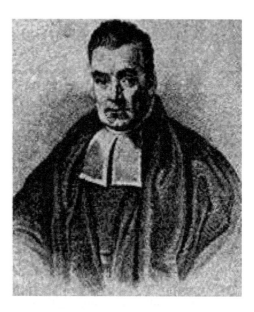

Figure 1. A drawing, commonly believed to be the Reverend Thomas
Bayes. Reprinted from www.bayesian.org/bayesian/bayes.html
with the permission of Dr. Stephen Stigler.

The mystery our determined detective-reader uncovers deepens upon learning that
the Reverend never submitted the paper for publication in the first place. In fact, the
manuscript languished among Bayes other writings and notes after his death. Waiting to be absorbed by the infinite urn of time, never to be read by others, they were
identified and resuscitated by his friend Richard Price.

Similarities and differences mark the relationship of these two men. Both
were ministers. Born in 1702, Thomas was the son of the nonconformist minister
Joshua Bayes. Nonrebellious, he followed his father into the ministry, becoming a
Presbyterian minister in the village of Tumbridge Wells (about twenty-five miles
south of London) at the age of twenty-nine. He published only two papers during
the course of his life, the first focusing on the ministry.[*] His second written in 1736,
entitled, "An Introduction to the Doctrine of Fluxions, and a Defense of the
Mathematicians Against the Objections of the Author of the Analyst", was a gentle
defense of Newton's calculus, a publication many believed earned him entrance
into the prestigious Royal Academy of Science. However, once admitted, he remained quiet and unremarkable, never publishing again for the remaining twenty-
five years of his life.

The rebellious, articulate Richard Price, however, was quite another matter. Also born into a family of ministers, Price quickly rejected the strict religious

---

[*] In 1731, Bayes published "Divine Benevolence, or an Attempt to Prove that the Principal
End of the Divine Providence and Government Is the Happiness of His Creatures."

teachings of his family. Openly rejecting the prevalent Christian doctrines of original sin and eternal damnation, he earned the ire of many traditionalists.

Undaunted, he entered the ministry himself, and upon reaching the pulpit, shared his iconoclastic convictions with his parishioners. Contending that individuals had the obligation to use not just the Bible, but their own conscience and the best of their reasoning skills to resolve a moral dilemma made him the focal point of local criticism. Undaunted, he went on to argue against the deity of His Majesty the King (Figure 2).

This outspoken iconoclast and the insular, enigmatic Bayes had two things in common. One was the ministry, although no doubt their theological views differed. The second was an affection for mathematics. While very little is left of Bayes work (a notebook that contains some brief astronomical observation, a table of logarithms, and some musings in calculus), Price's intense interest in probability is well established. It was through mathematics that the activist Price and the reserved Bayes became friends.

Thus, it was no surprise that, upon Reverend Bayes' death in 1761, his bereaved family would call upon Reverend Price to examine and organize Bayes' papers and notebooks, leading Price to discover the scattered writing of his dead friend.

Price recognized the topic of the paper was probability. Maybe the two of them had some earlier conversations about the interesting notion of using the past to predict the future. Nevertheless, Price went about the task of revising Bayes' manuscript draft. Bayes had written an introduction — Price replaced it. In addition, Price added an appendix [4]. Others suggest that Price made other substantial changes, amplifying the use of probability in a revolutionary way. Finally, Price read the revised manuscript before the Royal Society on September 23, 1763, two years after Bayes' death, giving full credit to his friend. In 1765, two years after the manuscript was published, Price was himself admitted to the Royal Society for his own work on probability.[*]

The precise contributions of Bayes and Price in the 1763 manuscript remains a mystery. However, we can say that, while it was ultimately Bayes' bombshell, the hand that repacked the explosives and lit the fuse belonged to Reverend

---

[*] Price went on to publish several books including *Observations on the Nature of Civil Liberty, the Principles of Government, and the Justice and Policy of War with America in 1776*. His chapel was visited by such notables as John Howard, leader of an influential group of prison reformers, and John Quincy Adams, future President of the United States.

Price.* The paper itself, like a slowly burning fuse, languish unnoticed for a decade.†

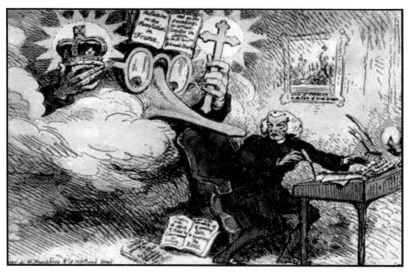

Figure 2. A figure of Richard Price, drawn by James Gillray in 1790. It depicts the Reverend's torment by an overbearing King, whom he advocated could be overthrown. Reprinted with permission from the website ww.spartacus.schoolnet.co.uk/PRprice.htm.

Trapped in a Bottle

The breakthrough manuscript, a result of the tag-team efforts of Bayes and Price was a difficult read. Arcane notation, complicated examples, and a new challenging concept combined to keep the manuscript well below the radar scope of eager, aggressive mathematicians of the time. However, despite its opaque presentations, the manuscript is the first coherent attempt to deal with a vexing problem — deducing cause from effect mathematically, a procedure that would come to be known as

---

* The posthumous publication of the works of others generates predictable controversy even in this century, as the recent appearance of unpublished drafts and fragments of poety of Elizabeth Bishop reveals. Among the most respected American poets, well known for her high standards, Bishop published approximately ninety poems in her lifetime. *The New Yorker*, one of the few widely read magazines that publishes poetry, edited and published her heretofore unseen works, including drafts and verse that Bishop herself crossed out in her own private notes. The magazine has in turn been excoriated for its decision to reveal these private writings by a second magazine, *The New Republic*. See Motoko Rick's article "Publish-After-Perish Controversy," in the *New York Times*, April 1, 2006, page A17.

† Steven Stigler, a leading historian of statistics, has even suggested that Bayes Theorem was really discovered by Nicolas Saunderson, a blind mathematician who was the fourth Lucasian Professor of Mathematics at Cambridge University. Stephen Hawking is the current holder of this chair.

inversion. The solution invoked both probability and philosophy in a new, contentious, but illuminating way.

By the mid 18th century, probability was an accepted, even respected branch of applied mathematics. Its users at the time were well acquainted with the binomial probability distribution, which computes from a sequence of n independent success-failure trials the probability that there are exactly k successes.[*] The use of this elementary probability model generated useful conclusions about the effects of a cause.

For example, a particularly virulent scourge of the time was diarrhea. While the effects of diarrheal disease were disabling in urban life, the disease could incapacitate an army. Racing through camps, it could bring huge segments of otherwise mobile units to a standstill, removing thousands of men from a battle at a critical moment. At the time, organized meal preparation was an unknown concept in the armies of Europe. Each man was responsible for bringing his own utensils, carrying his own food, and cooking his own meal over a group campfire. However, careful observers quickly noticed that, while diarrhea did not have just one cause, it appeared to be related to how a soldier's meal was prepared.[†] Specifically, diarrhea was more prevalent in soldiers who prepared their meals with unboiled water.

Probability built on this observation. For example, it was easy to compute how many soldiers out of twenty would be sick if only 10% of them boiled their water. Termed "reasoning from cause to effect," the process used knowledge of how common the habit of boiling water was to compute the "effect" of that habit i.e., predicting the number of soldiers expected to be sick. This was a straightforward, correct, and commonly helpful probability application.

However, suppose one reverses the logic. An observer is confronted with twenty soldiers, six of whom are ill. How likely is it that un-boiled cooking water is the cause of the illness? In this circumstance, the public health worker is compelled to reason "backward" from the effect (i.e., the sick soldiers) to the cause of their illness. This reversal of the deduction process would come to be known as "inversion" (Figure 3).[‡]

The concept of inversion was groundbreaking, requiring new thought in two dimensions. The first concept was the mathematical one of "reversing the given." One can compute the probability of a particular number of sick soldiers when you know that they did not boil their water. Now, one wishes to compute the probability that they didn't boil their water, given the number of sick soldiers. It is this reversal of condition for which Bayes is known, his work encapsulated in Bayes Theorem. In modern terms, it states that the probability of the hypothesis given the evidence can be computed from the probability of the evidence given the hypothesis, or

---

[*] We will have much more to say about the binomial distribution in Chapter One.

[†] Other causes were spoiled food, wounds, and sepsis.

[‡] Knowledge of one conditional probability does not imply knowledge of the probability with the conditions inverted or reversed. In a modern day context, the probability that given the car is a Ferrari, a male is driving is high. However, the inverse probability, i.e., the probabilty that given the male is a driver, the car that he is driving is a Ferrari is low.

$$P[\text{Hypothesis} \mid \text{Evidence}] = KP[\text{Evidence} \mid \text{Hypothesis}] * P[\text{Hypothesis}] \quad (1)$$

where K is a proportionality constant. One starts with a collection of hypotheses; each of which is assigned a plausibility. Evidence is then used (e.g., the conduct of an experiment to examine the plausibility of these experiments). The result is a new or updated set of plausibilities (Figure 4).

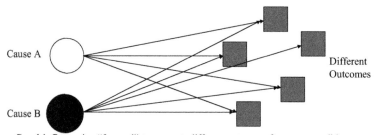

Panel 1: Reasoning "forward" to compute different outcomes from two possible causes.

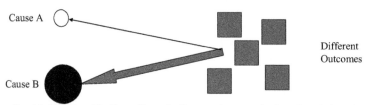

Panel 2: Inversion: The Bayes "inversion" approach reasons backwards to deduce that Cause B is more likely than Cause A based on the outcomes.

Figure 3. The classical approach (Panel A) of predicting outcomes from cause. The Bayes approach (Panel B) uses mathematics to deduce cause from outcome.

However, this process of inversion is not merely the clever use of probability formulas. Its discovery and adoption led to foundation shattering questions about the meaning of probability. Specifically, was probability objective or subjective?

To the probabilist of the time (and to many applied probabilists today), probability is defined as relative frequency. The probability of an event of interest is simply the ratio of the number of outcomes that comprise the event divided by the total number of possible outcomes. In the above example, we know that there is one soldier in ten who boiled their water, so the probability is simply $1/10 = 0.10$. This probability is used to identify the distribution of sick soldiers.

However to use the inversion process, Bayes and Price suggested that probability was subjective; it was a belief whose plausibility sometimes defied quantification. One had an idea of how likely it was that soldiers boiled water.

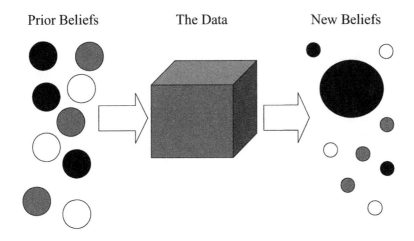

Prior Beliefs   The Data   New Beliefs

Figure 4. The Bayes procedure in operation. The plausibility of a set of prior beliefs (circles) is altered by the data, increasing the likelihood of one of those beliefs, while decreasing the plausibility of others.

One then considered the evidence (i.e., the number of observed sick soldiers) and changed or updated their original idea. To Bayes and Price, probability wasn't a mere mathematical fraction; it was the degree of truth in an event.

While the "degree of truth" definition was liberating to Bayes and Price, it was unnerving to many others, upending the relative frequency applecart. To the relative frequentists, probability (like the fraction representing relative frequency) must be trapped between zero and one. To the Bayesian, probability could have any metric, as long as it was consistently used. Also, the Bayes-Price approach could deal with probabilities that relative frequentists didn't dare touch, e.g., "What is the probability that the King is divine?" or "What is the probability that God is everywhere at once?" While both relative frequentists and Bayesians alike had opinions and beliefs about these fundamental events, only Bayesians dared deduce, dream of experiments, and update probabilities based on them. It is this disagreement about probability that would separate the (relative) frequentists from the Bayesians for hundreds of years.

Yet in 1763, the year of jubilation, these ideas lay dormant, trapped in the published, but unread paper like a gargantuan genie stuffed into a tiny bottle. It was Laplace, who yanked the cork out, releasing the Bayes approach on an unsuspecting world.

Unleashed!

In the 1760s the teenaged Simon Laplace had a problem. Born into a poor family with few resources, his parents consigned him to a safe, secure, but inconspicuous existence. However, incessantly pulled by the restless force of greatness, he struggled to walk another path. Yet that path required education, and education required money. With no money of his own, and his family unable to contribute, he turned to an unusual and untapped source — his neighbors!

Through his unique combination of force of personality, unshakeable will, and an uncanny knack to discern what people needed to hear, young Simon went from house to house, alternately asking, cajoling, and demanding that the different households, themselves poor, provide money for his training. The astonished neighbors acceded to his request, committing their hard earned money to his education.

Having acquired the funding, Laplace threw himself into his work. After completing some university training, he presented a well received paper before the French Academy of Science in 1773 in which he demonstrated the stability of planetary motion. He was twenty-four years old. Already a mathematical power-house, he followed this with the first of four works that rocketed the field forward into a perilous but promising future.

His manuscript, entitled *Mémoire sur la Probabilité des Causes par les Évènements* provided further justification for the use of what would become known as the prior distribution, establishing the legitimacy of the inversion approach. For this natural extension, we return to the example of infantry illness and food preparation, where one wishes to deduce the probability that a group of soldiers (among which k of them have developed diarrhea) have in fact boiled their water. For the Bayesian argument to contribute to the fund of knowledge, we must have an initial or prior estimate p for the probability that the soldiers first boiled their water, which we will use data to update. However one had to choose the initial value of p. There were no procedures in place to choose this probability.

Laplace rejected the belief that this probability of boiling water should be some fixed constant. Through a deft piece of mathematical reasoning, using the binomial distribution in combination with Equation (1), he deduced that p should not have a single value at all, but that it should have its own probability distribution.

This was the second of a one-two punch dealt to the established relative frequentists. They had not recovered from the Bayes-Price argument that probability needn't be a relative frequency when Laplace informed them that it was perfectly acceptable for probabilities to have their own probability distribution! To these workers, a relative frequency was a proportion. How could it have different values at different times? To many, applying a probability distribution to a probability was a pernicious abstraction, like playing a game by rolling a six-sided die when the probability that a particular face appears is not constant, but varies from roll to roll. The concept was mind boggling. Yet this is precisely what Laplace proved.

Consider a company of one hundred 18th century soldiers divided into ten groups. The soldiers act independently of one another, some boiling their water, others not. We might expect that in each of the ten groups, there will be different proportions of soldiers who boil their water before cooking it. Thus, if one were to focus on only one group of soldiers, the proportion of those boiling water would be a fixed, single number. However, by stepping back and examining the ten groups, we see that each group has its own proportion. It is easy to reflect this variability in p by producing the probability distribution of p (Figure 5).

Now, taking a step back, we can view the entire army as composed of hundreds of companies, and thousands of these ten-soldier groups. If we were to graph the distribution of p, its more complete distribution emerges. To a Bayesian, the variability of the values of p from group to group is not produced by the sample-to-sample variability, but by different values of the parameter itself. Thus, one can arrive at the concept of a "prior" probability distribution for p by reasoning from the relative frequency perspective.

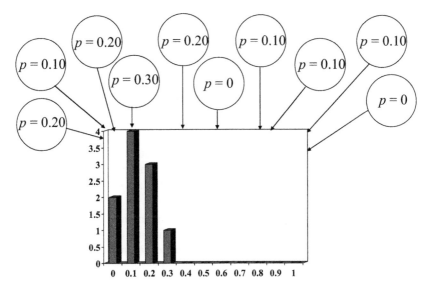

Figure 5. From individual values of p, the proportion of soldiers who boil their water, a distribution of the value of p emerges.

The relative frequentists hesitated as they struggled with this step into an uncertain future for the relative frequency argument. Laplace responded by shoving them forward, announcing the exact probability distribution of one should assume for p. His manipulation of equation (1) revealed that the distribution was one in which p was evenly distributed across all numbers between zero and one. This distribution was, in the eyes of Laplace, a completely fair one, not favoring one region of possible vales of p for another. In this distribution, intervals of equal length have equal probability (i.e., it was just as likely that p was between zero and 0.10 as it was to be between 0.90 and 1) (Figure 6).[*]

---

[*] This is known as the uniform probability distribution. Think of spinning a spinner on a circular board, with all the numbers between 0 and 1 a possible landing point for the spinner. Then the probabilty of the spinner landing in any one region of the board is as likely as it landing in any other region of equal area.

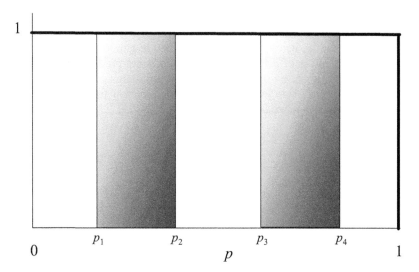

Figure 6. The uniform prior for a probability value. Under it, the probability that p is between p_1 and p_2 (shaded area) is the same as the probability that it is between p_3 and p_4 if the intervals are of equal length, i.e., $p_2 - p_1 = p_4 - p_3$.

The stage was now set for the first modern Bayes computation. What was the proportion of soldiers who boiled their water? The traditional computation was very easy. If out of 10 soldiers, three sickened with diarrhea, then the probability that a soldier boiled his water was simply 3/10 = 0.30. However, according to Laplace, the assumption of a uniform distribution of values for p, in accordance with equation (1) produced the surprising, counterintuitive answer of $(3+1)/(10+2) = 0.334$! The addition of one in the numerator and two in the denominator are a direct consequence of the uniform prior distribution.

Which calculation was right? Each was, according to its perspective. In the traditional argument, where the proportion of soldiers who boil their water is fixed, and one wishes to estimate that proportion in only the collection of ten soldiers who have data, then the value 0.30 is correct. However, from the Bayes perspective, since the proportion of soldiers boiling their water differs from group to group, a different estimator should be used that takes this variability into account. In the Bayes paradigm, one is not trying to simply estimate the proportion of soldiers who boil their water among these ten fighting men, but the overall proportion, among all soldiers, recognizing that the proportion varies from group to group.

Laplace also asserted that different prior distributions generated different updated values of p. For example, if we assume that the prior distribution of p was not evenly (or uniformly) distributed between zero and one, but instead favored smaller values of p, then the updated value of p would be neither 0.30 (the frequentists estimate), nor 0.334 (the Bayes estimate with a uniform prior), but 0.174 (Figure 7). The smaller "posterior" value of *p* reflects the prior "belief" that smaller values of *p* are more likely than larger ones.

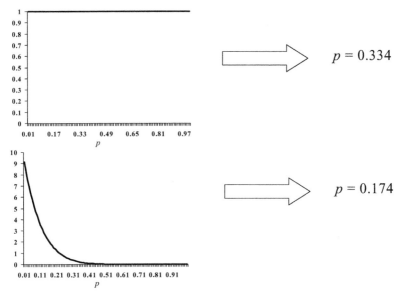

Figure 7. Two different prior probability distributions produce different estimates of *p*, the probability a soldier boils his cooking water.

As colleagues shook their heads in puzzlement at these different answers to the same simple question, "what proportion of soldiers boiled their water?" Laplace revealed the inner mechanism of this new probability generating machine. It wasn't just that the final value of *p* was altered. This final value came from a final distribution or *posterior distribution* of *p*. Laplace argued that this made perfect sense. One began with a prior distribution. Then one obtained data. The prior distribution was combined with the data to produce a posterior distribution. The posterior distribution wasn't a new distribution it was the updated prior. The prior distribution was updated to a posterior distribution though incorporation of the data. It was this posterior distribution that provided updated estimates for *p*. (Figure 8).

These circumstances raised the specter of different prior distributions producing different posterior estimates from the same data. If there was to be one right answer to the question of what is the proportion of soldiers who boil their water, then one would have to select the right prior distribution. But exactly how does one do that?

Laplace had opened a door into either a lush valley of intellectual and philosophical fruit, or a sharp precipice that would tear the young field of probability apart on the jagged shards of contradiction. And he did this without ever using Bayes' paper! The stark differences between his derivations and those of Bayes make it unlikely that he relied on Bayes initial work. However, Laplace's

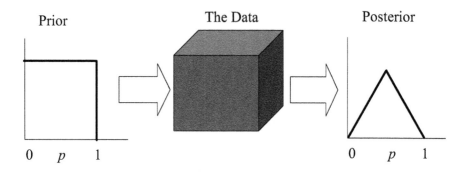

Figure 8. Converting a prior distribution to a posterior distribution. This was a common practice of statisticians in the 19th century.

legendary, regrettable tendency to pirate and then disparage the work of others forces us to keep this an open question.

Even his warmest admirers acknowledged Laplace's vanity and selfishness. He was contemptuous of the benefactors of his youth, ungrateful to his policial friends, and his appropriation without acknowledgment of the work of others was reprehensible. Those who subsequently rose in favor, such as Legendre and Fourier, never forgot the mistreatment of their work by Laplace. In all fairness, Laplace was straightforward and honest about his religious, philosophical or scientific views. He was also very protective and generous toward his students. In one case, he suppressed a paper of his own in order that a pupil might have the sole credit of the investigation [5].

At this point, Laplace was not the only mathematician eager to explore the process and implications of inversion. Other great minds of the time, such as Lagrange, and James Bernoulli grappled with inversion theory. It was clear that something new was brewing in probability, and the atmosphere was exciting. It was not unlike watching the early PC industry in the 1980's. As Apple, IBM, and Osborne, competed, no one knew who would win, but one thing was clear – the time was right for a critical advance. This was the case in probability in the late 18th century.

Laplace laid the groundwork, expanding the ideas of inversion, overturning staid ideas in probability, demonstrating the stunning richness of the theory. Workers now explored the entire family of possible prior distributions. Interrogation of the use of the posterior distribution was demanded; new converts to the field responded. Laplace's work was order shattering. Regardless of whether his colleagues agreed with everything Laplace wrote or not, one thing was sure; his home-town's initial investment in him was amply rewarded.

Holy Grail

The period of Laplace-generated probability storms was followed by a relative pe-riod of calm as probabilists caught their breath, taking the time to absorb both the astonishing finding of Bayes, and its Laplaceian implications.

Many of the most renown mathematicians of the time entered the field, beginning to patiently explore the differences between "objective" or relative fre-quency probability, versus the newer "subjective" probability, generated by Bayes. Poisson (known for the Poisson distribution), Bolzano (discoverer of Bolzano's constant in chemistry and physics), Ellis, Fries, Mill, and Counot made contribu-tions to the roots of probability [3] in discussions that were more philosophical than mathematical. In addition, Boole, Veenn, and Chrystal continued Laplace's work on distinguishing inverse probability and objective probability.

Prior distribution identification vexed the most capable minds at the time. To a Bayesian, ignoring the prior distribution was as disastrous as ignoring the data itself. Laplace had shown that, at least mathematically, any probability distribution could serve as a prior distribution. However, his work begged the question, "Which probability distribution serves as the best prior?" Enunciation of the "indifference principle" i.e., the idea that the prior distribution should express no bias toward one set of values over another, affirmed the belief of Laplace. However, while this prin-ciple set the goal, it didn't say how the goal could be achieved. Laplace revealed one solution. Were there others? Despite the dedicated work of many, little useful progress was made as every step forward was shoved backward by the identifica-tion of new logical inconsistencies. The search for the non-preferential prior be-came increasingly desperate and despondent, taking on the look and feel of an Ar-thurian search for a Bayesian Holy Grail, continuing into the 20th and now the 21st century.

Despite these limitations, the use of subjective probabilities and the Bayes-Laplace perspective increased in popularity. It was common practice to complete the multistep process of 1) construct a prior distribution, 2) obtain the data, and 3) update the prior distribution to the posterior distribution during the 19th century [6,7] (Figure 8).

However, a new problem arose as everyone (relative frequentist and Bayes-Laplace converts alike) struggled with the concept of drawing accurate con-clusions from a small sample that would apply to the population at large, known as statistical inference. Hampered by their use of subjective probability, fledging Bayesian methods to draw conclusions about the population from the sample were halting, inconsistent, and confused.

Thus, the forward charge of Bayesians slowed at the beginning of the 20th century. William Gosset (who developed the *t*-test using the pseudonym Student) worked with prior and posterior distributions, but did not link them to the concept of inverse probability. Pearson, the father of the correlation coefficient, developed an entire collection of useful probability distributions but didn't examine the impli-cations of his work for the inverse thought process. And, even though eminent English statisticians, e.g., Edgeworth [3] integrated the inverse probability concept into their work, the movement hesitated. Keynes wrote about the use of subjective probability, but conceded that the degree of belief might not be quantifiable [8], a major stumbling block in the application of the procedure. After winning the hearts and minds of eminent mathematicians at the beginning of the 19th century, the Bayesian-Laplace approach was trapped between,the unscalable mountain of the indifference principle on the one hand, and the unfordable river of statistical inference on the other.

Trapped there, it was all but routed by Ronald Fisher and the *p*-value, which captured the field of applied statistics, reversed the Bayesian logic, and nearly strangled the field.

Attack of the Frequentists

The subject approach existed amicably with the relative frequency perspective in the 19th and early 20th century, brokering a peaceful co-existence. Struggling against their own mathematical obstacles, they together fought for the recognition of statistics as a fully fledged, independent discipline from the other science fields [9]. In fact, the Bayes approach was so well accepted into the 1920s that it was a well accepted part of the academic curriculum of statistics departments. Ronald Fisher shattered this *modus vivendi*.

The figure of Ronald Aylvmer Fisher casts a long shadow over the development of statistical thinking in the 20th century. Born in East Finchley, London in 1890, Fisher finished his schooling at Gonville and Caius College in Cambridge, where he received instruction in the Bayesian approach to statistics. Working as a statistician at Rothamsted Experimental Station in 1919, he developed an interest in designing and analyzing agricultural experiments. Concentrating on the design and analysis of these experiments, Fisher recognized that better methods were necessary to deal with the natural variability of crop yields. It was during this period that he developed the randomization process, ensuring that differences in the plots of land (e.g., moisture or insect density) could not systematically influence the results. The advantage of this tool was self-evident to agriculturalists,[*] and Fisher's influence expanded.

Fisher's subsequent, order-shattering ideas on the link between statistical analysis and hypothesis testing galvanized many, while shocking others. Up until the 1920s the core principle of knowledge development was the scientific method. Its implementation began with a researcher's belief, known as the hypothesis, and ended with the execution of an experiment that would either verify or refute that scientist's idea. Fisher turned the world of statistics (both for the relative frequentists and the Bayesians alike) on its head, arguing from a postulate that he called the

---

[*] It took several more decades before clinical trial workers were comfortable embedding the random allocation of therapy as a concept in clinical experimentation.

likelihood principle.* While he agreed that data were necessary to assess a scientific theory, he argued that the true test of the theory was the likelihood of the data given the theory, not the likelihood of the theory given the data. To a Bayesian (and to much of the scientific world) this was backward thinking.

In the first edition of his 1925 book *Statistical Methods for Research Workers* [10], Fisher extended his thinking to incorporate an important and familiar mathematical implement; the indirect proof, or prove by contradiction. This tool requires the workers to turn their backs on what they believe to be true, accepting instead what they don't believe. They then argue logically from this fallacious belief until they arrive at a contradiction i.e., an untenable conclusion that is undeniably false. Since the arguments after the first assumption are logical and correct, the only possible conclusion is that the first assumption is false. This valuable device appears in all fields of mathematics, and fundamental findings (e.g., the proof of the existence of irrational numbers) are based on its clever use.

Fisher recognized that the proposition "if *a* occurs then *b* occurs" can be refuted by a single observation of *b* without the occurrence of *a*. He extended this to statistical inference, asking the question, "What is needed to refute the thesis 'if *a* occurs then *b*' occurs with probability *c*?" Clearly, this second assertion would not be refuted in the presence of many observations of *b* without *a*, since the proposition admits that *b* without *a* can occur. However, if the proportion of times that *b* occurs without *a* is greater than $1 - c$, then the hypothesis of "*a* then *b* with probability *c*" is suspect. Fisher believed that the worker should look at the likelihood of the data (i.e., how many times *b* occurred without *a*) evaluating if the number of these occurrences was "likely" based on the proposition. The hypothesis of *a* then *b* (called the null hypothesis) would be discarded if the likelihood of the data under the assumption of the hypothesis was small.

For the first time, scientists, used to dealing the likelihood of their hypothesis, now must grapple with the likelihood of the data.

In Fisher's scheme, the scientist begins with their question, e.g., is there a relationship between methamphetamine use and teeth grinding? However the beginning of the statistical evaluation requires the scientist to abandon her belief, assuming that the reverse is true; i.e., there is no such relationship between abuse of the drug and dentition. Fisher named this assumption the *null hypothesis*, since it was the hypothesis to be nullified by the data.

With null hypothesis in hand, the researcher then collects data and examines a measure of the data called a test statistic. Under the null hypothesis, the test statistic will follow a well-known probability distribution. Thus, some regions of test statistic will be highly probable while others remain improbable. If the test statistic falls in an improbable region, then the researcher concludes that the null hypothesis was incorrect.

This is the hallmark of the indirect proof applied to statistical inference. If the null hypothesis was true, then the *p*-value will be large. Therefore, since the *p*-value is small, the null hypothesis is false, and we reject it with an acknowledged

---

* The use of this term is ironic, since it was the development of the "likelihood principle" years later that would power the return of the Bayesians to the forefront of modern statistical thinking.

error rate (*p*-value) (Figure 9). The *p*-value, or the type I error rate, is the probability of falsely rejecting the null hypothesis when the null hypothesis is true.*

How small should the *p*-value be? In a short 1926 paper entitled "The arrangement of field experiments" [11], Fisher used an example from agronomy to motivate significance testing and introduce the 0.05 level. In his illustration, the crop yields of two neighboring acres of land, one treated with fertilizer, the other untreated, were to be compared. The fertilizer-treated plot produced a 10% greater crop yield than that of the non-treated plot, suggesting that the fertilizer increased the yield. Yet, Fisher knew that crop yields varied for a variety of reason. How could he be sure that the 10% increase was really due to the fertilizer, and not to chance alone? Fisher concluded that if there was only one in twenty chance that the play of chance would produce a 10% difference in crop yield then,

> "...the evidence would have reached a point which may be called the verge of significance; for it is convenient to draw the line at about the level at which we can say, 'Either there is something in the treatment or a coincidence has occurred such as does not occur more than once in twenty trials.' This level, which we may call the 5 per cent level point, would be indicated, though very roughly, by the greatest chance deviation observed in twenty successive trials." [11]

This casual statement birthed the significance level of 0.05 [12].

The Bayesians were caught completely by surprise with this approach. Through the clever adoption of the indirect proof, and the development of the level of significance or *p*-value, Fisher claimed that he had broken the back of the inference problem that bedeviled statistics for generations. And, he was quick to point out, he never had to rely on the concepts of subjective probability or prior distributions. The basis of Fisher's deductions was relative frequency, and the solution to the question of how one uses data from samples to infer results in larger populations lied squarely in the hands of the frequentists.

At last, a method was emerging that would provide formal and reproducible mathematical structure to the inference process. Fisher's work was followed by an avalanche of additional development in the field of statistical inference as workers became comfortable with this new mathematical structure. In the 1930s, Egon Pearson and Jerzy Neyman developed the formal theory of testing statistical hypotheses, introducing the concept of the alternative hypothesis [13], and then the likelihood test statistic [14]. This led to the use of hypothesis testing and inference as they are currently used. They also developed the theory for the confidence interval [15,16,17,18].

---

* In health care research that explores exposure-disease relationships, it is more useful to think of the *p*-value as the probability that a population in which there is no relationship between the exposure and the diesease produces a sample in which the relationship is present.

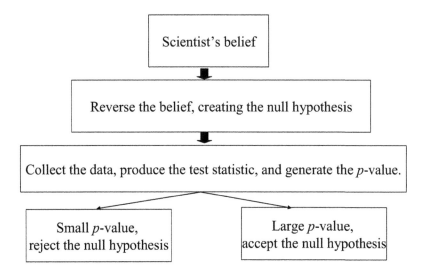

Figure 9. Fisher's approach was to assume the scientist's hypothesis is false, disproving this false "null" hypothesis with a small p-value.

In addition, these two statisticians codify the notion of significance testing by its formalization, leading to the first early sample size computations. Now, researchers had a formal, objective way to compute the size of their research effort, helping to adequately protect against both type I and type II errors. In doing so, they created what would come to be recognized as the reframe of the frequentist.

> "But we may look at the purpose of tests from another viewpoint. Without hoping to know whether each separate hypothesis is true or false, we may search for rules to govern our behavior with regard to them, in following which we ensure that, in the long run of experience, we not often be wrong." [16]

This clear statement points to the heart of the frequentist creed. Concern rests not with the result of the current experiment, but the long-term accuracy of the decision-making process, whether that proportion be the fraction of soldiers boiling their cooking water before a meal, or the proportion of experiments in which the test statistic leads to rejection of the null hypothesis when the null hypothesis is true. The metric of the frequentist is the long-term predictive ability of their decision rules. Even if the decision rule is obviously inferior for an individual experiment, the long term accuracy of the process to the frequentist justifies its use. The frequentist juggernaut, with a full head of steam was rolling now.

Total War

Reaction to Fisher's "significance testing" approach was immediate, and much of it was critical. Observationalists in science believed the significance testing scenario was dangerously counterintuitive. At the time, many reputable scientists abided by the time honor maxim of Karl Pearson, i.e., "After all, the higher statistics are only common sense reduced to numerical appreciation." Statistics was supposed to make sense. It should be the easy part of the research, not add new theoretical encumbrances.

To these critics, Fisher's work was complex, forcing the scientist to enter an unnatural process. Now, the researcher must replace the strong assertion of his own affirmative scientific hypothesis with the tepid alternative of disproving a hypothesis that he did not believe. To them, this reverse logic was just the type of unhelpful product generated by clueless mathematical workers who didn't leave their offices enough. The reaction of epidemiologist was particularly vitriolic. This field, already bruised by the two decade-old assault on its philosophical foundations by physicists and mathematical theorists [19], reacted quickly and sternly with comments that still resonate with life and power. One said,

> "What used to be called judgment is now called prejudice, and what used to be called prejudice is now called a null hypothesis … it is dangerous nonsense …" [20]

Fisher a spirited, tough minded, and sharp tongued debater, proved himself equal to the task of defending his ideas, with published papers by Berkson [21, 22] and Fisher [23] provide some feel for the repartee of the time. At one point, Fisher finally responded to one more Berkson critique by saying "It is not my purpose to make Dr. Berkson seem ridiculous nor of course for me to prevent him from providing innocent entertainment" [23]. The debates were tough, visceral, and personal. Unfortunately, they commonly producing more heat than light.

Bayesians were singled out for particularly tough treatment by Fisher, who patiently dismantled their arguments. About the posterior distribution, he stated,

> "It is important that the scientific worker introduces no cost functions for faulty decisions.…To do so would imply that the purposes to which new knowledge was to be put were known and capable of evaluation. If, however, scientific findings are communicated for the enlightenment of other free minds, they may be put sooner or later to the service of a number of purposes, of which we can know nothing." [24]

And, finally, Fisher rejected the use of inverse probability itself, formally characterizing the motives of its original author in his manuscript *Two New Properties of Mathematical Likelihood:*

"Indeed, we are told that it was his doubts respecting the validity of the postulate needed for establishing the method of inverse probability that led to his withholding his entire treatise from publication. Actually, it was not published until after his death." [25]

Fisher was saying that not only was the Bayes thought process worthless, but that the Reverend Bayes himself knew it! This was why the reverend suppressed the publication of his own work. According to Fisher, Price was the real villain, breathing the vestige of life into an expired idea that had died along with its creator.

It was difficult going for Bayesians in the early 20th century as the work of Fisher spread from agricultural research to other fields, e.g., psychology. While workers such as von Mises used Bayesian arguments to reveal foundation-level weaknesses in the confidence interval perspective [26], they engaged in an uphill fight against the frequentists. The advocates of subjective probability, while vigorously defending their perspective, were losing the hearts and minds of the practicing statisticians to Fisher's inference approach. Yet, a hero would be found, a geologist and astronomer who rallied the cause just before it was stampeded into the backwaters of mathematics.

Fighting Back

An English scientist, Harold Jeffreys emerged from training in 1914, having studied physics, chemistry, geology, and mathematics [27].[*] Moving to Cambridge, he studied earthquakes and atmospheric circulation, always focusing on the mathematical underpinnings of these physical sciences.[†] It was during his work in geology that he developed the notion of probability from one of relative frequency to a system based on "relative belief."

Jeffreys wanted to harness the force of probability to directly address important modern scientific questions, e.g., Einstein's breakthroughs "Could probability be used to test the theory of relativity?" [28,29]. This research question seemed to be outside the application of the relative frequency argument, residing wholly in the domain of scientific hypothesis testing. Jeffrey's appreciated the Bayes approach, recognizing its ability to update prior beliefs as the natural perspective for the problem. His criticism of the relative frequency point of view led him to debate Fisher over its utility in science [30,31,32,33,34,35,36]. Jeffrey's mild-mannered but sustained defense of the Bayes perspective persisted in the face of withering attacks of Fisher and others.[‡]

---

[*] Much of the discusion of Jeffreys comes from John Aldrish at the University of South Hampton The URL is www.economics.soton.ac.uk/staff/aldrich/jeffreysweb.htm

[†] As a result of his study of earthquake waves, Jeffreys became the first to claim that the core of the Earth is liquid.

[‡] As a lecturer Jeffreys had a poor reputation. A former student D J Finney recalls that "in 1937–8 ... Lawley and I were two young graduate mathematicians in Cambridge ... We began by attending a lecture course given by Professor Harold Jeffreys on probability. He was not the clearest of lecturers, and we were soon very confused. ... Jeffreys' personal charm and enthusiasm did not prevent a steady decline in attendance until Lawley and I

Undaunted by Fisher's disdain, Jeffreys enunciated in 1939 his own point of view in a text. Rejecting the recent frequentists arguments for statistical inference, Jeffrey's *Theory of Probability* [37] couched the Bayesian notion of subjective probability in modern mathematical language. This text, the first modern treatment of the Bayes perspective, demonstrated the sound mathematical underpinnings of the theory, while opening the field of physical sciences to its application.

This was a giant step forward for the Bayes philosophy, which was withering in the acidic soil of relative frequency. Moving forward, Jeffreys sunk his mathematical ax deep into the root of one of the most vexing problems Bayesian had faced, i.e., how to select the best prior distribution. Once Bayesians had accepted the notion of subjective probability, they were saddled with how to find the prior distribution. They had to begin somewhere, even if they had no prior information. Laplace's arguments while intuitive, had not yet been justified using modern mathematical thought. Through careful, persuasive mathematical argument, Jeffrey's developed the idea of the "vague" or "non-informative" prior distribution [38,39]. This work is the cornerstone of modern "objective" Bayesian analysis.

This, at long last was the solution Bayesians had sought. Jeffreys demonstrated how the Bayes approach would be productive, once it was "jumpstarted" with a vague prior distribution. The posterior distribution identified by initiating the work with the vague prior distribution would then be used as the first "informed" prior for the next experiment. Thus, prior distributions would evolve over time, produced from the posterior distribution of the previous experiment (Figure 11).

Jeffrey's breakthrough findings were cemented in place by the instructive, powerful arguments of L. J. Savage. A logical, skilled theoretician, his development of axioms of subjective probability sunk the roots of the Bayes approach even deeper into the mathematical soil [40,41]. It would be difficult for anyone to argue that subjective probability was ethereal after reading the mathematically precise, dense arguments of Savage. An implacable Bayes loyalist, he lashed out at its opponents, defending Jeffrey's advocacy of vague priors.

---

found ourselves the only survivors of an initial 15. There came a week when we were both prevented from attending, and the following week we found to our embarrassment that the lecturer had abandoned the course."

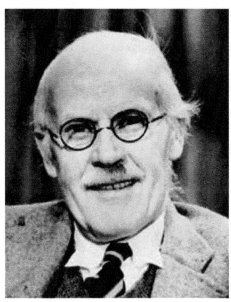

Figure 10. A photograph of Harold Jeffreys, 20th century scientist who Revitalized the Bayes approach. Taken from www-groups.dcs.st-and .ac.uk /~history/PictDisplay/Jeffreys.html

This was the frequentist-Bayesian fight at its worst. The relative frequentists led by the towering Fisher slashed the Bayesians for their undisciplined use of probability, their penchant for drifting prior distributions, and their unrepentant attitude in the face of persuasive "frequentist" arguments. Bayesian, struck back, lacerating the frequentists with new, detailed, and bruising mathematical arguments of their own. For the first time in decades, Bayesian, standing on the shoulders of Jeffreys and Savage could look to the future of their field with a spirit of boldness and confidence, prepared to take great leaps forward [42]. Yet when it came to the medical community, their first view of this promising new future shocked them. That community, it seems, had already made up its mind.

The Health Care Love Affair with P-Values

As the Bayesian-frequentist proponents hurled themselves at each other in the 1940s, medical research exploded onto the scene [43]. World War II generated military and civilian casualties at a rate never seen before in history, demanding immediate advances in medical care delivery. Millions of dollars poured into the small field of health care research, and the community responded with a blizzard of new ideas and avenues to pursue. Research teams, including the renowned Medical Research Council (MRC) of England, developed new research methodology, including the first early clinical trials. As young investigators hurled themselves into the exciting field of research, they soon exhausted available grant resources, and the avalanche of their manuscripts buried the small number of peer reviewed journals available to publish them. Harried grant administrators together with over-worked journal reviewers and editors were overwhelmed by demands for their di-minished resources. Each group struggled with how to separate the research "wheat from the chaff." They chose the p-value as the filter.

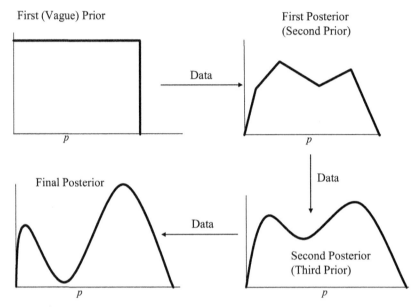

Figure 11. Jeffreys envisioned a sequence of Bayes analyses, starting with the vague prior and sequentially updating it, with the posterior from the preceding experiment becoming the prior for the next.

While this decision has been much maligned in retrospect, it was not un-dertaken maliciously. Grant administrators and journal editors strove to fund and ultimately publish the best research, fueled not just by scientific enthusiasm, but, in this time of global conflict, by a spirit of national survival. Yet, the absence of a traditional discriminator thwarted their determined efforts to separate the actual scientific evidence from an author's exorbitant claims buttressed by imaginative calculations.

Therefore, this powerful oversight collection of granting agencies and journal editors chose to require objective statistical analyses. This, they believed, would force all data to be analyzed using the same types of procedures, and re-ported the same way, using the p-value. This data-based, readily available, easily computed tool, incorporated sample size, effect size, variability, and sampling er-ror, while insulating itself from investigator subjectivity [44]. At the time, the p-value appeared to be the perfect tool for the job.

Thus, not only would the p-value be the basis of grant awards and manu-script publication, but it would also be the best basis for therapeutic options and determining government health policy. The threshold for all analyses, would be

Fisherian — $p < 0.05$. Adaptation of these rules would bring all health care research, from surgery to psychiatry, under one rubric, governed by one metric. Moving on this conclusion, these administrators quickly required that research grant applications and manuscripts must include formal statistical hypothesis testing in general, and p-values in particular. The embrace of p-values by granting agents and academia was followed by their wholesale acceptance by the regulatory industry and consequently, the pharmaceutical industry.

Uniformity was sought, and (for better and for worse) uniformity was achieved.

Circling Two Suns

The frequentist sun reached in zenith in health care research in the 1970s as the research community accepted the requirement of "$p < 0.05$" as its mantra. However, its blinding light was part of the problem. Obsession with small p-values commonly excluded other methodologic concerns, leading to comments, e.g. "Since the study found a statistically significant relative risk...the cause relationship was considered established."[45].

The determination of causality can be complex, requiring that features, e.g., strength of association, dose response relationships, challenge-dechallenge-rechallenge experiments, biologic plausibility, and consistency be simultaneously considered [46]. Frequentists in health care research had, it seemed developed their own Holy Grail — p-value < 0.05. Epidemiologists who never ended their determined fight against the p-value hegemony rose again to do battle, debating the use of this much used and abused tool in the literature [47,48,49,50,51]. Finally, in 1987 the prestigious *American Journal of Public Health* solicited an editorial calling for a ban on all p-values in manuscripts submitted for peer review.

Meanwhile, a new technical fuel fed the Bayesian engine as advanced computing generating a new level of its application to applied health care statistics. Moving away from simple problems involving mathematically undemanding prior distributions, Bayesians could now tackle complex problems using computers that were for the first time readily available in the researchers' offices.

Powered by these computational devices and new generation of dynamic investigators, Bayes procedures are now readily available in health care research. For example, there are now papers that deal with how to compute sample size both in the absence [52] and presence [53] of event misclassification.

While continuing to sustain criticism, e.g., the amusing critique of Feinstein [54], infusion of the Bayesian perspective has introduced a new level of insight and imagination into complicated research issues, offering refreshing alternatives to the frequentist approach. The role of adaptive randomization in clinical trials, i.e., permitting the trends in treatment effect within the trial itself to influence the proportion of patients who are allocated treatment is useful in the practice of Phase II clinical trials [55]. Other writers focus on the use of Bayesian procedures in assessing causal nature of the exposure disease relationship when clinical preference drives the exposure [56].

Another area of inference is the role of Bayes procedures in the statistical monitoring of clinical research. The link between Bayesian tools and statistical monitoring of clinical research was explored in the 1980s [57,58,59]. This philosophy has generated discussion [60] and the development of additional methodology [61,62]. Bayes procedures are also being applied to observational studies [63,64], and a particular series of useful analysis on missing data [65].

　　　　While one can't say that the sun is setting on the frequentist approach. All appearances suggest that the Bayesian perspective, evolving and maturing over the past 140 years, is here to stay. Applied statistics will be governed by two suns for the foreseeable future.

References

1.　Morrison S.E. (1972). *The Oxford History of the American People. Vol 1*. New York and Scarborough, Ontario. Mentor Books. pp. 224–225.
2.　Bayes T. (1763). "An Essay Towards Solving a Problem in the Doctrine of Chances." *Philosophical Transactions of the Royal Society of London,* **53**:370–418.
3.　Fienberg S.E. (2006). When did bayesian inference become "bayesian? *Bayesian Analysis* **1**:1–40.
4.　Stigler S.M. (1986). The History of Statistics: The Measurement of Uncertainty before 1990. Cambridge, London. The Belknap Press of Harvard University Press. p. 98.
5.　Ball W.W. Rouse (1960). *A Short Account of the History of Mathematics (4th Edition*. New York: Dover Publications.
6.　Zabell S. (1989). R.A. Fisher on the History of Inverse Probability. *Statistical Science* **4**:247–256.
7.　Zabell S. (1989). R.A. Fisher on the History of Inverse Probability. Rejoinder. *Statistical Science* **4**:261–263.
8.　Keynes J.M. (1921). A Treatise on Probability, Vol 8. New York. St. Martins Press.
9.　Moyé L.A. (2006). Statistical Reasoning in Medicine. The Intuitive P-value Primer 2nd Edition. New York. Springer.
10.　Fisher R.A. (1925).　*Statistical Methods For Research Workers.* Edinburg. Oliver and Boyd.
11.　Fisher R.A. (1926). The arrangement of field experiments. *Journal of the Ministry of Agriculture.* 503–513.
12.　Owen D.B. (1976). On the History of Probability and Statistics. New York. Marcel-Dekker.
13.　Neyman J., Peason E.S. (1933). On the problem of the most efficient tests of statistical hypotheses. *Philosophical Transactions of the Royal Society (London) Se A* **231**: 289–337.
14.　Neyman J., Pearson E.S. (1933). On the use and interpretatin of certain test criteria for purposes of statistical inferences: parts I and II. *Biometrika* **20**:175–240: 263–294.
15.　Pytkowsi W. (1932). The dependence of the income in small farms upon their area, the outlay and the capital invested in cows, (Polish, English summaries), Monograph no. 31 of series Bioblioteka Pulawska, publ. Agri. Res. Inst.

Pulasy, Poland. Wald. A. (1950) *Statistical Decision Functions*, New York, Wiley.

16. Neyman J. (1937). Outline of a theory of statistical estimation based on the classical theory of probability. *Philosophical Transactions of the Royal Society (London) Ser A* **236**:333–380.

17. Neyman J. (1938). L'estimation statistique traitée comme un problème classique de probabilité. Actual. Sceint. Instust. **739;** 25–57.

18. Neyman J., Peason E.S. (1933). On the problems of most efficient tests of statistical hypotheses. Philos Trans Roy Soc A **231**:289–337.

19. Moyé L.A. (2003). Multiple Analyses in Clinical Trials. Fundamentals for Investigators. New York. Springer.

20. Edwards A. (1972). *Likelihood.* Cambridge, UK: Cambridge University Press.

21. Berkson J. (1942). Experiences with tests of significance. A reply to R.A. Fisher. *Journal of the American Statistical Association* **37**: 242–246.

22. Berkson J. (1942). Tests of significance considered as evidence. *Jounal of the American Statistical Association* **37**:335–345.

23. Fisher R.A. (1942). Response to Berkson. *Journal of the American Statistical Association* **37**:103–104.

24. Fisher R.A. (1956). *Statistical Methods and Scientific Inference*, New York. Hafner.

25. Fisher R.A. (1934). Two new properties of mathematical likelihood. *Proceedings of the Royal Society A*, **144**:285–307.

26. von Mises (1942). On the correct use of Bayes' formula. *Annals of Mathematical Statistics* **13**:156165.

27. O'Conno J.J., Robertson EF. Harold Jeffreys www-groups.dcs.st-andrews.ac.uk/~history/Mathematicians/Jeffreys.html.

28. Wrinch D., Jeffreys H. (1919). On Some Aspects of the Theory of Probability, *Philosophical Magazine* **38**, 715–731.

29 Wrinch D., Jeffreys H. (1921/23). On Certain Fundamental Principles of Scientific Inquiry (Two Papers), *Philosophical Magazine* **42**:369–390, **45**:368–374.

30. Fisher R.A. (1932). Inverse Probability and the Use of Likelihood, *Proceedings of the Cambridge Philosophical Society* **28**:257–261.

31. Jeffreys H. (1933). On the Prior Probability in the Theory of Sampling, *Proceedings of the Cambridge Philosophical Society* **29**: 83–87.

32. Jeffreys H. (1932). On the Theory of Errors and Least Squares, *Proceedings of the Royal Society, A* **138**:48–55.

33. Fisher R.A. (1933). The Concepts of Inverse Probability and Fiducial Probability Referring to Unknown Parameters, *Proceedings of the Royal Society, A* **139**:343–348.

34. Jeffreys H. (1933a). Probability, Statistics, and the Theory of Errors, *Proceedings of the Royal Society, A* **140**:523–535.

35. Fisher R.A. (1934.) Probability, Likelihood and the Quantity of Information in the Logic of Uncertain Inference, *Proceedings of the Royal Society, A* **146**:1–8.

36. Jeffreys H. (1934). Probability and Scientific Method, *Proceedings of the Royal Society, A* **146**:9–16.

37. Jeffreys H. (1931). *Scientific Inference*, reprinted with additions in '37 and with new editions in '57 and '73, Cambridge: Cambridge University Press.
38. Hartigan J.(1964). Invariant Prior Distributions, *Annals of Mathematical Statistics* **35**:836–845.
39. Dawid P., Stone M., Zidek J.M. (1973) Marginalization Paradoxes in Bayesian and Structural Inference (with discussion). *Journal of the Royal Statistical Society B* **35**:189–233.
40. Savage L.J. (1951). The theory of statistical decision. *Journal of the Ameridan Statistical Association* **46**:55–67.
41. Savage L.J. (1954). *The Foundations of Statistics*. New York. Wiley (1972 edition).
42. Tales of Statisticians. L.J. Savage. (1917–1971). From www.umass.edu/wsp/statistics/tales/savage.html.
43. Moyé L.A. (2005). *Statistical Monitoring of Clinical Trials: Fundamentals for Investigators*. New York. Springer.
44. Goodman, S.N. (1999). Toward Evidence–Based Medical Statistics. 1: The *p*-value fallacy. *Annals of Internal Medicine* **130**:995–1004.
45. Anonymous. (1988). Evidence of cause and effect relationships in major epidemiologic study disputed by judge. *Epidemiology Monitor* **9**:1.
46. Hill B.A. (1965). The environment and disease: association or causation? *Proceedings of the Royal Soceity of Medicine* **58**:295–300.
47. Walker A.M. (1986). Significance tests represent consensus a and standard practice (Letter) *American Journal of Public Health.***76**:1033. (See also *Journal erratum* **76**:1087.
48. Fleiss J.L. (1986). Significance tests have a role in epidemiologic research; reactions to A.M. Walker. (Different Views) *American Journal of Public Health* **76**:559–560.
49. Fleiss J.L. (1986). Confidence intervals versus significance tests: quantitative interpretation. (Letter) *American Journal of Public Health* **76**:587.
50. Fleiss J.L. Dr. Fleiss response (Letter) (1986). *American Journal of Public Health* **76:**1033–1034.
51. Walker A.M. (1986). Reporting the results of epidemiologic studies. *American Journal of Public Health* **76**:556–558.
52. Moyé L.A. (1997). Sizing Clinical Trials with Variable Endpoint Event Rates. *Statistics in Medicine* **16**:2267–2282.
53. Rahme E., Joseph L., Gyorkos T.W. (2000). Bayesian sample size determination for estimating binomial parameters from data subject to misclassification. *Applied Statistics* **49** (Part I):119–128.
54. Feinstein A. (1977). The haze of Bayes, the aerial palaces of decision analysis, and the computerized ouija board. *Journal of Clinical Pharacology and Therapeutics* **21**:482–96.
55. Berrry D.A., Eick S.G. (1995). Adapative assignment versus balanced randomization in clinical trials — a decision analysis. *Statistics in Medicine* **14:**231–246.

56. Korn E.L., Baumrind S. (1998). Clinician preferences and the estimation of causal treatment differences. *Statistical Science* **13**:209–235.
57. Spiegelhalter D.J., Freedman L.S., Balckburn P.R. (1986). Monitoring clinical trials. Conditional or predictive power? *Controlled Clinical Trials* **7**:8–17.
58. Freedman L.S., Spiegenhalter D.J. (1989). Comparison of Bayesian with group sequential methods for monitoring clinical trials. *Controlled Clinical Trials.* **10**:357–367.
59. Freeman L.S., Spoiegelhbalter D.J., Permar M.K. (1994). The what, why, and how of Bayesian clinical trial monitoring. *Statistics in Medicine* **13**:1371–1383.
60. Berry D.A. (1993). A case for Bayesianism in clinical trials (with discussion). *Statistics in Medicine* **12**:1377–1404.
61. Carlin B.P., Louis T.A. (2000). *Bayes and Empirical Bayes Data Analysis* Boca Raton. Chapman and Hall/CRC Press.
62. Parlmar M.K., Frittiths G.O., Speigelhalter D.J., Souhami R.L., Altman D.G., van der Scheuren E. CHART Steering Committee. (2001). Monitoring of large randomized clinical trials: a new approach with Bayesian methods. *Lancet* **358**:3785–381.
63. Ashby D., Hutton J., McGee M. (1993). Simple Bayesian analysis for case-control studies in cancer epidemiology. *The Statistician* **42**:385–397.
64. Dunson D.B. (2001). Practical advantages of Bayesian analysis of epidemiologic data. *American Journal of Epidemiology* **153**:1222–1226.
65. Kmetic A., Joseph L., Berger C., Tenenhouse A. (2002). Multiple imputation to account for missing data in a survey: estimating the prevalence of osteoporosis. *Epidemiology* **13**:437–444.

1

Basic Probability and Bayes Theorem

1.1 Probability's Role

Questions propel us through life. Instinctually driven tens of thousands of years ago, the search for their solution may now be more cerebral, but their irresistible tug is unchanged. Be they questions of personal survival in primitive cultures ("Where will my next meal come from? Will I be attacked? Will my baby survive?"), questions of agriculture ("Will our crops be raided by the enemy? Will there be enough rain?"), modern national security ("Will our enemy attack? When will that be? Will we be ready?"), society is besought with questions. Personal questions are no less demanding (Will I graduate? Can I find a good job? Will I survive this car accident? Can I pay for the damages?). The consuming capability of emotional questions ("Will he ever leave me? Does she really love me? Will my death be long and painful?") speaks to their own personal power. Our survival seems destined to depend on questions, and our life's character is shaped by the search for their answers.

From thousands of years ago to the present day, man believed the answers to questions were found wholly in the supernatural. Later, society learned to appreciate its own role in shaping its own history ("the answers lie not in the stars, Brutus, but in ourselves," Shakespeare's character Cassius reminded 16th century audiences in *Julius Caesar*).

Yet, whatever the source of the final truth, we are unwilling (and many times cannot afford) to wait until the answer is self-evident. We seek an early view to the future so that we can influence that future (e.g., abandon the development of a new drug that will not be very effective and cause dangerous adverse events). The goal is accurate predictions. Accurate predictions generate precise redirections of our actions, changing the future and perhaps ourselves. Whether it is a general trying to predict the movement of his enemy or a gambler discerning the next card he'll be dealt in blackjack, the goal is the same, to change the course of the future. Ultimately, we desire to shape, and not be shaped by events that could have been predicted.

There are many such predictive tools, but they can in general be classified into two schemas: objective versus subjective probability. The Prologue developed the rise and occasional conflict between these two perspectives. Here we will examine the role of each.

1.2 Objective and Subjective Probability

Each of these tools seeks the same goal, the future prediction of events. However, in their purest forms, they rely on wholly different skill sets.

Objective probability is mathematical. It relies on calculations that are explicit, based on a specific assumption set that can be examined and either verified or rejected. Subjective probability, in its purest form, is not statistical. Using no mathematics, it is the result of a complex ensemble of experience, impressions, as well as hopes and fears about the future.

Examples concerning each's role in the clinical sciences. For example, the Survival and Ventricular Enlargement Trial (SAVE) examined the role of angiotensin-converting enzyme inhibitor (ACE-i) in the late 20th century. Using modern numerical methods, this investigation demonstrated that patients with weakened heart function would on average live longer while taking ACE-I therapy. The magnitude and plausibility of this effect were widely reported [1], its narrow confidence interval and small p-values nailing down the effect magnitude with an irresistible air of certainty.

However, suppose you are an experienced cardiologist at the bedside of a patient with congestive heart failure. Your patient is somewhat weaker than those patients in the clinical trial. She is also experiencing a small amount of renal impairment, a finding that kept patients out of the SAVE study. The patient is reluctant to be placed on yet one more new medication, given the bad reaction to a medication you previously tried. Yet her family, anxious to arrest the declining health of their loved one, is forcefully demanding that you intervene with the ACE-I therapy. Everyone wants the patient to improve, but what action will produce the improvement?

Objective probability, its reliance of relative frequency generating the commonly used relative risks, confidence intervals, and p-value fails here. This situation requires the collection of 1) experience with the patient, 2) expertise with acceptable heart failure treatment strategies, 3) costs, and 4) anticipated patient and family emotional reactions be combined into an ensemble that generates the appropriate decision. The process is decidedly nonnumeric. It is also individual, permitting different cardiologists with similar training and experience to draw different conclusions about the same patient.

1.3 Relative Frequency and Collections of Events

Probability relates *action* to *outcomes*. The action is known to produce several (perhaps many, and in some cases, an infinite) number of outcomes or events. Uncertainty blocks our view of the actual outcome to be produced. We know that any outcome is possible. We would like to know how frequently a particular event will occur. The notion of relative frequency is particularly constructive because it allows the creation of a collection of rules permitting us to compute the probability of interesting and relevant events. Define probability as

$$P[\text{event of interest}] = \frac{\text{outcomes that comprise event of interest}}{\text{total number of events}}. \quad (1.1)$$

This reduces probability to an issue of counting. Sometimes the process of counting is straightforward while other times it is more complex, but from the relative frequency perspective, the central issue is always one of counting.

Example 1.1. Probability as Relative Frequency: There are fifty-five patients scheduled to be seen in surgery clinic today. The demographic breakdown of these fifty-five patients is as follows; African-American – 15; Asian – 10: Caucasian – 10; Hispanic – 20. Out of the fifty-five patients selected, the probability that the first patient is Caucasian is simply

$$P[\text{first patient is Caucasian}] = \frac{\text{number of Caucasian patients}}{\text{total number of patients}} = \frac{10}{55}.$$

To compute the probability the first patient is Caucasian or Asian, we compute

$$P[\text{first patient is Caucasian or Asian}]$$
$$= \frac{\text{number of Caucasian or Asian patients}}{\text{total number of patients}} = \frac{20}{55}.$$

More complex events require more complicated counting devices. For example, computing the probability the second patient will be Caucasian demands an additional element, requiring us to know something about the identity of the first patient. If the first patient was Caucasian, then the probability that the second will also be Caucasian is 9/54. Alternatively, if the first patient was not Caucasian, the probability that the second will be Caucasian is 10/54. We will discuss how to combine these estimates to get the final solution shortly.

1.4 Counting and Combinatorics
To develop another useful way of counting, let's try to find the probability that the first three patients selected are Caucasian. We might anticipate that this will be an infrequent occurrence. There are many different ways to select three patients from fifty-five, and, since most patients are not Caucasian, choosing three from this group to the exclusion of the other groups would not occur often.

In this case we must select three Caucasians from among ten. This number would reside in the numerator of the probability. The denominator consists of the number of ways to select three individuals from the total fifty-five patients.

Focusing first on the numerator, imagine that there are three slots to fill, one for each of the three patients to be selected. For the first slot, there are ten possibilities, because there are ten Caucasians from whom we can select. Having selected one of these patients for the first slot, we find that there are nine remaining patients for the second slot. Proceeding, we have eight patients left from which the third must be chosen. Thus, there are $(10)(9)(8) = 720$ possible ways to select these patients. Define for any positive integer n, n-factorial, or $n!$.[*] Then

$$n! = n(n-1)(n-2)(n-3)...(2)(1). \tag{1.2}$$

Using this notation, the number of ways to select three Caucasians from ten is

$$\frac{10!}{(10-3)!} = (10)(9)(8) = 720. \tag{1.3}$$

However, a close inspection of how we produced this reveals that there is some "double counting" involved. For example identify the individual Caucasians as c_1, c_2, c_3, ...,c_{10}. Then equation (1.3) counts the following outcomes $\{c_4, c_8, c_{10}\}$, $\{c_8, c_{10}, c_4\}$, $\{c_{10}, c_4, c_8\}$, $\{c_4, c_{10}, c_8\}$, $\{c_{10}, c_8, c_4\}$, and $\{c_8, c_{10}, c_4\}$, as different "events." However, for our purposes, they each constitute the same event, since they involve the same three patients c_4, c_8, and c_{10}. Therefore, we must decrease our count so that equivalent events are not double-counted. We do this by dividing by 3!. Thus the number of ways to select 3 individual patients from 10, written as $\binom{10}{3}$ is

$$\binom{10}{3} = \frac{10!}{3!(10-3)!} = \frac{10!}{3!7!} = \frac{(10)(9)(8)}{(3)(2)(1)} = 120. \tag{1.4}$$

which is substantially less than the 720 from equation (1.3) and is the computation we require.

The solution to the probability of selecting three Caucasians is

$$P[3\text{ Caucasians}] = \frac{\binom{10}{3}}{\binom{55}{3}} = \frac{120}{26235} = 0.00457,$$

---

[*] It is no surprise that $1! = 1$. However, the assertion that $0! = 1$ is surprising. This equation is more a definition than a result, and is quite useful, if not essential.

a small number which confirms our intuition. In general, the number of ways to select r subjects from n when order matters is called a *permutation*, $P(n, r)$, where

$$P(n,r) = \frac{n!}{(n-r)!} \tag{1.5}$$

A *combination* is the number of ways to select r objects from n (colloquially expressed as "n choose r") when order does not matter, and is expressed as

$$\binom{n}{r} = \frac{n!}{r!(n-r)!}. \tag{1.6}$$

Example 1.2. Language Translator for the Clinic

In the clinic scenario developed in this section, assume that Dr. K. one of the physicians on duty, will see ten of the fifty-five patients. New to the country, Dr. K. has never seen Hispanic patients before, and will need a translator if required to evaluate any of these twenty patients. What is the probability that Dr. K. requires a Spanish translator for at least part of the day?

Since the call for a translator is made if Dr. K. sees any Hispanic patient, we must compute the probability that Dr. K. will have Hispanic patients in his collection of ten patients. If H is the number of Hispanic patients that Dr. K will see, then H could be any integer value from 0 to 10. We need the probability that Dr. K sees at least one Hispanic patient. This is the sum of the probabilities that he sees exactly one, or exactly two, or exactly three (up to exactly ten) Hispanic patients. Since we would use the same procedure to compute any of these probabilities, we will compute one of them first $\left(\text{i.e., } P[H = 4]\right)$, then proceed to compute the remaining ones, analogously.

Recall that there are twenty Hispanic patients, and thirty-five non-Hispanic patients. Requiring the doctor to see four Hispanic patients, obligates him to see six non-Hispanic patients. How many ways can one do this? Dr. K must have selected four from twenty Hispanic patients, and selected the remaining six patients from the thirty-five non-Hispanic patients. We know how to compute the number of possible selections, namely

$$\binom{20}{4}\binom{35}{6} = (4,845)(1,623,160) = 7,864,210,200,$$

revealing a mind boggling number of ways to select four Hispanic patients in a sample of ten. The denominator of the probability is the number of ways to select ten patients (regardless of their individual race/ethnicity) from the total of 55 patients, or $\binom{55}{10} = 29,248,649,430$. We can now compute the probability that Dr. K

sees exactly four Hispanic patients in a sample of ten as

$$P[H = 4] = \frac{\binom{20}{4}\binom{35}{6}}{\binom{55}{10}} = \frac{7,864,210,200}{29,248,649,430} = 0.269. \qquad (1.7)$$

We require the probability that Dr. K. sees at least one, or the sum of the probabilities that he sees, $1, 2, 3, \ldots 10$. We can write this as

$$P[H \geq 1] = \sum_{i=1}^{10} P[H = i] = \sum_{i=1}^{10} \frac{\binom{20}{i}\binom{35}{10-i}}{\binom{55}{10}}. \qquad (1.8)$$

The summand on the right-hand side of expression (1.8) will be complicated to compute as it requires nine computations analogous to that in expression (1.7). However, a little study reveals an alternative approach for the problem. We know that H can only be one of the integers from zero to ten. Since the sum of these probabilities must be one, then the probability that he sees at least one Hispanic patient is one minus the probability that he sees none. This we can compute easily as

$$P[H \geq 1] = 1 - P[H = 0] = 1 - \frac{\binom{20}{0}\binom{35}{10}}{\binom{55}{10}}$$

$$= 1 - \frac{(1)(183,579,396)}{29,248,649,430} \qquad (1.9)$$

$$= 1 - 0.00628$$

$$= 0.994.$$

This is a much easier calculation, clearly demonstrating Dr. K's pressing need for a translator.

∎

1.5 Simple Rules in Probability
The previous example provided more than just a new way to count events. It revealed a strategy that reformulates complicated outcomes in terms of a simpler

event whose probability we could more easily find. This is a recurring motif in probability, requiring us to develop familiarity and flexibility with event manipulation.

1.5.1 Combinations of Events

Consider E_1, E_2, E_3, ..., E_n as a collection of outcomes whose probabilities can be computed. For example, E_i could be the event that i^{th} patient has an abnormal brain imaging study. In this scenario, assume we can compute the probability of any of these events as a relative frequency, using equation (1.1). While this may be easy to do, there are other events that, while more complicated, are of interest as well. For example, the event that both patient 5 and patient 6 have abnormal brain imaging may be of interest. Or, the probability that patients seven through twelve have abnormal imaging results. Likewise, the probability that neither patient seventeen or eighteen have abnormal imaging tests could be of value.

These latter events, although more complicated than the events signified by E_1, E_2, E_3, ..., E_{100}, are nevertheless related to them. We will describe these relationships, and then show how to compute the probabilities of these more complicated events by reducing them to combinations of simpler ones.

1.5.2 Joint Occurrences

A central component of both objective, and subjective probability is the assessment of joint events. Therefore the ability to successfully understand and manipulate probabilities of joint occurrences is critical to understanding both frequentist and Bayesian probability. There will be some mathematical notation, but the concept is simple.

The joint occurrence of events E_1 and E_2 simply means that the two events occur together. It is a compound event, involving knowledge of the occurrence of two (and sometimes more than two outcomes). The compound event requiring both to occur is known as an *intersection,*[*] and is written as $E_1 \cap E_2$. Probabilities of these joint events are simply called *joint probabilities*. For example, the probability that both patient 7 and patient 12 have abnormal brain imaging results is depicted as $P[E_7 \cap E_{12}]$. The inclusion of either is not sufficient; both must be present.

How we compute probabilities of these joint events depends on the relationships between the events. Events can either be mutual exclusive, or not. If they are not mutually exclusive, then they can be independent or dependent. The definitions of these properties are straightforward.

1.5.3 Mutual Exclusivity

Mutual exclusivity is a property of events. Two events A and B are mutually exclusive if the occurrence of one precludes the occurrence of the other. For example, if A is the occurrence of a six on one roll of a die, and B is the occurrence of 5, then the two events A and B are mutually exclusive. Since the occurrence of both is impossible, the probability of the joint occurrence must be zero, and we write

---

[*] Probabilists frequently state this as "E_1 intersect E_2".

$P[A \cap B] = 0$. Thus, computing the probability of joint events is trivial when the events are mutually exclusive.

If the events are not mutually exclusive, we must then explore their relationship, determining if they are independent or not.

1.5.4 Independence

One of the most useful properties of event relationships is the notion of independence. Events can be independent or dependent. They are independent if the occurrence of one event tells us nothing about the occurrence of the other. Dependent events are events where the occurrence of one event allows us to adjust the probability of the occurrence of the other event. In general, while dependent relationships are the most informative, their probabilities are more complicated to compute.

Although we have a general understanding of the concept of independence and dependence, its central role in the Bayesian paradigm requires us to take a moment to examine its properties and implications.

The descriptors "independence" or "dependence" are properties not of events, but of relationships between events. We don't ask if the occurrence of acute tubular necrosis is "independent." But rather if the occurrence of acute tubular necrosis is independent of the patient's gender. This property is one of relationships.

Independent events do not affect the occurrence of each other. Specifically, the occurrence of one of them does not affect in any way the occurrence of the other, and an observer who notes the occurrence of one event learns nothing about the occurrence of the second event if the two events are independent. Consider the thought process of a doctor who is examining a patient suffering from a bowel disorder that his physician believes may be ulcerative colitis. During the examination, the doctor may notice and record the patient's height. However, the observation that the patient is six feet tall does not influence the likelihood that the patient is suffering from ulcerative colitis. Height simply does not inform the diagnostic process. We say that the two events of ulcerative colitis and height are independent of each another [2]. Independent events are denoted by the " $\perp$ ", and we denote the independence of events E_1 and E_2 as $E_1 \perp E_2$.

Identifying the joint probability of independent events is straightforward. If $E_1 \perp E_2$, then $P[E_1 \cap E_2] = P[E_1]P[E_2]$. When the events are independent, then the probability of their joint occurrence need not be zero, but simply the product of the probabilities of the independent events. Thus, when flipping a fair coin twice, and E_1 be the event of a head on the first toss, and E_2 the probability of a head on a second toss, then we compute

$$P[E_1 \cap E_2] = P[E_1]P[E_2] = \left(\frac{1}{2}\right)\left(\frac{1}{2}\right) = \frac{1}{4}.$$

The computation of the joint event probability when the events are independent is typically quite simple – just multiply the probabilities of the individual occurrences. Researchers take advantage of this property when they draw random samples of subjects from a larger population. Allowing each subject to have the same probability of being selected from the sample all but ensures that the sample sub-jects' measurements are independent of each other. Thus, identifying probabilities of joint events reduces to simply multiplying probabilities of the individual events. This work is the foundation on which the formulas for commonly used statistical estimators (e.g., means, variances, and incidence rates) are computed.

1.5.5 Dependence

The computation of the probability of two events' joint occurrence is relatively simple if they are mutually dependent or independent. However, matters become much more interesting, and somewhat complex when it comes to dependent out-comes. It is on this scenario that we will focus much of our attention in this book.

The dependence property implies that knowledge of the occurrence of one informs us about the likelihood of the other's occurrence. We may rely on one to tell us about the occurrence of the other. However, in order to utilize this property, the nature of the relationship must be clarified. Specifically, the scientist must know exactly how to update her assessment of the occurrence of one event when another dependent event has been generated. This updated assessment is the *conditional probability*.

Physicians commonly use conditional probability each day in their prac-tices perhaps without being formally aware of it. Patients admitted to the hospital suspected of having a stroke are commonly administered tissue plasminogen acti-vator factor (tPA) to limit the extension of the stroke. However, because of its ten-dency to produce intracerebral bleeding, it is best to give tPA within three hours of onset of symptoms, requiring 1) the rapid identification of the ill patient, 2) their rapid delivery to the hospital, and 3) the rapid administration of tPA.

A patient, their anxious family waiting just outside the exam room, under-goes a swift evaluation as the doctor rapidly works to identify the cause of the pa-tient's symptoms. Are they conscious? Does the patient have new difficulty con-trolling her eye movements, and do her pupils react appropriately to light? Are there new facial asymmetries? Does she have sudden, lasting difficulty controlling the movement of her limbs. Does anyone in the family know if she has diabetes, or hypertension? Has she (or anybody in her family) had a stroke? Each of these ques-tions has a well-deserved place in the evaluation of the patient, because each is be-lieved to alter the probability that a patient has had a stroke. The rapidly closing window of whether the patient can receive tPA requires the physician to ask the most informative questions. The answers to these questions alter and update his assessment of the likelihood the patient has suffered a stroke.

Conditional probability is also useful because it is commonly difficult to specify the nature of the dependency persuasively and completely using other quan-titative approaches. Consider, for example, the relationship between health care access and cultural background. It has been well established that some cultures in the United States visit physicians and health care providers more commonly, re-ceive prescriptions at a greater frequency, and are more likely to receive prenatal care than others. However, the precise nature of the connection is unknown, and there is no equation that precisely depicts the relationship. Conditional probability allows us to formulate the relationship by computing different probabilities of

health care access for different cultural backgrounds. The differences in these probabilities are one of the best descriptors of the nature of the relationship between
culture and health care access. They delineate the magnitude of the relationship
without having to elucidate the dependency's nature.

We may specifically denote the probability of an event A when the event B
has occurred as $P[A\,|\,B]$. This probability may be computed as

$$P[A\,|\,B] = \frac{P[A \cap B]}{P[B]}. \qquad (1.10)$$

This formula may appear mysterious, but is actually quite intuitive when viewed
graphically (Figure 1.1).

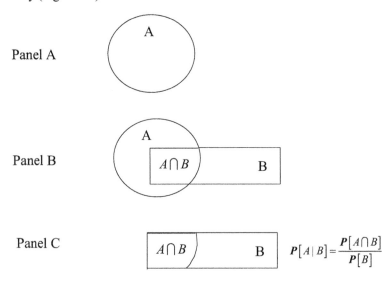

Figure 1.1 Development of conditional probability.

In Figure 1.1, Panel A represents an event A, whose probability, $P[A]$ is
measured by the area of the circle. In Panel B, we introduce the event B, whose
probability, $P[B]$ is represented by the area of the rectangle. Since events A and B
overlap, we denote the segment of overlap, $P[A \cap B]$ signifying that in this region,
both A and B occur.

We can understand the formula (1.10) by first recognizing that the event
$A \cap B$ resides wholly in B (Panel C). The event A given B begins with the occurrence of event B, asking what fraction of the time that event A also occurs. This is

relative proportion of the time that A occurs in B, which is $\dfrac{P[A \cap B]}{P[B]}$. We

can use the same reasoning to see that $P[B \mid A] = \dfrac{P[A \cap B]}{P[A]}$.

Since $P[A \mid B]$ is the relative probability of $A \cap B$ to B, this conditional probability's value can not be deduced from simply knowing that the probability of B (sometimes referred to as the marginal probability of B) is large or small.

Thus, we have three circumstances in which we can compute the probability of the joint event, $A \cap B$ (Figure 1.2). We first determine if the events are mutually exclusive, independent or dependent. If mutually exclusive, then $P[A \cap B] = 0$. If the events are independent, then $P[A \cap B] = P[A]P[B]$. Finally, if we find the events are dependent, and we can compute conditional probabilities, then $P[A \cap B] = P[A \mid B]P[B] = P[B \mid A]P[A]$.

1.5.6 Unions of Events

Computing the probability of events in health care requires us to be able to deconstruct complex events into simpler events whose probabilities are easier to find. One such tool in this deconstruction is the intersection. A second useful tool is the union.

As with the intersection, the concept of the union is simple. The union of two events A and B is simply the event that at least one of them occurs. We write this as $A \cup B$, stating it as "A union B," or "A and/or B." Computing the probability of this event follows directly from examination of the possible ways that this can occur (Figure 1.3).

If we desire the probability of $A \cup B$, the probability that at least event A or event B occurs from Panel A of Figure 1.3, we simply add the probability of A to the probability of B. In this case, $P[A \cup B] = P[A] + P[B]$. However, the circumstance is more complex in Panel B, where the two events C and D are not mutually exclusive. Here, writing $P[C \cup D] = P[C] + P[D]$ is incorrect, because it double counts the region of intersection, $C \cap D$. To correct this, we must remove one of these redundant components. Thus $P[C \cup D] = P[C] + P[D] - P[C \cap D]$.

If A and B are mutually exclusive

$$P[A \cap B] = 0.$$

If A and B are independent

$$P[A \cap B] = P[A]P[B].$$

If A and B are dependent

$$P[A \cap B] = P[A \mid B]P[B] = P[B \mid A]P[A].$$

Figure 1.2 Computing the probability of joint events. First determine if the events are mutually exclusive, independent, or dependent.

1.5.7 Complements

One final useful feature in constructing events of interest is the use of complements. Any element that is not in the set A is in the complement of A. The complement of a set is its opposite. The complement of the set A is the set A^c, termed "A complement" or "Not A." In general, $P\left[A^c\right] = 1 - P[A]$. We used this calculation to complete Example 1.2.

1.5.8 Probabilities and the Differential Effect of Gender: CARE

We can apply some of these concepts to the Cholesterol and Recurrent Events (CARE) clinical trial [3]. The trial was designed to determine the effect of the (HMG-CoA) reductase inhibitor pravastatin on the occurrence of clinical endpoints in patients with normal levels of low-density lipoprotein (LDL) cholesterol. CARE patients were randomized to receive pravastatin or placebo, and followed for approximately five years to assess the effect of this LDL lowering strategy on the combined endpoint of fatal and/or nonfatal coronary artery disease. The study reported the event rates for the overall cohort by gender (Table 1.1).

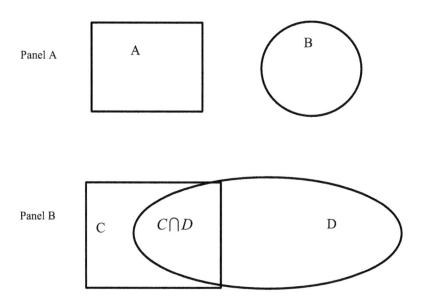

Figure 1.3. Examination of the union of two events.

We may use this table to compute some useful properties using the concepts of relative frequency, union, intersection, complements, and conditional probability. For example, the probability that a patient is a female in CARE is $\frac{576}{(576+3583)} = 0.139$, and the probability that a patient is a male is $1 - 0.139 = 0.861$. The probability a patient has an endpoint is $\frac{(126+853)}{4159} = \frac{979}{4159} = 0.235$.

To compute the probability that a patient has an endpoint given that they are female, we first compute

$$P[\text{female} \cap \text{endpoint}] = \frac{126}{4159} = 0.0303,$$

and then write

$$P[\text{endpoint} \mid \text{female}] = \frac{P[\text{female} \cap \text{endpoint}]}{P[\text{female}]} = \frac{0.0303}{0.139} = 0.219,$$

Table 1.1 Distribution of Primary Endpoints by Gender in CARE

		Placebo	Active	Total
Female	Endpoint	80	46	126
	No Endpoint	210	240	450
	Total	290	286	576

		Placebo	Active	Total
Male	Endpoint	469	384	853
	No Endpoint	1319	1411	2730
	Total	1788	1795	3583

The primary endpoint is the combined incidence rate of fatal and nonfatal coronary artery disease, or coronary revascularization.

which can be verified by a direct inspection of Table 1.1 which demonstrates that

$$P[\text{endpoint} \mid \text{female}] = \frac{126}{576} = 0.219.$$

We can go through the analogous computation for males to find

$$P[\text{endpoint} \mid \text{male}] = \frac{P[\text{male} \cap \text{endpoint}]}{P[\text{male}]} = \frac{0.205}{0.861} = 0.238.$$

Thus the frequency of endpoints is slightly greater among men than women.

1.6 Law of Total Probability and Bayes Theorem

These simple tools of intersection, union and conditioning permit us to solve the inversion problem, a solution first proposed by Bayes and Price.[*] For an example, we return to the CARE trial. In this study, there were 4159 patients randomized to the trial, 2078 recruited to the placebo group, and 2081 to the active group. Out of this entire cohort, 486 patients experienced the primary endpoint of fatal or nonfatal coronary artery disease (CHD). Let E^+ be the event that a patient experienced a primary endpoint, and E^- be the complimentary event that they did not have an endpoint, where $P[E^+] + P[E^-] = 1$. We also define A as the event that a patient was recruited to the active group, and C that they were recruited to the control group, where $P[A] + P[C] = 1$.

---

[*] See the Prologue for a discussion of the collaboration of these two colleagues and friends.

In CARE, the proportion of patients who had a primary endpoint in the active group was 0.102, or $P[E^+ \mid A] = 0.102$. Similarly, the proportion of control group patients with an event $P[E^+ \mid C] = 0.132$. We are interested in determining the probability that a patient is in the control group given the patient had a primary endpoint, or $P[C \mid E^+]$.

This probability requires that we reverse the conditions we were provided, a problem historically known as "inversion," as is exactly the style of problem that the Bayes-Price paper attempted to solve.[*] The modern development of this solution is as follows.

Recognizing that $P[C \mid E^+]$ is a conditional probability, we can write it as

$$P[C \mid E^+] = \frac{P[C \cap E^+]}{P[E^+]}. \tag{1.11}$$

We need the two components; $P[C \cap E^+]$ and $P[E^+]$ which we do have directly. However, these can be computed from the available probabilities. Recall that we were given $P[E^+ \mid C]$, which is defined as

$$P[E^+ \mid C] = \frac{P[C \cap E^+]}{P[C]},$$

which we can write as $P[C \cap E^+] = P[E^+ \mid C] P[C]$, recognizing the values of both quantities to the right of the equal sign are known. Thus, we may rewrite (1.11) as

$$P[C \mid E^+] = \frac{P[E^+ \mid C] P[C]}{P[E^+]}. \tag{1.12}$$

We can find the denominator by observing that the probability of an event is the probability of an event in the control group plus the probability of an event in the active group. Thus we write this as

$$P[E^+] = P[E^+ \cap C] + P[E^+ \cap A].$$

---

[*] The development of this work and its subsequent "rediscovery" by Laplace is described in the Prologue.

This simple statement is known as the *Law of Total Probability*. It states that the overall probability of an event is the sum of the probability of the event in mutually exclusive domains where the domains make up all possible outcomes (in this case, active patients or placebo patients).

But we know that $P\left[E^+ \cap C\right] = P\left[E^+ \mid C\right]P[C]$, and we may also write analogously that $P\left[E^+ \cap A\right] = P\left[E^+ \mid A\right]P[A]$. Therefore,

$$P\left[E^+\right] = P\left[E^+ \cap C\right] + P\left[E^+ \cap A\right]$$
$$= P\left[E^+ \mid C\right]P[C] + P\left[E^+ \mid A\right]P[A]$$

Substituting this into the denominator of (1.12) reveals

$$P\left[C \mid E^+\right] = \frac{P\left[E^+ \mid C\right]P[C]}{P\left[E^+ \mid C\right]P[C] + P\left[E^+ \mid A\right]P[A]}. \tag{1.13}$$

This is the statement of Bayes Theorem. Derived from simple manipulation of conditional probability, it expresses combinations of known conditional probabilities into the inverse probability (i.e., the probability with the condition reversed). In our example, the probability that a patient is in the control group given that an endpoint has occurred is

$$P\left[C \mid E^+\right] = \frac{P\left[E^+ \mid C\right]P[C]}{P\left[E^+ \mid C\right]P[C] + P\left[E^+ \mid A\right]P[A]}$$
$$= \frac{(0.132)(0.50)}{(0.132)(0.50) + (0.102)(0.50)}$$
$$= 0.564.$$

Example 1.3: Cause of Death

Modern controlled clinical trials currently sit atop the pinnacle of evidence based medicine. Use of the *random allocation of therapy* assigns patients to receive either the intervention to be tested or the control therapy such that patient personal characteristics play no role the therapy assignment [4]. Thus, in clinical trials, the only difference between patients taking the therapy and those who do not is the therapy itself. This makes it easier to attribute differences between the intervention and control groups occurring at the end of the study to the intervention itself. In addition, where practically and ethically possible, patients and investigators in the study are not permitted to know who has received the intervention and who has been randomized to control. This *blinding feature* distributes the biases that patients and investigators bring to the study about the intervention's effect across the intervention and control group [5].

Having reduced the role of bias, and ensuring that the only difference between subjects receiving the intervention and those who do not is the intervention itself, well-conducted clinical trials wield tremendous influence in the medical community. Prominent examples are the Cholesterol and Recurrent Events (CARE) trial in atherosclerotic cardiovascular disease [6], and the Anti-Hypertension and Lipid Lowering Heart Attack Trial (ALLHAT) in preventing the clinical sequela of essential hypertension [7].

Investigators who design clinical trials take great care in choosing the patients who are accepted in the study, and in deciding what will be the primary analysis variable, known as the *primary endpoint*. However, matching the intervention, the characteristics of the subjects, and the endpoint can be a delicate business. Essentially the clinical trial must recruit enough patients who in turn will generate a large enough number of endpoints in order to determine if the intervention affects the occurrence of these endpoints. For example, a clinical trial that will evaluate an intervention's effect on the death rate in people who have had a heart attack must not only recruit patients who have had a heart attack, but patients who are likely to die from that heart attack.

In this kind of study, the clinical trial's investigators must have a mechanism in place to identify the cause of death. This mechanism is known as an *endpoint's committee*. The task of this committee is to review each death in the trial to determine if the cause of death allows it to be counted as a primary endpoint. These committees commonly work in a blinded fashion, i.e., they review an patient's record without knowing to which therapy the patient was assigned, therefore keeping the endpoint committee member from applying any bias they may have about the effectiveness of therapy to their determination of cause of death.

Suppose a clinical trial is designed to determine the effect of therapy on deaths due to an arrhythmia, or unusual heart rhythms. From the inclusion/exclusion criteria of the study, it is an anticipated that 20% of patients will die from an arrhythmia. Another 55% will die from other cardiac causes (e.g., heart attacks, or congestive heart failure), and 25% will die from non-cardiac causes (e.g., cancer, or stroke). It is known that if someone has a non-cardiac illness, the probability they will die during the duration of the study is 0.10. If they have an arrhythmia, there is a 70% probability that they will die in the study. If they have some other cardiac disease, the chance that they will die in the study is 35%.

However, when the endpoint committee meets, they know only that the patient has died in the study. What we wish to compute is the probability that the patient has died of an arrhythmia given that we only know they have died. This is an example of "inversion." Here, we have the probability of death given the underlying disease. However, the endpoint committee's task is to compute the probability of the underlying disease given that death has occurred.

Bayes theorem may be applied here, introducing just a little notation to help us succinctly formulate the problem. Let Θ be the cause of death. Then we can easily allow Θ to have three values.

If patient dies of an arrhythmia, then $\Theta = 1$
If patient dies of another cardiac cause, then $\Theta = 2$
If patient dies of non-cardiac cause, then $\Theta = 3$

The conditions of the problem tell us that $P[\Theta = 1] = 0.20$, $P[\Theta = 2] = 0.55$, and $P[\Theta = 3] = 0.25$.

Now, define X as the vital status of the patient, i.e., let $X = 0$ denote that the patient is alive and $X = 1$ mean that the patient has died. We are told that:

$$P[X = 1 | \Theta = 1] = 0.70$$
$$P[X = 1 | \Theta = 2] = 0.35$$
$$P[X = 1 | \Theta = 1] = 0.10$$

The endpoint committee wishes to know the probability that given a patient has died, what is the probability their death was arrhythmogenic (i.e., caused by the arrhythmia). This is $P[\Theta = 1 | X = 1]$. To compute, we simply apply Bayes theorem, writing

$$P[\Theta = 1 | X = 1] =$$
$$\frac{P[X = 1 | \Theta = 1]P[\Theta = 1]}{P[X = 1 | \Theta = 1]P[\Theta = 1] + P[X = 1 | \Theta = 2]P[\Theta = 2] + P[X = 1 | \Theta = 3]P[\Theta = 3]},$$

and the solution is as simple as using the given values of these probabilities

$$P[\Theta = 1 | X = 1] = \frac{(0.70)(0.20)}{(0.70)(0.20) + (0.35)(0.55) + (0.10)(0.25)} = 0.392.$$

Notice how the updating process worked. Without knowledge of a patient's death, the probability that a patient died an arrhythmic death was 0.20. This has now been doubled in the presence of a death to 0.39.

However, we must also admit that, while this was a doubling of the probability of an arrhythmic death, it appears strange that, in a clinical trial designed to detect the effect of an intervention an the risk of arrhythmic death, there is a relatively low yield of such events.

An examination of Bayes theorem suggests a possible mechanism to increase the proportion of patients who are classified as having deaths due to arrhythmia. By altering the inclusion and exclusion criteria of the study, they can increase the $P[\Theta = 1]$. If, for example, they accept more patients with worse arrhythmic disease at entry into the study and fewer patients with milder forms of other cardiac disease, they can increase the probability of death due to an arrhythmia from 0.20 to 0.40, and decrease the probability of death from other cardiac causes from 0.55 to 0.35. Using these revised estimates, we again compute using Bayes Theorem

$$P[\Theta = 1 | X = 1] = \frac{(0.70)(0.40)}{(0.70)(0.40) + (0.35)(0.35) + (0.10)(0.25)} = 0.683,$$

improving the yield of arrhythmic deaths.

Bayes theorem may be used to graphically depict the relationship between the prior and posterior probabilties of arrhythmic deaths.(Figure 1.4). It is this type of relationship depiction that is most useful to investigators as they plan their study. Since the number of patients they are required to recruit is based on the probability of an arrhythmic death, they can use Figure 1.4 to compute the most helpful prior probability of an arrhythmia, and use their collection of patient inclusion and exclusion criteria to produce this proportion of patients. ∎

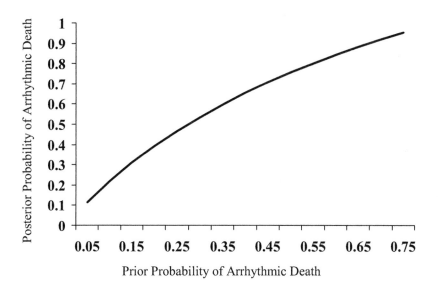

Figure 1.4. Posterior probability of an arrhythmic death increases as the prior probability grows.

Example 1.4: Market Share

Different pharmaceutical companies commonly manufacture and market products for the same conditions, each competing to have their product become the most popular among physicians, pharmacists, and patients. This hypothetical example demonstrates the use of Bayes theorem in computing the relative popularity of two fictitious drugs for the treatment of commonly occurring arthropathies in the United States.

A common cause of chronic pain in adults is arthritis. There are two dominant forms of this condition: rheumatoid arthritis and osteoarthritis. The hallmark of rheumatoid arthritis is inflammation, as the body's immune system systematically destroys the thin, delicate covering of cartilage that lines and protects the ends of the bone within the joint space. On the other hand, osteoarthritis is a disease of degeneration in which the cartilage, degraded by years of joint use (and sometimes, abuse) is frayed and fragmented, sometimes producing painful spikes of new and distorting painful bone growth known as spurs. Each of these conditions generates chronic pain requiring the use of chronic pain therapy in addition to physical therapy, and sometimes surgery.

Two pharmaceutical companies each legally market a compound for the treatment of each of these conditions. Company A markets compound A, and company B markets compound B to the physicians, in a tough and competitive environment in which millions of dollars are spent to gain dominance.

A stock market analyst wishes to compute the probability that the patient who has either osteoarthritis or rheumatoid arthritis is on drug A. Let RA denote whether a patient has rheumatoid arthritis or not (i.e., $RA = 1$ means the patient has rheumatoid arthritis; if the patient does not have rheumatoid arthritis, then $RA = 0$). Similarly, OA denotes whether the patient has osteoarthritis ($OA = 1$ means the patient has osteoarthritis, $OA = 0$ means no osteoarthritis). For this example, we will ignore the relatively small proportion of patients who have both. Similarly, we define

$$\Theta = A \text{ means the patient is on Company A's drug}$$
$$\Theta = B \text{ means the patient is on Company B's drug}$$

Then, the analyst needs to know $P[\Theta = A \mid RA = 1 \ \cup \ OA = 1]$. This is known as the percent of the market (of patients who have either rheumatoid arthritis or osteoarthritis who are on Company A's drug. This probability is known as Company A's *market share*. The greater the market share, the stronger the performance of the company's product, the greater the value of the company's stock, *ceteris paribus*.

A survey of physicians reveals that 40% of the use of Company A's product is for rheumatoid arthritis, i.e., $P[RA = 1 \mid \Theta = A] = 0.40$. In addition, the probability that Company A's medication is used for osteoarthritis is 0.55. Similarly, Company B's compound is used 60% of the time for rheumatoid arthritis and 20% for osteoarthritis. Let $P[\Theta = A] = 0.60$, and $P[\Theta = B] = 0.50$. Invoking Bayes theorem we find

$$P[\Theta = A \mid RA = 1 \ \cup \ OA = 1]$$
$$= \frac{P[RA = 1 \ \cup \ OA = 1 \mid \Theta = A] P[\Theta = A]}{P[RA = 1 \ \cup \ OA = 1 \mid \Theta = A] P[\Theta = A] + P[RA = 1 \ \cup \ OA = 1 \mid \Theta = B] P[\Theta = B]}. \quad (1.14)$$

To solve this, we break these seemingly complicated conditional probabilities into some simpler components. Remembering our assumption that rheumatoid arthritis and osteoarthritis occur in different patients, we can write

$$P[RA = 1 \cup OA = 1 | \Theta = A] = P[RA = 1 | \Theta = A] + P[OA = 1 | \Theta = A]$$
$$= 0.40 + 0.55 = 0.95.$$

Analogously,

$$P[RA = 1 \cup OA = 1 | \Theta = B] = P[RA = 1 | \Theta = B] + P[OA = 1 | \Theta = B]$$
$$= 0.60 + 0.20 = 0.80.$$

We now substitute these values into equation (1.14) to find

$$P[\Theta = A | RA = 1 \cup OA = 1] = \frac{(0.95)(0.60)}{(0.95)(0.60) + (0.80)(0.50)} = 0.587,$$

and Company A's market share is 59%. The market share of Company B is similarly computed as

$$P[\Theta = B | RA = 1 \cup OA = 1] = \frac{(0.80)(0.50)}{(0.95)(0.60) + (0.80)(0.50)} = 0.444.$$

∎

Example 1.5: Sensitivity and Specificity

As a final and commonly used example of Bayes Theorem, we will consider the development of a biomarker to predict the presence of multiple myeloma.

One of the most exciting lines of investigation in genetics is the science of proteomics, or the process by which proteins are identified in the blood that indicate the early presence of disease. Our researchers have examined a combination of proteomic markers that they believe indicate the early presence of multiple myeloma. The identification of these measures is clinically important, since early detection of cancer can lead to the initiation of early therapy and increase the likelihood of cure.

There are many cells that are involved in the body's ability to fight off infection. Some cells (e.g., neutrophils, basophils, eosinophils, and macrophages) don't repel invaders – they digest them. Migrating their way to the sight of injury or infection, these cells close in on the aliens, and release a sequence of caustic enzymes that, if alive, will kill the invader. These lytic enzymes also dismember

1

the physical infrastructure of the alien, allowing its constituents to be either absorbed or expelled.[*]

However other cells are involved in a molecular warfare. They manufacture protein complexes called antibodies, whose shapes match those of the invader. These antibodies are attracted to the alien, and after combining with its outer core, begin to dismantle the foreign object. B-lymphocytes are crucial antibody generators.

Multiple myeloma is a cancer of the immune system specifically affecting the B-lymphocyte, affecting 0.02% (0.0002) of the population. These B-lymphocytes usually produce antibodies to bacteria, viruses, and other foreign substances. In multiple myeloma, they dramatically increase in number and become aberrant, sometimes attacking the body. After a quiet phase of the cancer's development (known as the indolent period), the immune system becomes increasingly erratic and dysfunctional. In the end, rather than generating mature, functioning antibodies that help destroy infectious agents, e.g., bacteria and virus, the distorted B-cells form an amorphous, dysfunctional protein known as amyeloid that is laid down in the gastrointestinal tract, heart and lungs. It is the interruption of the function of these vital organs that is commonly the cause of death in patients with multiple myeloma.

After years of work, the investigators have identified new proteins in the blood of patients that they believe will help detect patients who'll have multiple myeloma. These investigators have produced two assays, A_1 and A_2. With great excitement, the molecular biologists seek the help of a group of oncologists specializing in cancer of the lymphoid system to evaluate the assays. These doctors carry out the tests in a group of patients who they know definitely have multiple myeloma (denoted as M^+) and in a second group of patients without the disease (M^-).

The results are moderately successful for test A_1. Denote a positive test for A_1 as A_1^+. Then the quantity $P\left[A_1^+ \mid M^+\right]$ is known as the *sensitivity* of the test. The higher the sensitivity, the greater the utility of the tests for clinicians. However, since high sensitivity would be ensured by simply having the test be positive in all patients whether they had multiple myeloma or not, we must also be concerned about the probability that the test is negative when the patient does not have multiple myeloma, or $P\left[A_1^- \mid M^-\right]$. This second quantity is known as the *specificity* of the test. Accepting the oncologists' results from each test, the biologists compute the sensitivity and specificity for both A_1 and A_2 (Figure 1.5).

Figure 1.5 reveals that A_1 has moderate sensitivity and specificity, being positive in most patients with multiple myeloma, and negative in most patients without the disease. However, the performance characteristics of assay A_2 are substantially better than A_1.

---

[*] Unfortunately, this process can be self-destructive. For example, the pain of gouty arthritis is ascribed to the damage these enzymes do to the vulnerable and tender membranes that line joint surfaces as errant urate cystals are identified and dissolved.

Test	Sensitivity	Specificity
A_1	$P\left[A_1^+ \mid M^+\right] = 0.75$	$P\left[A_1^- \mid M^-\right] = 0.65$
A_2	$P\left[A_2^+ \mid M^+\right] = 0.99$	$P\left[A_2^- \mid M^-\right] = 0.99$

Figure 1.5. The sensitivity and specificity of test A_2 is superior to that of test A_1.

However, the clinicians, while initially excited about the promising results of these two tests, cannot directly assess the utility of these tests in their practices. When asked why, they explained sensitivity and specificity probabilities while interesting, are not the probabilities they need. In a diagnostic circumstance, the clinicians is not "given the disease." Instead, they are "given the test result." Thus, for example, while $P\left[A_1^+ \mid M^+\right]$ is intriguing, the probability of the disease given the test result, or $P\left[M^+ \mid A_1^+\right]$ would be more useful to the practitioner. This probability is known as *positive predictive value* or *PPV* of the test. We will also denote the negative predictive value as the probability that the patient is myeloma free given the test is negative, or $P\left[M^- \mid A_1^-\right]$. Thus, the clinicians need to see $PPV(A_1)$, $NPV(A_1)$, as well as the analogous quantities for the second assay.

Fortunately, each of the predictive values are available through the use of Bayes Theorem. For example, for $PPV(A_1)$, we write

$$\mathrm{PPV}\left(A_1\right) = P\left[M_1 \mid A_1^+\right] = \frac{P\left[A_1^+ \mid M^+\right] P\left[M^+\right]}{P\left[A_1^+ \mid M^+\right] P\left[M^+\right] + P\left[A_1^+ \mid M^-\right] P\left[M^-\right]},$$

and, substituting values for the sensitivity and specificity of A_1 as well as the prevalence of multiple myeloma, this becomes

$$PPV\left(A_1\right) = P\left[M^+ \mid A_1^+\right] = \frac{(0.75)(0.0002)}{(0.75)(0.0002)+(0.35)(0.9998)} = 0.00043.$$

$PPV(A_1)$ appears shockingly low. One hundred thousand positive tests would produce only 43 cases of multiple myeloma. The overwhelming number of false positives stigmatizes test A_1 as relatively worthless to the clinicians. Knowing that A_2 has superior sensitivity and specificity to A_1, they excitedly turn to its predictive value computation:

$$PPV(A_2) = P[M^+ | A_2^+] = \frac{(0.99)(0.0002)}{(0.99)(0.0002)+(0.01)(0.9998)} = 0.019. \quad (1.15)$$

While the stunning low $PPV(A_1)$ was somewhat predictable, the shockingly low positive predictive value of test A_2, is a profound disappointment to the clinicians. How, they complain, can clinicians possibly use a test in which, out of 1000 positive assays, only 19 will have multiple myeloma?

    The molecular biologists, themselves shocked by the findings, react defensibly to the dissatisfied clinicians. They point out that test A_2 has provided an important increase in identifying patients with multiple myeloma. While the clinicians may scoff at the $PPV(A_2)$ of 0.019, this is 95 times greater than the prevalence of multiple myeloma without carrying out A_2. "Much more needs to be done," they respond, "but much has been accomplished so far." How, they will ask, can we expect to develop a test with greater sensitivity and specificity than 99%?

    They also note that the sensitivity and specificity of A_2 is substantially higher than anything developed before. In fact the testing characteristics of assay A_2 are far superior than other early cancer detection tests that the oncologists use for other diseases (e.g., colon cancer). If, the molecular biologists ask, the oncologist's colleagues are satisfied with assays producing more moderate sensitivities and specificities, then why will they not themselves accept the superior characteristics of A_2? is more reliable than many acceptable tests for other diseases on the market.

    The genesis of the low predictive value of A_2 is perplexing. The issue lies not so much with the test's characteristics, but with the low prevalence of the disease. One way to see this is from the mathematics of Bayes Theorem, writing it as

$$PPV = \frac{\text{Sensitivity} * \text{Prevalence}}{\text{Sensitivity} * \text{Prevalence} + (1 - \text{Specificity}) * (1 - \text{Prevalence})}. \quad (1.16)$$

The second product in the denominator becomes very large for very small prevalence, even in the presence of high specificity. This was what occurred for the prevalence of test A_2 as revealed in equation (1.15).

    However, it is more revealing to allow figures to provide insight into what has happened in this case of low prevalence (Figure 1.6). In Figure 1.6, all patients are depicted within the area of the large square. The upper right-hand corner of the square identifies the small number of patients (signified by M^+) who have multiple myeloma, with the rest of the area of the larger square filled by patients who do not have multiple myeloma (M^-).

In this setting, we can now overlay the results of test A_2 (Figure 1.7). In Figure 1.7, we see that if we confine ourselves to the small square in the upper right- hand corner, the overwhelming majority of patients with multiple myeloma have a positive test, reflecting the high sensitivity of test A_2. Similarly, the overwhelming number of patients who do not have multiple myeloma have a negative test. This is in keeping with the known testing characteristics assay A_2. However, even though the vast majority of people who don't have multiple myeloma are A_2^-, there remain many M^- people with positive tests.

This is the key to understanding the low *PPV*. The low prevalence permits (1) the overwhelming number of people without multiple myeloma to test negative on A_2, driving up the specificity, while (2) simultaneously permitting a large number of people without the disease to test positive on A_2. It is not as though low prevalence undermines the test. It is simply that high specificity is not high enough, permitting substantial numbers of patients without the disease to also have a positive test, and thereby reduce the *PPV*. Thus, when one computes the predictive value, looking at only those patients who test positive on A_2 (i.e., those patients in the ellipse) most do not have multiple myeloma.

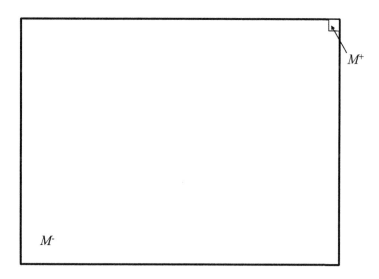

Figure 1.6. The prevalence of multiple myeloma (M^+) is small.

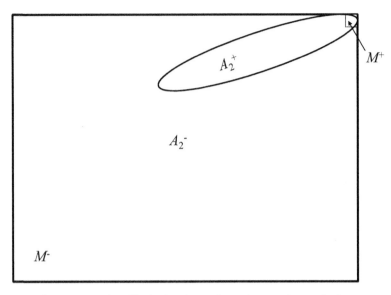

Figure 1.7. Adding test A_2. The elliptical region reflects those patients who have a positive response to A_2 (A_2^+). The region outside the ellipse containing patients who test negative (A_2^-).

References

1. Pfeffer M.A., Braunwald, E, Moyé L.A., Basta L., Brown E.J., Cuddy T.E., Davir B.R., Geltman E.M., Goldman S., Flaker G.C., Klein M., Lamas G.A., Packer M., Rouleau J., Rouleau J.L., Rutherford J., Wertheimer J.H., Hawkins C.M. on behalf of the SAVE Investigators (1992). Effect of Captopril on mortality and morbidity in patients with left ventricular dysfunction after myocardial infarction — results of the Survival and Ventricular Enlargement Trial. *New England Journal of Medicine* **327**:669–677.
2. Moyé L. (2003). *Multiple Endpoints in Clinical Trials: Fundamentals for Investigators*. New York. Springer.
3. Pfeffer M.A., Sacks F.M., Moyé, L.A. et al. for the Cholesterol and Recurrent Events Clinical Trial Investigators (1995). Cholesterol and Recurrent Events (CARE) trial: A secondary prevention trial for normolipidemic patients. *American Journal of Cardiology* **76**:98C–106C.
4. Friedman L., Furberg C., and DeMets D. (1996). *Fundamentals of Clinical Trials*. Third Edition. New York. Spinger.
5. Moyé L.A. (2003). *Multiple Analyses in Clinical Trials. Fundamentals for Investigators*. New York. Springer.

6. Sacks F.M., Pfeffer M.A., Moyé L.A., Rouleau J.L., Rutherford J.D., Cole T.G., Brown L., Warnica J.W., Arnold J.M.O., Wun C.C. Davis B.R., Braunwald E. for the Cholestrol and recurrent Events Trial Investigators. (1996). The effect of pravastatin on coronary events after myocardial infarction in patients with average cholesterol levels. *New England Journal of Medicine,* **335**:1001–9.
7. The ALLHAT Officers and Coordinators for the ALLHAT Collaborative Research Group. (2002). Major outcomes in high-risk hypertensive patients randomized to angiotensin-converting enzyme inhibitor or calcium channel blocker vs diuretic. The Antihypertensive and Lipid-Lowering Treatment to Prevent Heart Attack Trial (ALLHAT). *Journal of the American Medical Association,* **288**:2981–2997.

2

Compo nding and the Law
of Total Probability

2.1 Introduction

Just as physicians cannot diagnose a disease of which they have never heard, bio-statisticians and epidemiologists cannot predict the likelihood of events that they do not recognize or comprehend.[*] Thus, quantitative health care workers must understand the nature of the events they wish to predict. Fortunately, many useful and relatively simple probability models in health care are available. The traditional paradigms are very helpful, and several of these models will be introduced in this chapter.

However, we must acknowledge that the Bayesian perspective requires a more flexible application of these models. To the Bayesian, a probability computation is only as good as the accuracy of the prior information, information which is most useful if it truly reflects subjective impressions. If subjective probability is taken at its face value, that is, its foundation in the nonmathematical, intuitive impressions of several observers, then the incorporation of these strong but non-quantifiable belief systems into easily understood mathematical calculations would be problematic (setting aside the frequentists' claim that any attempt to incorporate them is inappropriate). Traditionally, probability calculations flowed smoothly when tightly confined to the tenets of relative frequency.

However, work by Jeffreys [1,2] , Savage [3], and Berger [4] had demonstrated how the subjective component of probability can be incorporated within a mathematically rigorous thought process. This integration, using the same rules we developed in Chapter One for probability calculations, leads to precise, interpretable results. In this chapter, we will introduce easily understood notational devices that permit this integration.

A useful starting point for the incorporation of subjective, prior information into commonly used traditional probability models is the discussion begun in Chapter One on the Law of Total Probability. After this law is briefly reviewed, we will introduce some basic probability models and reveal how the use of prior in-

---

[*] For example, one cannot compute the probability of drawing "three of a kind" in a poker game if you don't understand the composition of a deck of playing cards.

formation through the Law of Total Probability produces unanticipated predictions. The ensuing explanations will reveal the role and power wielded by the rigorous incorporation of subjective probability computations.

2.2 The Law of Total Probability: Compounding

The Law of Total Probability is quite simple. It only states that, if we have the joint probability of two sets of outcomes X and W, then we can find the probability of X by summing over the probabilities of W. Thus.

$$P[X = x] = \sum_{W} P[X = x, W = w]: \quad P[W = w] = \sum_{X} P[X = x, W = w].$$

Alternatively, the probability of W can be found by summing over all probabilities of X. This intuitive result is readily seen from a description of the findings from a clinical trial (Survival and Ventricular Enlargement or SAVE) designed to demonstrate the effect of the therapy captopril on the death rate in patients with cardiac left ventricular dysfunction in [5] (Table 2.1).

Table 2.1 Mortality distribution by age and treatment in SAVE

	Placebo		Captopril		Total
	Deaths	Percent	Deaths	Percent	
Age <= 55	54	0.1074	52	0.1034	
Age 56 to 64	77	0.1531	69	0.1372	
Age > 64	144	0.2863	107	0.2127	
Total	275	0.5467	228	0.4533	503

Table 2.1 provides the number and proportion of deaths that occur in each of eight treatment groups – age strata. The percent dead is computed from the total number of deaths in that cell divided by the total number of deaths in the study (503).

The numbers and proportions of deaths sum down the rows. For example, if we let X be the therapy group and W be the age group, then from the Law of Total Probability, we can see that to get the overall probability of death for a patient assigned to the placebo group, we simply add the probabilities of death for each of the age ranges in the placebo group (within rounding). We can obtain the five probabilities, (1) probability of death in the placebo group, (2) probability of death in the captopril group (3) probability of death for patients with ages ≤ 55, (4) probability of death for patients in the 56–64 age range, and (5) probability of death for patients greater than 64 years of age. Because these probabilities lie at the margins of the table, they are colloquially called *marginal probabilities*. Each is obtained by taking the sum of the joint probabilities in the appropriate row or column of the table.

The Law of Total Probability will be most useful when one of the events represents a value of a parameter θ. In this case, this law may be written as

$$P[X = x] = \sum_{\theta} P[X = x, \Theta = \theta]. \tag{2.1}$$

However, we know from the definition of conditional probability that

$$P[X = x, \Theta = \theta] = P[X = x \mid \Theta = \theta] P[\theta].$$

Thus, we may rewrite equation (2.1) as

$$P[X = x] = \sum_{\theta} P[X = x \mid \Theta = \theta] P[\theta]. \tag{2.2}$$

It is this format of the Law of Total Probability that will be most useful to us, revealing how one can go from a distribution that is conditional on the value of θ to a distribution which is completely free of this parameter. A marginal distribution $(P[X = x])$ becomes available through the manipulation of a conditional distribution $(P[X = x \mid \Theta = \theta])$ and another marginal $(P[\theta])$. This process, which will be an important emphasis of this chapter and the next is historically known as *compounding*.

2.2.1 The Role of Compounding in Bayes Procedures

We will see that the compounding process reveals interesting and useful results of its own accord. However, it is an intermediate result on the path to a complete Bayes solution.

Recall that, in the Bayesian framework, we are interested in posterior information about the parameter θ, based on a collection of measurements. We want to learn of θ's value (e.g., probability of death experienced by patients in a research effort) when we have data symbolized by $x_1, x_2, x_3, \ldots x_n$. Recall that we called this probability distribution of θ conditional on the data the posterior distribution of θ (because it was obtained after or posterior to the available data) and noted it as $\pi(\theta \mid x_1, x_2\, x_3, \ldots, x_n)$. Initially, we only had an idea or impression of the location of θ, denoted by a prior distribution or $\pi(\theta)$. We use the distribution of the data itself $f(x_1, x_2\, x_3, \ldots, x_n \mid \theta)$ to link the prior information $\pi(\theta)$ with the posterior distribution $\pi(\theta \mid x_1, x_2\, x_3, \ldots, x_n)$ (Figure 2.1). We accomplish this by conversion of prior to posterior information through the equation

$$\pi(\theta \mid x_1, x_2\, x_3, \ldots, x_n) = \frac{f(x_1, x_2\, x_3, \ldots, x_n \mid \theta) \pi(\theta)}{m(x_1, x_2\, x_3, \ldots, x_n)} \tag{2.3}$$

where the denominator is the probability distribution of x_1, x_2, x_3, ... x_n uncondi-tional on θ.

It is the Law of Total Probability that tells us how to compute $m(x_1, x_2\, x_3,...,x_n)$, the marginal distribution of the set of x_1, x_2, x_3, ... x_n. Specifi-cally, $m(x_1, x_2\, x_3,...,x_n) = \sum_{\theta} f(x_1, x_2\, x_3,...,x_n \mid \theta)\pi(\theta)$, a device that permits us to write Equation (2.3) as

$$\pi(\theta \mid x_1, x_2\, x_3,...,x_n) = \frac{f(x_1, x_2\, x_3,...,x_n \mid \theta)\pi(\theta)}{\sum_{\theta} f(x_1, x_2\, x_3,...,x_n \mid \theta)\pi(\theta)}. \qquad (2.4)$$

Thus, the Law of Total Probability is a pivotal point in obtaining the posterior dis-tribution of θ, representing a reformatting of the denominator of equation (2.4). In this chapter and Chapter Three, we will focus solely on the denominator of the right-hand side of Equation (2.4)

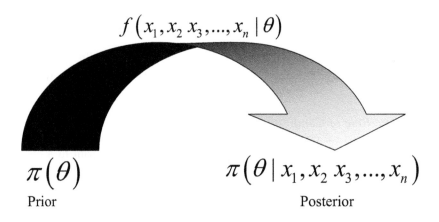

$$f(x_1, x_2\, x_3,...,x_n \mid \theta)$$

$$\pi(\theta)$$
Prior

$$\pi(\theta \mid x_1, x_2\, x_3,...,x_n)$$
Posterior

Figure 2.1. Using data to update prior to posterior information about a parameter θ.

We will first develop the probability model, and then show how the process of compounding can increase the utility of that model in the presence of uncertain information.

2.3 Proportions and the Binomial Distribution

We turn to a contemporaneous problem to develop a simple and useful probability model. An assisted living facility houses the elderly who can no longer care for themselves. We are interested in predicting the number X of patients who die of a particular disease in a year. There are n total patients in the apartment complex. Let a patient's probability of death be θ, and the probability that a patient survives the year is simply $1-\theta$.

Assume we have selected $X = k$ subjects from the total number of n elderly patients. It is reasonable to believe that the fate of one individual does not affect the likelihood that any other will die. In this circumstance, we can compute the probability that the k individuals die and the remaining $n - k$ survive as simply $\theta^k (1-\theta)^{n-k}$.

This probability is correct for any collection of k elderly individuals out of the total of n; however, we know that there are many ways to select k patients from our sample. For example, we could select the first k patients, or the last k observed. Thus, we need to count the number of ways we can select k subjects from n. From Chapter One, we know this is $\binom{n}{k}$.

We are ready to put the final distribution together now. For each selection of k individuals, we've determined that the probability that the k subjects chosen die and the remaining $n - k$ survive is $\theta^k (1-\theta)^{n-k}$. We also know that there are $\binom{n}{k}$ ways to select them. Thus the probability that out of n patients k die is simply

$$P[X = k] = \binom{n}{k} \theta^k (1-\theta)^{n-k}. \tag{2.5}$$

This is the *binomial distribution*. The binomial distribution is one of the most useful distributions in biostatistics or epidemiology. It requires that the event of interest be dichotomous (i.e., it either occurs or does not occur). In addition, subjects should experience the event independently of each other, and the probability of the event must be the same for each subject.[*]

From this distribution we can compute a measure of central tendency or the *mean*, as well as two measures of dispersion of the possible values, (1) the *variance* and (2) the *standard deviation*. In the case of the binomial distribution, the mean μ (also denoted as the expected value of X, or $E[X]$) is $n\theta$. Similarly, we can compute a measure of dispersion or variance as $\sigma^2 = n\theta(1-\theta)$, and the standard deviation as $\sigma = \sqrt{n\theta(1-\theta)}$.

Example 2.1

A clinical investigator is interested in determining the distribution of rehospitalizations for infections within one month following surgical amputation of a lower extremity. If he knows the probability of a repeat admission for this condition, he can readily compute the probability that out of 40 patients, k patients are rehospitalized for any value of k between zero and forty (Figure 2.2).

---

[*] Events that meet these three critiea are known as *Bernoulli trials*.

Note that the probability distribution of the number of patients hospitalized is critically dependent on the value of θ, the probability of readmission. The
results are very intuitive. When θ is small ($\theta = 0.10$), lower values of k have the
greatest probability; for θ large ($\theta = 0.90$), higher values of k predominate.

This intuition applies to the mean and standard deviations of these distributions as well. For $\theta = 0.10$, the mean number of readmissions is $\mu = (20)(0.10) =$
2.0 with standard deviation $\sigma = \sqrt{(20)(0.10)(0.90)} = 1.34$. For $\theta = 0.50$, the mean
increases to $(20)(0.50) = 10.0$. The variance also changes, in this case, increasing to
$\sigma = \sqrt{(20)(0.50)(0.50)} = 2.24$.

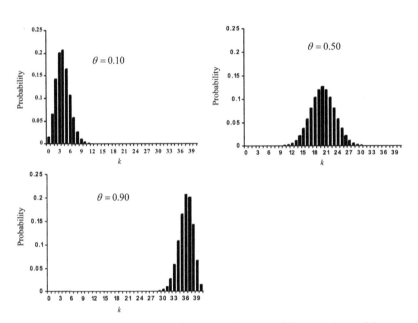

Figure 2.2 Graph of the binomial distribution for three different values of θ.

In this circumstance, the distribution of the likely values of k are available
when the investigator is provided values of n and θ. However, what would the circumstance be if the investigator was uncertain of the value of θ? For example, assume that the investigator expected the value of θ to be any one of 0.10, 0.50, or
0.90, but didn't know which value was the correct one. Can the investigator identify the distribution of the number of post-amputee readmissions in the face of this
uncertainty?

The answer is yes, if she knows something about the probability of these
alternative values of θ. For example, assume the following probability distribution
for θ, which we will call simply $\pi(\theta)$;

$$\pi(\theta) = \begin{array}{l} 0.60 \text{ if } \theta = 0.10 \\ 0.30 \text{ if } \theta = 0.50 \\ 0.10 \text{ if } \theta = 0.90 \end{array} \qquad (2.6)$$

We can graphically display the $\pi(\theta)$ easily (Figure 2.3).

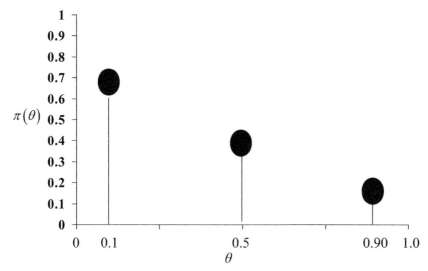

Figure 2.3. Probability distribution of θ. It can take on only three values 0.10, 0.50, or 0.90.

The relative probabilities for the different values of θ are reflected in the heights of the three bars in Figure 2.3. The solid balls at the top of each bar simply denote that probability is assessed only for one value of θ and not an interval of values, for example, $P[0.05 \le \theta \le 0.15] = P[\theta = 0.10] = 0.60$. This is an example of *point-mass* probability, i.e., we assign a "mass" of probability to a particular "point."[*]

This probability distribution of θ, $\pi(\theta)$, is a legitimate distribution, and we can compute probabilities for any range of values of θ. For example, $P[0 \le \theta \le 0.50] = P[\theta = 0.10] + P[\theta = 0.50] = 0.90$. We can symbolize this by using the summation sign, writing, $\sum_{\theta=0.0}^{0.50} \pi(\theta) = 0.90$.

---

[*] This is not the first time we use the concept of point-mass probability. The binomial distribution, which assigns probability to only the integers between 0 and n also utilizes this concept, applying probability to individual values. This is a property of any discrete probability distribution function.

A more succinct way to write the probability distribution $\pi(\theta)$ is through the use of *indicator functions*. Indicator functions are easy-to-understand, useful devices to appreciate the discrete values a probability distribution can take.

If we wanted to denote the fact $\pi(\theta) = 0.60$ when $\theta = 0.10$ and zero elsewhere we write $\pi(\theta) = 0.601_{\theta=0.10}$. The function $1_{\theta=0.10}$ is simply one when $\theta = 0.10$ and zero elsewhere. Using this notation, our probability distribution function for θ, $\pi(\theta)$, can be written as

$$\pi(\theta) = 0.601_{\theta=0.10} + 0.301_{\theta=0.50} + 0.101_{\theta=0.90}. \tag{2.7}$$

We can verify that $\sum_{\theta=0}^{1} \pi(\theta) = 1$ by carefully accumulating probability as θ increased from 0 to 1. Starting at $\theta = 0$, we accumulate or measure no positive probability until $\theta = 0.10$ when we suddenly accumulate 0.60 probability. Continuing to increase θ beyond 0.10, we accumulate no additional probability until $\theta = 0.50$, when we accumulate an additional 0.30 probability. This brings the total probability to 0.90. The process continues, adding no additional probability until $\theta = 0.90$, when the final 0.10 probability is added, bringing the total to 1.00 (Figure 2.4).

We are now in a position to answer the original question, what is the distribution of the number of post-amputee readmissions when the value of θ, the probability of a post amputee readmissions is unknown. Using our notation from the previous chapter, we have

$$P[X = k \mid \theta] = \binom{40}{k} \theta^k (1-\theta)^{n-k}. \tag{2.8}$$

Note that we write this probability as a conditional probability, since we have to be given the value of θ to compute it.[*] However, we also have the distribution of θ, $\pi(\theta)$.

These are the only tools required to compute the unconditional distribution of k, since. From Chapter One's discussion of the Law of Total Probability we know that $P[X = k] = \sum_{\theta=0}^{1} P[X = k \mid \theta] \pi(\theta)$. Thus,

$$
\begin{aligned}
P[X = k] &= \sum_{\theta=0}^{1} P[X = k \mid \theta] \pi(\theta) \\
&= \sum_{\theta=0}^{1} \binom{40}{k} \theta^k (1-\theta)^{n-k} \pi(\theta) \\
&= \sum_{\theta=0}^{1} \binom{40}{k} \theta^k (1-\theta)^{n-k} \left(0.601_{\theta=0.10} + 0.301_{\theta=0.50} + 0.101_{\theta=0.90} \right)
\end{aligned}
\tag{2.9}
$$

---

[*] We will ignore for a short period the fact that this conditional probability distribution is also a function of n, since n will be a constant throughout this problem.

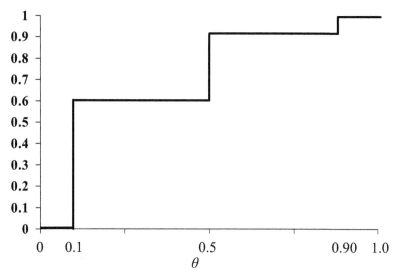

Figure 2.4. The accumulation of probability for $\pi(\theta)$.

This last equality from expression (2.9) we can write as

$$
= 0.60 \sum_{\theta=0}^{1} \binom{40}{k} \theta^k (1-\theta)^{n-k} \mathbf{1}_{\theta=0.10} + 0.30 \sum_{\theta=0}^{1} \binom{40}{k} \theta^k (1-\theta)^{n-k} \mathbf{1}_{\theta=0.50}
$$
$$
+ 0.10 \sum_{\theta=0}^{1} \binom{40}{k} \theta^k (1-\theta)^{n-k} \mathbf{1}_{\theta=0.90}.
$$

$$(2.10)$$

This expression is easy to identify if we take these three terms one at a time. Beginning with the expression $0.60 \sum_{\theta=0}^{1} \binom{40}{k} \theta^k (1-\theta)^{n-k} \mathbf{1}_{\theta=0.10}$, we evaluate the sum as we did $\pi(\theta)$, accumulating values of $\binom{40}{k} \theta^k (1-\theta)^{n-k} \mathbf{1}_{\theta=0.10}$ as θ is allowed to increase continuously from 0 to 1. However the indictor function tells us that the function $\binom{40}{k} \theta^k (1-\theta)^{n-k} \mathbf{1}_{\theta=0.10}$ is zero for all values of θ except when $\theta = 0.10$.

When $\theta = 0.10$, then $\binom{40}{k} \theta^k (1-\theta)^{n-k} 1_{\theta=0.10} = \binom{40}{k}(0.10)^k (0.90)^{n-k}$. Thus the

sum of values of $\binom{40}{k} \theta^k (1-\theta)^{n-k}$ collapses to just one value, and we can write

$$0.60 \sum_{\theta=0}^{1} \binom{40}{k} \theta^k (1-\theta)^{n-k} 1_{\theta=0.10} = 0.60 \binom{40}{k}(0.10)^k (0.90)^{n-k}.$$

Applying this reasoning to the other two terms in expression (2.10), we may write

$$P[X = k] = 0.60 \binom{40}{k}(0.10)^k (0.90)^{n-k} + 0.30 \binom{40}{k}(0.50)^k (0.50)^{n-k}$$

$$+ 0.10 \binom{40}{k}(0.90)^k (0.10)^{n-k}, \tag{2.11}$$

and we have arrived at our goal, the unconditional probability distribution of the values of k.

We started with the probability distribution of $P[X = k \mid \theta] = \binom{40}{k} \theta^k (1-\theta)^{n-k}$. This provided the distribution of value of k, but required us to know θ. However, although we don't know θ, we do have knowledge about possible values of θ and the probabilities of these values as summarized in $\pi(\theta)$. We then used the Law of Total Probability to convert $P[X = k \mid \theta]$ to $P[X = k]$. Thus, the θ was summed out of the distribution of k, removing its overt presence from formula (2.11), but imprinting its identity, embedding information about its possible values into $P[X = k]$. The appearance of the distribution is instructive (Figure 2.5).

A comparison of Figures 2.2 (demonstrating $P[X = k \mid \theta]$ for different values of θ) with Figure 2.5 (showing the unconditional probability distribution of k) reveals these distributions have the same general appearance. However it is the probability of the values of θ reflected in $\pi(\theta) = 0.601_{\theta=0.10} + 0.301_{\theta=0.50} + 0.101_{\theta=0.90}$ that produces the different amplitudes of the probability assignments for the different values of k. If we were to change the distribution of θ to $\pi(\theta) = 0.151_{\theta=0.10} + 0.701_{\theta=0.50} + 0.151_{\theta=0.90}$ a different shape for the unconditional distribution of X emerges (Figure 2.6).

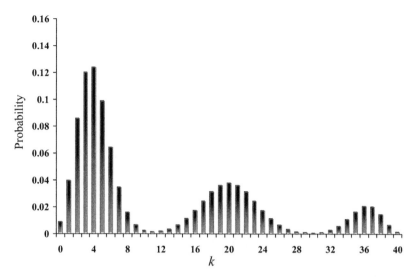

Figure 2.5. The unconditional (or marginal) distribution of k after removing or "summing out" possible values of θ.

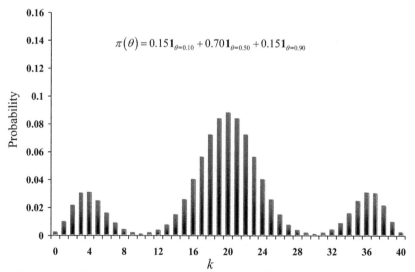

$$\pi(\theta) = 0.151_{\theta=0.10} + 0.701_{\theta=0.50} + 0.151_{\theta=0.90}$$

Figure 2.6. Change in the distribution of values of k, the number of patients rehospitalized after changing $\pi(\theta)$.

Thus, specific information about the probability distribution of θ directly affects the distribution of the number of re-hospitalized patients.

Note the contribution compounding made in this circumstance. Uncertainty about the parameter θ did not preclude us from using the binomial probability distribution as long as that uncertainty could be mathematically captured.

2.4 Negative Binomial Distribution

The use of repeated sequences of Bernoulli trials (that is, independent events which can be characterized as having two states, are independent, and have the same probability from trial to trial) is one of the most useful applications of probability and biostatistics to epidemiology. The binomial distribution, which produces the number of successes in n Bernoulli trials, is one such useful application.

However, suppose we reversed the question, and asked how many trials it takes to reach the kth success. In this case the number of trials, and not the number of successes is random. In the binomial distribution, we fixed n, and determined the distribution of k, where $0 \le k \le n$. Now, we wish to fix k, and allow n to vary.

To start, we know that n can be no less than k (since one must have at least k trials to have k successes occur). In this paradigm it doesn't matter how the first k – 1 successes occurred. However, the kth success must appear on the nth trial.

The mathematical development is straightforward. First we compute the probability of $k-1$ successes in $n-1$ trials. This is

$$P[k-1 \text{ successes in } n-1 \text{ trials}] = \binom{n-1}{k-1} p^{k-1} (1-p)^{n-k}.$$

An additional success would mean that the kth success occurred on the nth trial. Thus,

$$P[n^{th} \text{ trial holds the } k^{th} \text{ success}] = \binom{n-1}{k-1} p^k (1-p)^{n-k}. \quad (2.12)$$

The similarity between the binomial and negative binomial distribution can be confusing. In the binomial distribution, the number of trials is fixed, and it is the number of successes that are the random element. For the negative binomial distribution, the number of successes is fixed, and the number of trials are random.[*] Another helpful formulation is

$$P[k \text{ failures before the } r^{th} \text{success}] = \binom{k+r-1}{r-1} \left(\frac{\alpha}{(\alpha+t)}\right)^r \left(\frac{t}{(\alpha+t)}\right)^k. \quad (2.13)$$

---

[*] If X is the number of trials until the first success, then $P[X = k] = q^k p$ for k = 0, 1, 2, 3,… . This is commonly known as the geometric distribution.

This is the probability that in a sequence of independent success-failure trials there are k failures before the rth success, The mean of this distribution is r/p, and its variance is rq/p^2.

Example 2.2

Gastroenteritis-inducing viruses (e.g., the Norwalk virus) is an ever present threat to communities with little fresh water and poor sanitation. As a result of the Hurricane Katrina disaster that struck New Orleans in August 2005, tens of thousands of evacuees (many of them children) were transported 300 miles west to Houston, Texas for treatment and shelter. Over 1,000 buses arrived in Houston during the first two weeks of September. Large numbers of survivors arrived having had no fresh water or food for 72 hours. Weakened by chronic exposure, acute malnourishment and dehydration, they were susceptible to diarrhea producing viral infections. Assume that the overall probability an individual is infected with one of these viruses is $\theta = 0.28$.

Assume that a bus contains 50 survivors, and the workers wish to know the probability that at least 15 of these people are infected. Since in this case, the number of survivors at risk of the infection is fixed at $n = 50$ and the question is about the number of individuals out of that fixed number who are infected, we use the binomial distribution. The probability that exactly k out of the 50 survivors are infected is

$$P[\text{exactly } k \text{ of 50 survivors are infected}] = \binom{50}{k}(0.28)^k (0.72)^{50-k}.$$

To find the probability that least 15 of the survivors are ill, we write

$$P[\text{at least 15 of 50 survivors are infected}] = \sum_{k=15}^{50} \binom{50}{k}(0.28)^k (0.72)^{50-k}$$

$$= 1 - \sum_{k=0}^{14} \binom{50}{k}(0.28)^k (0.72)^{50-k}$$

$$= 1 - 0.571$$

$$= 0.429.$$

Note the use of the complement argument to ease the computation of this probability.[*]

However, other pressing questions require use of the negative binomial distribution. A major concern among health care workers was the threat of tuberculosis, a lung infection that, if left untreated, affects every organ of the body and is

---

[*] Computer programs such as Excel make computations based on standard probability distributions easier.

fatal. Assume the probability of infection is 0.015. What is the probability that 200 people must be screened (i.e., receive a chest x-ray) in order to identify 4 cases of tuberculosis.

In this case the number of cases is fixed at 4, and we must compute the distribution of the number of patients from whom cases will be discovered. This requires use of the negative binomial distribution.

$$P\left[200^{th} \text{ patient represents the } 4^{th} \text{ case}\right] = \binom{199}{3}(0.015)^4 (0.985)^{196} = 0.00339.$$

The probability that between 200 and 300 survivors have to be screened to identify four cases is

$$\sum_{n=200}^{300}\binom{n-1}{3}(0.015)^4 (0.985)^{n-4} = 0.310.$$

However, this combination is based on the probability of infection is 0.015. If we assume that there is some controversy about the probability of infection, with workers evenly divided between the probability, the rate of infection is 0.015 on the one hand, and 0.030 on the other. In this case, we can write the distribution of θ, the probability of infection as

$$\pi(\theta) = (0.50)\mathbf{1}_{\theta=0.015} + (0.50)\mathbf{1}_{\theta=0.030}. \tag{2.14}$$

We then can compute the probability that between 200 and 300 patients must have chest x-rays to identify four cases of tuberculosis as

$$\sum_{\theta}\sum_{n=200}^{300}\binom{n-1}{3}\theta^4 (1-\theta)^{n-4}\left((0.50)\mathbf{1}_{\theta=0.015} + (0.50)\mathbf{1}_{\theta=0.030}\right)$$

$$= (0.50)\sum_{n=200}^{300}\binom{n-1}{3}(0.015)^4 (0.985)^{n-4} + (0.50)\sum_{n=200}^{300}\binom{n-1}{3}(0.030)^4 (0.970)^{n-4} \tag{2.15}$$

$$= 0.310 + 0.130 = 0.440.$$

One moves from the first to the second line of expression (2.15) by simply summing over the values of θ as we did in the previous section. ∎

Each of the binomial and negative binomial distributions are important predictive tools in applied biostatistics. The common application for them both is to assume that the probability of the event, θ is constant from trial to trial. However, even though this probability is constant we have seen two circumstances where its value is uncertain. While the assumption of a constant probability from subject to subject has been upheld, it can be unclear just what that constant value is. In these circumstances, where the precise value of θ is unknown, but there is some information about the possible values that it can take, we use the Law of Total Probability to find the unconditional distribution of either the number of events (binomial distribution) or the number of trials until a given number of events (negative binomial distribution) have occurred.

2.5 The Poisson Process

Assume that a new subdivision has just been completed and is now attracting home owners to buy a house and live there. Most adult male family members do not have angina pectoris, the crushing, substernal pain that commonly presages a heart attack. However, there are men who come to live in this community with this non-contagious disease. Assume that angina pectoris inflicted men arrive in the community at the rate of $\lambda = 6.6$ patients with angina pectoris per year.

With this development it is easy to compute the expected number of patients living in the subdivision who arrived with angina by simply multiplying the arrival rate λ by time. For example, in one year, we would expect on average 6.6 men in the community to be suffering from and need treatment for angina pectoris. However, this is only an average, and commonly we are interested in the distribution of the number of patients with this disease in a given time period t as X_t. If we also assume that these men arrive into the community independently of each other, then the probability distribution of the number of men with angina pectoris who arrive in the community over a given time t is

$$P\left[X_t = k\right] = P_k\left[t\right] = \frac{\left(\lambda t\right)^k}{k!}e^{-\lambda t} \qquad (2.16)$$

for $k = 0, 1, 2, 3, \ldots$. Both its mean and variance are λ. The Poisson distribution, was named for Siméon Denis Poisson, a French mathematician (Figure 2.7).[*]

---

[*] Poisson's biography is a tribute to the vicissitudes of life. As a child, he was left hanging in clothes that were nailed high on the wall of his home because of his nurse's inordinate fear that he would be eaten by animals. Left swinging for most of the day, he developed a life-long interest in the study of swinging objects, particularly pendulums. Later, forced to enter training to be a physician, he left medicine for the field of mathematics after a patient died after he applied a hot blister to them (an accepted medicinal treatment at the time). Poisson is best remembered for the probability distribution that bears his name; however, he was most valued by his eighteenth century contemporaries for his work in physics, and mechanics, which became the foundation of the subsequent work by Riemann. See Ball R. (1908) *A Short Account of the History of Mathematics 4th Edition*. New York: Dover Publications.

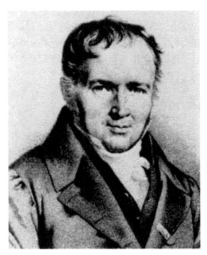

Figure 2.7. Figure of Siméon Denis Poisson, French mathematician who developed the Poisson distribution. From www-history.mcs.st-andrews.ac.uk/BiogIndex.html.

Example 2.3: Using the scenario introduced in this section, the probability that in one year, 8 men arrive with angina pectoris is $P[X_t = 8] = (6.6)^8 e^{-6.8}/8! = 0.122$. Is we assume that the arrival rate is the same for each of three years, then we can compute the exact probability that 30 patients arrive in three years as $P[X_t = 30] = (3(6.6))^{30} e^{-3(6.6)}/30! = 0.0075$. Thus, as long as the arrival rate remains homogeneous, the Poisson distribution may be applied to events that occur over different time intervals. If there are, at time $t = 0$, a_0 men with angina pectoris, then the probability that there are k men with angina at time t, where $k \geq a_0$ is the probability that there were $k - a_0$ arrivals by time t or

$$P[X_t = k - a_0] = \frac{(\lambda t)^{(k-a_0)}}{(k-a_0)!} e^{-\lambda t}.$$

∎

The Poisson distribution may appear to be esoteric, but its development is actually quite straightforward. We can begin a brief examination by evaluating the arrival rate assumption. The argument that arrivals to the community are constant over a period of time is reasonable. However, to develop the concept of "Poisson arrivals" from first principles, let's assume that we can adjust the "time-clock," slowing time down until we can observe what happens in a very small period of time, i.e., the interval from time t to time $t + \Delta t$. We continue to slow the passage of time down, making Δt so small that only one arrival can take place in this tiny time interval. The probability of an anginal patient's arrival in this infinitesimal interval is simply $\lambda \Delta t$.

Let's now focus on the probability of having no patients with angina in the system at time $t + \Delta t$. There is only one way that this can happen; there must be no patients in the system at time t, and there are no anginal patient arrivals in the system from time t to time $t + \Delta t$. Thus we write

$$P_0[t, t + \Delta t] = P_0[t](1 - \lambda \Delta t). \tag{2.17}$$

We can write equation (2.17) as

$$\frac{P_0[t, t + \Delta t] - P_0[t]}{\Delta t} = -\lambda \tag{2.18}$$

We now examine what happens as Δt become very small. The left side of equation (2.18) is the range of change of $P_0[t]$ over the time Δt. As Δt gets very small, approaching zero, the left side of equation (2.18) gets closer and closer to the instantaneous rate of change of $P_0[t]$. This is also known as the derivative of $P_0[t]$, which can be written as $dP_0[t]/dt$. Thus, by taking the limit of equation (2.18) as Δt approaches zero, the equation reduces to a very simple differential equation $dP_0[t]/dt = \lambda t$, the solution to which is $P_0[t] = e^{-\lambda t}$. This matches the value of $P_0[t]$ from equation (2.16) when $k = 0$. An analogous evaluation for each value of k produces the probability distribution of equation (2.16).

The Poisson distribution is one of the most ubiquitous probability distributions in use. All that is required for the Poisson distribution to be applied is that there are random occurrences which occur independently of one another with the same arrival rate. This collection of conditions is known as the *Poisson process*. An entire field of probability, known as stochastic processes (i.e., processes that are probabilistic in time), subsumes this and related procedures.

Example 2.4
Assume that the arrival of patients to a suburban emergency room (ER) follows a Poisson process with hourly arrival rate θ, and the ER physicians wish to know the distribution of the number of arrivals in four hours. Dr. G., when interviewed, suggested that, in his estimation, the average arrival rate of patients was four per hour. Using formula (2.16) and Dr. G's estimate, they compute

$$P[X_4 = k] = P_k[4] = \frac{(4\lambda)^k}{k!} e^{-4\lambda} \tag{2.19}$$

for different value of k (Figure 2.8).

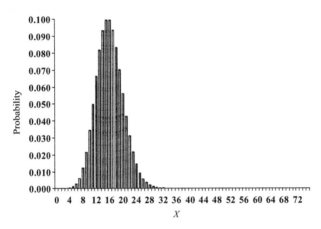

Figure 2.8. Distribution of number of emergency room visits, X for a 4 hour period from a Poisson distribution with mean $\lambda = 4$ arrivals per hour.

On average, they would expect 16 patients over a four hour period. They can easily compute the probability that more than 40 patients are seen in this four hour period as

$$P\left[X_4 \geq 40 \mid \lambda = 4\right] = \sum_{k=40}^{\infty} \frac{\left((4)(4)\right)^{40}}{40!} e^{-16} = 1 - \sum_{k=0}^{40} \frac{\left((4)(4)\right)^{40}}{40!} e^{-16} \approx 0,$$

a conclusion quickly confirmed by an examination of Figure 2.7. In fact, from this figure they would not expect to see less than four patients in four hours nor more than 32 patients during this time period.

However, later, when other physicians are interviewed, a disagreement about the average hourly patient arrival rate ensues. Most other ER workers take issue with Dr. G.'s perspective on the average hourly rate. Several workers are convinced that the average hourly patient arrival rate is larger than four, and some think it is substantially higher than this initial estimate. After a series of discussions, the distribution of the arrival rate is characterized as

$$\pi(\lambda) = 0.151_{\lambda=4} + 0.251_{\lambda=9} + 0.601_{\lambda=13}, \tag{2.20}$$

reflecting the belief that $\lambda = 4$ with probability 0.15, $\lambda = 9$ with probability 0.25, and $\lambda = 13$ with probability 0.60. Note that uncertainty about the arrival rate has been converted into a probability distribution for the arrival rate λ. The probability distribution of the number of patients who visit the emergency room in four hours is profoundly altered when variability in the arrival rate is introduced (Figure 2.9).

The distribution of the number of arriving patients with this more complex consideration of the arrival rate is much more complicated. In fact, the distribution of the number of arrivals that was based on Dr. G's simple assumption of a 4 patient per hour arrival rate is present, and in fact visible in Figure 2.8. However, the distribution has a new, complicated component that reflects the possibility of higher arrival rates as incorporated in equation (2.20).

Based on this more intricate arrival rate considerations, the clinic physicians still wish to compute the probability that they will see more than 40 patients in 4 hours. The uncertainty about the value of λ requires that they incorporate $\pi(\lambda)$ into their calculation. Following the development from the previous section, they write

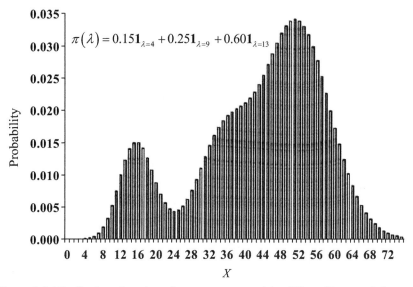

Figure 2.9. Distribution of number of emergency room visits, X for a 4 hour period produced from a mixture of Poisson distributions according to $\pi(\lambda)$.Note the shift to a greater number of ER visits.

$$P\left[X_4 \geq 40\right] = P\left[X_4 \geq 40 \mid \lambda\right]\pi(\lambda)$$

$$= 1 - \sum_{k=0}^{39} \frac{(\lambda t)^{40}}{40!} e^{-\theta t}\left[0.151_{\lambda=4} + 0.251_{\lambda=9} + 0.601_{\lambda=13}\right]$$

$$= 1 - \left(0.15\sum_{k=0}^{39} \frac{((4)(4))^{40}}{40!} e^{-16} + 0.25\sum_{k=0}^{39} \frac{((9)(4))^{40}}{40!} e^{-36} + 0.60\sum_{k=0}^{39} \frac{((13)(4))^{40}}{40!} e^{-52}\right)$$

$$= 0.375,$$

a value that is substantially greater than the approximate value of zero based on Dr. G's arrival rate assumption.

The mean arrival rate is $(0.15)(4) + (0.35)(9) + (0.60)(13) = 10.65$. One could produce the distribution of ER arrivals based on a single Poisson distribution of 10.65 and compare that to the rate based on $\pi(\lambda)$ (Figure 2.10).

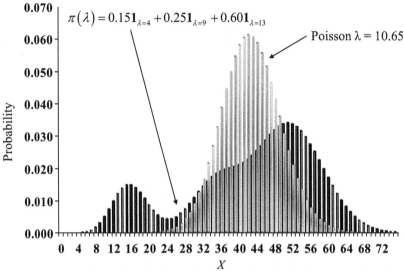

Figure 2.10. Comparison of the distribution of the number of arrivals when produced from the computed mean arrival rate, versus that previously computed from $\pi(\lambda)$. Building the distribution based on $\pi(\lambda)$ provides substantially more variability in the distribution of the number of patient arrivals.

The distribution of the arrival rate based on the single Poisson distribution with one assumption for the arrival rate ($\lambda = 10.65$) is substantially tighter than the distribution for the number of ER arrivals based on $\pi(\lambda)$. Some insight into the difference is revealed by the process by which the distribution were built. The use of $\pi(\lambda)$, a mix of different estimates of λ, reflects the absence of a real consensus about the value of λ. Thus, there are two sources of variability, (1) the value of λ, and (2) the number of arrivals given the value of λ. These two unknowns increase the variability of the distribution. When working from the single Poisson distribution, there is no longer variability about the value of λ. Thus, its variability is less than that derived from the mixture.

2.5.1 Compound Poisson Process
The previous example invoked the Poisson process when its parameter λ was not constant, but varied according to a distribution $\pi(\lambda)$. However, there are circum-

stances in which the Poisson process captures the variability of a parameter in another distribution.

As a simple example, consider an outcome X whose probability follows a binomial distribution with parameters n and θ. We assume that θ will be constant throughout this example. From what we know about the binomial distribution, X must take on an integer value between 0 and n. However assume n follows a probability distribution itself.

We know how to solve the problem if we allow n to have a distribution with that has a finite number of discrete values, e.g., $\sum_{j=1}^{J} p_j 1_{n=n_j}$, where

$\sum_{j=1}^{J} p_j = 1$. However, there are other useful assumptions. One is to allow n to follow a Poisson distribution with parameter λ. In this circumstance, using the Law of Total Probability, Appendix 1 reveals that the marginal distribution of X follows a Poisson distribution with parameter $\lambda\theta$.[*]

Example 2.5: Cold Checks

When one member of a family has a cold, the mother will commonly bring not just the one child into the clinic for an examination, but will bring her other children with them, each to be examined and perhaps treated. From the mother's perspective, the absence of the symptoms of infection in a child simply means the child does not have a cold yet, raising the optimistic hope of early and perhaps preventive treatment. Thus, commonly in clinics, entire families request evaluations for "cold checks."

Assume that the number of children who are actually showing signs of infection in a family with n children follows a binomial distribution where θ is the probability that a child has symptoms. In this particular season $\theta = 0.65$. However, the number of children in a family is not fixed, but follows a Poisson distribution with parameter λ. The ER administrator is interested in the distribution of the number of symptomatic children in a family. From earlier in this section, we know that the unconditional distribution is Poisson with parameter $\lambda\theta = (3.8)(0.65) = 2.47$ (Figure 2.11).

Figure 2.11 depicts two Poisson distributions. The distribution of the number of children in the family follows a Poisson distribution with parameter 3.8, while the distribution of the number of colds in a family follows a Poisson distribution with parameter 2.47. This satisfies our intuition since not every child examined is expected to have a cold.

The wide distribution in the family size has implications for the time required to treat these families. While most times, physicians will conduct between one and five child examinations, occasionally they may have to examine as many

---

[*] We will take the tack of abrogating more complicated mathematical developments to the Appendices of this book. This allows the general reader to follow the main discussion without being sidetracked by unneccessary mathematical encumbrances, while making the complexity of the derivations available to the more advanced reader.

as ten children. These examinations will increase the likelihood that the physician will themselves become infected.

There is substantial sensitivity of these evaluations to the value of the parameter θ from the binomial distribution, which reveals a substantial reduction in the yield of colds when θ is reduced from 0.65 to 0.20 (Figure 2.12).

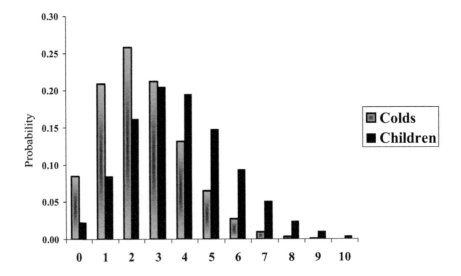

Figure 2.11. Probability distribution of number of children in a family, and the number of "colds" among children in a family based on the combination of a binomial and Poisson distributions.

2.6 The Uniform Distribution

This probability distribution is one of the most useful to probabilists in general, and to Bayesians in particular. Its assignment of probability in a non-preferential way is particularly attractive to Bayes probabilists in their construction of prior distributions.[*] The use of the uniform distribution and other related probability assignment strengthens our capability to implement Bayes procedures, but first, we must alter how we measure probability.

2.6.1 Measuring Probability

Whether the action was the toss of a coin, or observing the race/ethnicity of a clinic patient, or counting the number of children in a family, we assigned probability to a single number. We did this successfully whether there were a finite number of points, e.g., the number of successes observed from the binomial distribution, or whether the number of points was infinite, as in the number of trials until a fixed number of successes occurs (i.e., the negative binomial distribution). When we combine events using the algebra of unions, intersections, and complements, we

---

[*] This was one of the major contributions of Harold Jeffries as discussed in the Prologue.

add or subtract the probabilities of these points. However, there are circumstances where we need to assign probability differently, changing our metric to capture the probability accurately.

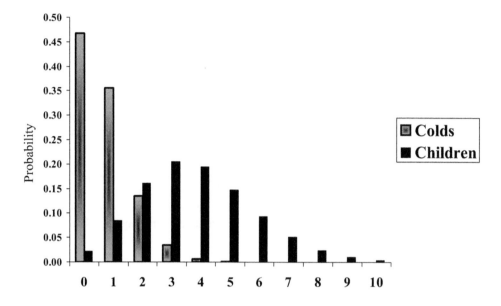

Figure 2.12. Probability distribution of number of children in a family, and the number of "colds" among children in a family based on the combination of a binomial and Poisson distributions when the probability of a cold is substantially reduced.

This is neither uncommon or unusual in everyday life. For example, consider an environmental scientist tasked with measuring the annual available water in a community. It is natural for her to start with a simple gauge that measures rainfall. Her use of this accurate instrument allows her to accumulate the total precipitation in the community. At the end of the year, she knows how much rain fell.

However, rainfall is not the only available water in the community, as her survey of the area with its two clean, freshwater lakes reveals. She cannot rely on her reliable rainfall gauge to estimate the volume of these large lakes, and must use a different instrument to measure this source of water. Since the purpose is to measure the total available water accurately and not use the same measuring tool, the act of switching instruments poses no theoretical obstacle.

But the metric she uses for measuring rainfall, as well as the separate measure used to gauge lake depth fails to measure the volume of water trucked in from surrounding communities in the midst of a summer drought. So, in order to get a final tally of the available water, she must use yet a third measuring instrument, summing up the volume of water contained by each truck. Again, one tool doesn't work for all.

This is what we must do in accumulating probability. Many times, the probability assignment system we have developed thus far, i.e., placing probability on each individual point, makes no sense. While the underlying mathematics can be complicated, it boils down to the observation that there are so many points that one cannot assign positive probability to each one and still have the total probability add to one.[*] Thus, like the hydrologist who cannot use the rain gauge to measure all of the available water in a community, we must develop a different tool to measure probability. One that is most useful is the concept of *probability as area*.

2.6.2 Probability as Area

Choose a number between 0 and 1. If that number was chosen randomly, any number in this range would be equally likely. However, since there are too many numbers to count in this interval, we say that we will not assign probability to any one of them; instead we will assign probability to an interval of numbers. The probability will simply be the length of the interval. Thus the event to which we assign probability is not that "$X = 0.20$," but is instead, the event that "X lies in the interval $[0, 0.10]$". The probability of this event is simply $0.10 - 0 = 0.10$. Similarly, the probability that X lies in $[0.90, 1]$ is 0.10. The probability of any interval is simply the length of the interval, and intervals of equal length have equal probability (Figure 2.13).

Figure 2.13 demonstrates how easy it is to compute probabilities of events which are uniformly distributed on the $[0, 1]$ interval. We are also free to use the rules of unions, intersections, and complements from Chapter One.

To denote this dispersal of probability, we will use the notation as $f(X) = 1_{X \in [0,1]}$. This adaptation of our previous notation tells us how to accumulate probability for the uniform distribution as X moves from 0 to 1. In fact, it is in general more useful to consider this process as assigning probability not so much to an interval, but instead to an area under a curve (Figure 2.14).

In the case of the uniform distribution, we wish to assign probability to a region that is bounded above by the line $f(x) = 1$ between $x = 0$ and $x = 1$. The region under this curve between 0.40 and 0.60 is simply a rectangle of unit height

---

[*] While one can assign probability to all of the integers in a way that the sum of all of these probabilities is 1 (such as for the Poisson distribution), we cannot assign positive probability to all of the numbers between 0 and 1. That vast collection of rational and irrational numbers overwhelms any assignment of positive probability to each of them. No matter how we assign the probability, its sum will be infinite.

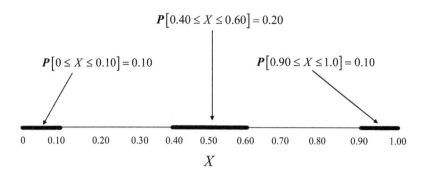

$$P[0 \le X \le 0.10] = 0.10 \quad P[0.40 \le X \le 0.60] = 0.20 \quad P[0.90 \le X \le 1.0] = 0.10$$

In addition,

$$P[0 \le X \le 0.10 \cup 0.90 \le X \le 1.0] = P[0 \le X \le 0.10] + P[0.90 \le X \le 1.0] = 0.20$$

$$P[0 \le X \le 0.10 \cup 0.40 \le X \le 0.60] = P[0 \le X \le 0.10] + P[0.40 \le X \le 0.60] = 0.30$$

Figure 2.13. For the uniform distribution, probability is simply the length of The interval, and intervals of equal length have the same probability.

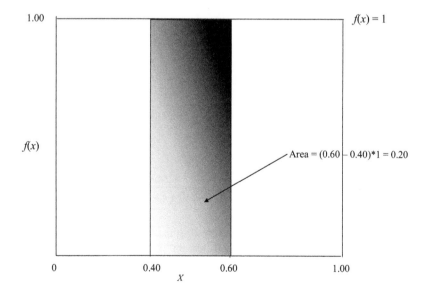

Figure 2.14. The probability that $0.40 = X = 0.60$ is the shaded area under the curve.

and width 0.20, so the area is 0.20. While finding these areas will involve looking up their values in tables for more complex probability distributions, the process of computing probabilities based on interval assignments will be the same.

2.6.3 Compounding with the Uniform Distribution

This adaptation of probability can be put to work at once. For example, assume that a health worker is interested in the probability that patients have rhinovirus infections. A frequent cause of the common cold, these viral infections sweep through families and communities, producing illnesses that last between three to ten days. She would like to know the probability that among n patients, k of them have disease.

Since the total size of the sample is fixed, she wishes to use the binomial distribution, computing $P[X = k] = \binom{n}{k} \theta^k (1-\theta)^{n-k}$. However, she doesn't know the value of θ, and unlike in previous examples, she has no prior estimates for its value. With no additional information, and no idea whether θ is close to 0 or near 1, she would like to use the uniform distribution to express her lack of knowledge about the possible value of θ.

Using the Law of Total Probability, she writes,

$$
P[X = k] = \sum_{\theta} P[X = k \mid \theta] \pi(\theta) = \sum_{\theta} \binom{n}{k} \theta^k (1-\theta)^{n-k} 1_{\theta \in [0,1]}
$$

$$
= \binom{n}{k} \sum_{\theta} \theta^k (1-\theta)^{n-k} 1_{\theta \in [0,1]}. \tag{2.21}
$$

However, the last summation in expression (2.21) is complicated to evaluate, being the area under the curve $f(\theta) = \theta^k (1-\theta)^{n-k}$ for $0 \le \theta \le 1$. Appendix B reveals this area to be simply $\dfrac{k!(n-k)!}{(n+1)!}$. Thus, placing this result in the last line of expression (2.21) she finds her final solution to be

$$
P[X = k] = \binom{n}{k} \frac{k!(n-k)!}{(n+1)!} = \frac{n!}{k!(n-k)!} \frac{k!(n-k)!}{(n+1)!} = \frac{n!}{(n+1)!} = \frac{1}{n+1}. \tag{2.22}
$$

This finding is quite illuminating, demonstrating the transforming effect a distribution for the parameter θ can have. Recall that the probability distribution of $X = k$ given θ was binomial. We have seen earlier in this chapter that this probability distribution generates different probabilities for different values of k. However, with no knowledge of the value of θ, she incorporated the uniform distribution on [0, 1] into her calculations. Using this distribution for θ, she finds that the unconditional distribution for $P[X = k]$ is a fixed constant, independent of the value of k. For example, if she were to identify 20 people for her evaluation, this unconditional probability distribution for $X = k$ reveals that, assuming a uniform distribution for θ,

$$P[X = 0] = P[X = 1] = P[X = 2] = P[X = 20] = \frac{1}{21}.$$ Essentially, the uncondi-

tional distribution of X has become "uniform" itself in the sense that it assigns equal probability to every possible value of X.

Now, suppose our investigator improves her knowledge about θ slightly, now learning that θ must be less than 0.90. She doesn't know what value it has, and from this health care worker's point of view, any region in the interval [0, 0.90] is as likely as any other region of equal length. She would like to use a uniform distribution, not on [0, 1], but on [0, 0.90]. This probability distribution for θ can easily be denoted as $\pi(\theta) = (1.11)\mathbf{1}_{\theta \in [0,0.90]}$, the leading value of 1.11 required to be sure that the sum of the probabilities is equal to one.[*]

She now must compute

$$P[X = k] = \binom{n}{k}\sum_{\theta}\theta^k(1-\theta)^{n-k}(1.1)\mathbf{1}_{\theta \in [0,0.90]} = (1.1)\binom{n}{k}\sum_{\theta}\theta^k(1-\theta)^{n-k}\mathbf{1}_{\theta \in [0,0.90]}.$$

The Table in Appendix C provides the values that she needs. For example, if she wishes to identify the probability of 6 positive assays out of 10, she computes

$$P[X = 6] = (1.1)\binom{10}{6}\sum_{\theta}\theta^6(1-\theta)^{10-6}\mathbf{1}_{\theta \in [0,0.90]} = 0.101.$$

It is instructive to examine the probability distribution of k for different values of the upper bound of θ (Figure 2.15).

Figure 2.15 demonstrates how sensitive the probability distribution of $X = k$ is to the assumptions we place on the distribution of θ, the probability of success. In each of the four cases in this figure, θ follows a uniform distribution. Yet, the shape of the unconditional distribution of k changes as the range of values over which θ can range widens. When θ is permitted to range between 0 and 0.20 only, solely the small values of k have large probability. However, the larger the maximum value of θ, the wider the distribution of values of θ becomes, the more uniform becomes the probabilities of the different values of k.

---

[*] In general, if we wish to denote the distribution of X where X is uniformly distributed between the values a and b, then $f(x) = \frac{1}{b-a}\mathbf{1}_{x \in [a,b]}$.

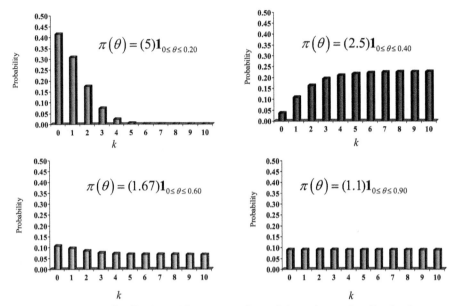

Figure 2.15. The distribution of k successes in n trials varies as the distribution of θ permits a larger range of variables.

2.7 Exponential Distribution

The uniform distribution served as our introduction to a combination of events and probability where probability was assigned not to individual points but to intervals. While this stands in contrast to discrete distributions, i.e., distributions that provide probabilities to individual points, sometimes discrete and continuous distributions are closely related.

For example, consider a health care worker interested in tracking the arrival of patients with a noncontiguous connective tissue disorders to a community served by a single emergency room. He expects these patients to arrive independently of one another, with the same arrival rate λ. If X_t signifies the number of patients who have arrived by time t, then the probability that $X_t = k$ follows a Poisson distribution, i.e.,

$$P[X_t = k] = \frac{(\lambda t)^k}{k!} e^{-\lambda t} \mathbf{1}_{k=0,1,2,3,\dots} \tag{2.23}$$

If she is interested in computing the probability that there are no arrivals of patients with connective tissue disorder by time t, she simply uses formula (2.23), to compute $P[X_t = 0] = e^{-\lambda t}$.

However, this event may be viewed in two ways. We have chosen to take an arrival-oriented perspective, i.e., the number of arrivals in time $[0, t]$ is zero. We could just as easily consider this event not as a matter of arrivals, but as a matter of time. Let T be the time until the first patient arrives. Then T is a continuous variable, taking any value from $T = 0$ to infinity. The probability that no patient arrives by time t, or $P[X_t = 0]$ is also the probability that the first patient arrives after time t, or $P[T \geq t]$.

From this alternative point of view, the probability that the first arrival occurs before time t is simply $1 - e^{-\lambda t}$. If we wanted to find the probability that the first arrival time is between time t_1 and t_2, we simply compute

$$P[t_1 \leq t \leq t_2] = P[t \leq t_2] - P[t \leq t_1] = \left(1 - e^{-\lambda t_2}\right) - \left(1 - e^{-\lambda t_1}\right) = e^{-\lambda t_1} - e^{-\lambda t_2}. \quad (2.24)$$

This is the characterization of the distribution of interarrival times between events, and is commonly known as the *negative exponential* distribution. For this probability assignment, we say $f(t) = \lambda e^{-\lambda t}$. Like the uniform distribution, it assigns probabilities not to individual points, but to intervals. However, unlike the uniform distribution, probability is not assigned equally to equal intervals (Figure 2.16). Its mean is $\frac{1}{\lambda}$, and its variance is $\frac{1}{\lambda^2}$.

If the epidemiologist is uncertain of the value of λ, but has information about what its values might be, he can still compute the probability that the interarrival time is in an interval of interest as illustrated by the following example.

Example 2.6
Assume the emergency room is in the midst of a diagnostic equipment upgrade, a process that will take 12 days to complete. The epidemiologist has been asked how likely it is that patients with connective tissue disorders will be seen within 12 days. She is told the arrival rate λ is 6 patients per 100 days or 0.06. Then, from equation (2.24), she computes

$$P[0 \leq t \leq 12] = 1 - e^{-\lambda t} = 1 - e^{-(0.06)(12)} = 0.513,$$

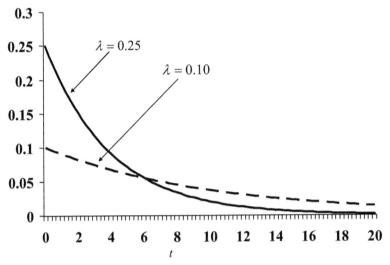

Figure 2.16. Probability distributions of inter-arrival times of patients with connective tissue disorders for two different arrival rates using the exponential distribution.

revealing that it is more likely than not that the equipment will be required before it is ready. However, uncertainty about the value of λ requires her to build a probability distribution that admits another possible value for this parameter. She chooses $\pi(\lambda)$, where

$$\pi(\lambda) = p\mathbf{1}_{\lambda=0.005} + (1-p)\mathbf{1}_{\lambda=0.06}, \qquad (2.25)$$

where p is chosen such that $0 \le p \le 1$. This distribution considers two possible values for λ, using the value p to reflect the preference for one value over another. When $p = 0$, the distribution selects only λ = 0.06, while choosing $p = 1$ permits only λ = 0.005. Intermediate values of p allow intermediate values of λ such that $0.005 \le \lambda \le 0.06$ (Figure 2.16, dotted line).

Having selected $\pi(\lambda)$, the worker can compute $P[0 \le t \le 12]$. She knows $P[0 \le t \le 12 \mid \lambda] = 1 - e^{-12\lambda}$, and now uses the Law of Total Probability to write

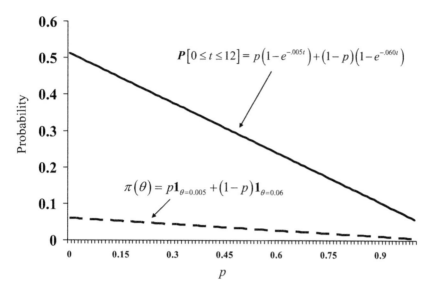

Figure 2.17. Probability of an arrival within twelve hours of each other as a function of p in the distribution of θ.

$$P[0 \le t \le 12] = \sum_{\lambda} P[0 \le t \le 12 \mid \lambda] P[\lambda]$$

$$= \sum_{\lambda} (1 - e^{-\lambda t})(p\mathbf{1}_{\lambda=0.005} + (1-p)\mathbf{1}_{\lambda=0.06}) \qquad (2.26)$$

$$= p(1 - e^{-.005t}) + (1-p)(1 - e^{-.060t}).$$

This final probability that an arrival will occur within 12 days is a function of p, the preference for either of the two values of λ. Figure 2.17 reveals that as the preference for the value of p increases, preference is shifted away from the larger value of λ to the smaller value of 0.005 (dotted line). This decline in the value of the arrival rate decreases the likelihood that a patient with a connective tissue disease will be seen in the first 12 days (solid line). Thus, preferences as expressed in the probability distribution of the parameter (in this case for the patient arrival rate) are directly reflected in the probability of arrivals within 12 days.

     This useful relationship allows the worker to gauge the sensitivity of the final solution to the preference expressed for the actual arrival rate. In this circumstance, the wide range of values of $P[0 \le t \le 12]$ is too wide to be very helpful, spurring additional effort to generate a more precise measure of either the arrival rate itself, or at least a narrower range for realistic values of p.

     The next chapter will incorporate the Law of Total Probability in more complicated scenarios involving clinical trials.

Problems

1. Verify the Law of Total Probability by computing the overall probability of death in each of the three age ranges in Table 2.1.

2. During the 1980s many physicians and public health workers believed the scourge of tuberculosis was a disease of the past. Factors including immigration policy and poverty have led to a resurgence of the disease. There are several classes of mycobacteria: *Mycobacterium tuberculosis, Mycobacterium avium, Mycobacterium intracellulare,* and *Mycobacterium leprae.* Each is more likely to affect patients with a compromised immune system. Close contact with an infected individual is the major source of the infection. Commonly this individual is a family member.

    The probability an individual is infected given close contact with an infected family member are as follows;

    $$P[tuberculosis\ infection\mid contact]=0.85$$
    $$P[avium\ infection\mid contact]=0.025$$
    $$P[intracellulare\ infection\mid contact]=0.35$$
    $$P[leprae\ infection\mid contact]=0.19$$

    The probability that a family member is infected with each of *M. tuberculosis, M. avium, M. intracellulare,* and *M. leprae* are respectively 0.09, 0.15, 0.11, and 0.005. Compute each of the following probabilities

    a) The probability that a family member has tuberculosis, given the patient has TB.
    b) The probability that a family member has the avium infection given the patient is infected with *M. avium.*
    c) The probability that a family member has the intracellulare infection, given the patient is infected with *M. intracellulare* avium.
    d) The probability that a family member has the leprae infection, given the patient is infected with *M. leprae.*

3. Creutzfeldt-Jacob encephalopathy (mad cow disease) is a condition that produces long-term delirium and dementia in patients exposed to prions, the causative agent in tainted beef. Assume that out of 30 cattle selected from herds believed to be at risk of the disease, the probability that k are infected with the prions follows a binomial distribution with parameter θ, the probability that an individual cow is infected. There is confusion about the value of θ. The workers decide to treat θ as a variable, following a uniform distribution on the [0, 0.10] real line. Compute the probability that at least three cows are infected.

4. An infant has been injured in a motor vehicle accident. She requires a blood transfusion but has an uncommon blood type. Individuals with blood types independent of one another must be tested to see if they can be donors for the injured child.
    a) Compute the probability that at least 10 individuals must be screened if the probability that a potential donor has a matching blood type is 0.010.
    b) Compute the probability that at least 10 individuals must be screened if the probability that a potential donor has a matching blood type follows a uniform distribution on [0, 0.30] real lines.

5. From June to November, cities and towns along the gulf coast of the United States turn to the Gulf of Mexico, ever watchful for signs of hurricanes. Assume that given that there are n hurricanes in a given year. The probability that k of them make U.S. landfall follows a binomial distribution.
    a) Assume that the parameter $\theta = 0.70$. If $n = 8$, compute the probability that at least five storms have a U.S. landfall.
    b) Now assume that n follows a Poisson distribution, parameter $\lambda = 8$. Compute the probability that at least five storms have a U.S. landfall.
    c) Assume now that $n = 8$, and θ is equal to .65 with probability 1/3, 0.70 with probability 1/3, and 0.80 with probability 1/3. Compute the probability that at least five storms have a U.S. landfall.
    d) Assume that $n = 8$, and θ follows a Uniform [0, 0.60] distribution. Compute the probability that at least five storms reach U.S. land.

6. Assume that patient arrivals to a coronary care unit follow a Poisson process with arrival rate λ. Assume that λ is equal to 0.50 patients per day with probability ½, and equal to 1.9 patients per day with probability ½. Compute the probability that there are seven arrivals to the CCU in a week.

References

1. Jeffreys H. (1933). On the Prior Probability in the Theory of Sampling, *Proceedings of the Cambridge Philosophical Society* **29**: 83–87.
2. Jeffreys H. (1931). *Scientific Inference*, reprinted with additions in '37 and with new editions in '57 and '73, Cambridge: Cambridge University Press.
3. Savage L.J. (1954). *The Foundations of Statistics*. New York. Wiley (1972 edition).
4. Berger J.O. (1980). *Statistical Decision Theory. Foundations, Concepts, and Methods*. New York: Springer-Verlag.
5. Pfeffer M.A., Braunwald E., Moyé L.A. et al. (1992). Effect of Captopril on mortality and morbidity in patients with left ventricular dysfunction after myocardial infarction - results of the Survival and Ventricular Enlargement Trial. *New England Journal of Medicine* **327**:669–677.

3
Intermediate Compo nding
and Prior Distrib tions

3.1 Compounding and Prior Distributions

Chapter Two developed the notion of compounding distributions, or generating the unconditional distribution of x, $P[x]$, from combining the conditional distribution $P[x|\theta]$ and $P[\theta]$ using the Law of Total Probability, $P[x] = \sum_{\theta} P[x|\theta]P[\theta]$.

Bayes procedures commonly begin with this step, but use different notation. What we have termed the marginal distribution of θ is what Bayesians call the prior distribution of θ. Thus, from the Bayesian perspective, "compounding" is simply combining prior information about θ with current information about x (i.e., the conditional probability distribution of x) to obtain x's marginal distribution. To the Bayesian, obtaining $P[x]$ is not the end of the process, but is instead a way station or resting point, before one proceeds to finish the job by computing the posterior distribution of θ given x, or $P[\theta|x]$.

However, frequentists note that compounding is not "Bayesian" at all, but merely the simple use of conditional probability, producing marginal distributions of x that are of importance in their own right. Bayesians argue that the Bayesian approach subsumes compounding, and that the results held in such high regard by frequentists are merely the low hanging, easily plucked fruit from the Bayesian tree. In any event, recognizing the potential of compounding is a useful skill for the developing Bayesian statistician.

Several of the examples that will be provided in this chapter focus on the identification of effects from clinical research. While clinical practice provides the best of modern therapy for patients, it must evolve, and clinical research is the basis for that evolution. This influence is transmitted through the effects and effect sizes of clinical research. For example, how much lower is the infection rate using laproscopic aneurism resection than the traditional, invasive approach? Is there a larger reduction in low density lipid (LDL) cholesterol achieved through HMG-coA reductase inhibitor (statin) therapy than with simply diet and exercise? How much greater is the heart attack rate in patients taking cyclooxygenase (COX-2) inhibitors than in patients administered alternative analgesics for their pain?

It is the effect size that sways the medical community and galvanizes public health workers to action. Contemporary attention on Avian flu is not based on the fact that the virus's transformation to human infectivity provides insight into the adaptability of these minute quasi-living particles, but because it can potentially kill millions of people. Effect size is the force that moves communities.

There are several important ways to measure these effect sizes in clinical research and practice. Each is related to the research or clinical paradigm. After a brief introduction to epidemiology, this chapter focuses on effect measures in the clinical sciences, useful probability distributions that allow us to assess them, and how prior information can be used to provide new and useful information about their magnitude and variance through compounding. The tools developed in Chapter Two will be extremely helpful here.

3.2 Epidemiology 101

Modern textbooks define epidemiology as the discipline that identifies the determinants of disease. It may be easier to understand the role of this critical field as determining the true nature of an exposure-disease relationship. Consider the following example.

3.2.1 The Orange Juice or the Bee

A young, healthy but harried businesswoman held up by rain-snarled traffic finally arrives at the airport one hour before a flight that she must not miss. Grabbing her single overnight bag and her purse, she leaps from the back of the cab, hurrying across the two lanes of taxis, limousines, and vans busily emptying themselves of travelers. Jostled by co-passengers struggling to rapidly enter the narrow terminal entrance, our businesswoman squeezes through, walking briskly to the check-in area, tightly gripping her heavy overnight bag in her left hand, ignoring its sudden pinch on her ring finger. Sighing with relief as her boarding pass slides effortlessly in and out of the automatic check-in dispenser, she attaches herself to the end of the serpentine security line. Fifteen minutes later, she gathers her belongings and rushes to her plane.

With ten minutes before boarding time, her growling stomach reminds her that she has once again skipped breakfast. Seeing a kiosk, she quickly walks over where she mercifully drops her heavy bag to sit and enjoy a glass of orange juice, savoring its cold, full taste on this humid morning. Suddenly, she hears her flight called for boarding, and her last act after placing the empty plastic cup on the table is to wipe her mouth.

The airport police are called by the owner of the kiosk. Thirty seconds after they arrived, a panicked call goes out for a doctor. A passenger who is a physician arrives ninety seconds later, but it's too late. Our businesswoman is dead.

The sudden and unexpected death of a healthy adult woman calls for an investigation. However, once the police determine that there was no foul play and therefore no crime was committed, they turn the investigation over to epidemiologists.

Epidemiologists identify causes of disease, but more specifically, they work to get to the true nature of the exposure–disease relationship. In this case there are several possible exposures that may be considered. Could she have brought an infection to the airport that just happened to kill her there? Could the orange juice have been toxic? Or was it her reaction to a bee sting on her ring finger that produced the pinch she notices on her way into the terminal? Any of these could be the possible culprit.

Each culprit has been associated with the death, that is, occurred immediately preceding the death. *Association* is one property of an exposure–disease relationship, characterizing the two events as occurring "relatively simultaneously." Association is about time-proximity. However, epidemiologists seek something deeper and more powerful — a producing cause.

The *cause* of the disease is that exposure that excited the production of the disease. A causal relationship has directionality, force and power. In the absence of the exposure, the illness was not present. When the exposure arrives it works through a combination of mechanisms, some well understood, others unknown, to produce the disease.

The epidemiologic thought process that differentiates an associative versus a causal relationship between exposure and disease has been nicely elaborated by the eminent epidemiologist A. Bradford Hill [1]. In 1965, he outlined the nine criteria for causality arguments in health care. The common sense approach summarized by these nine tenets relies not on mathematics, but a clear, naturally intuitive understanding of the properties of a causal relationship. For example if we believe an exposure causes a disease, then there should be a greater clustering of disease in the exposed group than the unexposed group, i.e., there should be more disease cases in the exposed than in the unexposed group. This property is known as *strength of association*.

In addition, if the exposure causes a disease, then the greater the intensity of the exposure (either in dosage or duration), the greater the intensity of disease cases. This is known as *dose (or duration)–response relationship*, or *biologic gradient*.

While these two questions will be the focus of our discussion, there are other questions that Hill suggested that would explore the believability of the relationship. The nine Bradford Hill criteria are (1) strength of association, (2) temporality, (3) biologic gradient, (4) biologic plausibility, (5) consistency, (6) coherency, (7) specificity, (8) experimental evidence, and (9) analogy.

Finally to the degree that health care workers require the detective skills of careful observation and deductive reasoning in elucidating the relationship between cause and effect, we are all epidemiologists and can learn much from the disciplined use of the tools developed in this field.

Strength of association requires that we measure the proportion of patients with disease in the presence of an exposure, comparing this fraction to the proportion of patients with the disease in the absence of the exposure. This comparison is the basis of more complex and meaningful comparisons, e.g., odds ratios and relative risks. However, before we explore these concepts, and how the use of the Bayes perspective provides new insight into their utility, we first focus on the utility of proportions in some useful probability models.

3.3 Computing Distributions of Deaths

Bayesians consider every probability distribution to be a conditional distribution, i.e., conditional on its parameters, which themselves may have their own distributions. This is the heart of compounding. A useful rule of thumb for the Bayesian is to always consider the possibility of compounding when the observed distribution is not what one would expect from a simple examination of the nature of the event.

Example 3.1

Assume that an epidemiologist has identified n birds infected with the H5N1 influenza type A virus (avian flu). All of these birds are at risk of dying, and she is interested in determining the distribution of the number of their deaths. That is, she wishes to compute the probability of k deaths, or P_k out of n birds at risk of death.

Since the events are dichotomous (birds either live or die), a natural probability distribution to consider is the binomial distribution,

$$P_k = \binom{n}{k} p^k (1-p)^{n-k},$$

from which the computation of P_k is straightforward.

In this case, n is fixed. However, what should she do about the value of the parameter p? Clearly the utility of any value of P_k will depend on the value of p that she assumes. However, in this case, p is likely to be a function of time. The longer the birds live, the greater the likelihood that they will survive the infection. Thus the epidemiologist opens herself to the possibility that the probability of death might decrease as a function of time.

A commonly used model for this circumstance is a simple adaptation of the binomial distribution, known as the death model [2]. If we let k be the number of deaths that have occurred at time t, and assuming that deaths occur independently of one another, we may write.

$$P_k(t) = \binom{n}{k} \left(e^{-\upsilon t}\right)^k \left(1-e^{-\upsilon t}\right)^{n-k} = \binom{n}{k} e^{-k\upsilon t} \left(1-e^{-\upsilon t}\right)^{n-k}. \tag{3.1}$$

For fixed time t, this distribution has the same properties of the binomial distribution discussed in Chapter Two. However, it is slightly more complicated because the probability of death, $e^{-\upsilon t}$, is a function of t, and thus she computes not just P_k, but $P_k(t)$. Thus, for a fixed time, the probability that there are k deaths in n subjects is a simple binomial computation. However, as t increases, the probability of death decreases, thereby altering the distribution of deaths (Figure 3.1).

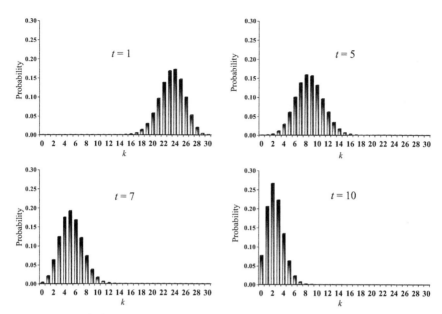

Figure 3.1. Distribution of number of avian flu deaths in 30 birds as a function of time, t.

Figure 3.1 depicts $P_k(t)$, the probability of k deaths having occurred in n susceptible at time t, as a function of time. For early times, there is a greater probability of death, and the number of dead birds is greater. However, for larger values of t, the probability of death diminishes, and the number of birds that have died tends to cluster closer to zero. Thus, as t increases, the distribution of deaths moves to the left, favoring a smaller number of early deaths.

The use of the death model, while more realistic, has not freed the epidemiologist from her parameter based concerns. Initially, she focused on the value of p. Use of $P_k(t)$ from equation (3.1) is now not a function of p, but of the parameter v. We might think of v as related to the survival rate of the birds. For a fixed time t, the larger its value the less likely birds are to die (Figure 3.2).

The survival parameter is of greatest interest to the investigator because she suspects that it is directly related to an immunity factor that she would like to identify, and hopefully propagate. Unfortunately, the birds are of different strains, and the immunity factor is not the same from bird to bird. She therefore suspects that the parameter v is not constant, but itself follows a probability distribution in the wild.

Here is where she uses the compounding process. She uses the exponential distribution to approximate the probability distribution of v, with parameter λ, writing $f_v(v) = \lambda e^{-\lambda v}$. The epidemiologist's task is to now compute the distribution of k unconditional on v.

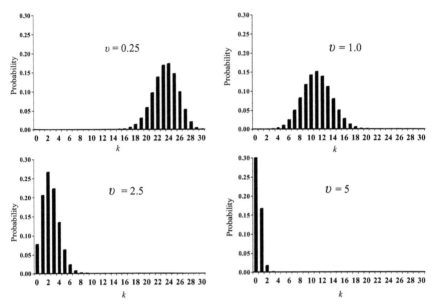

Figure 3.2. Distribution of number of avian flu deaths in 30 birds as a function of the survival parameter, v for $t = 1$.

Using the Law of Total Probability, she writes

$$P_k(t) = \sum_v P_k(t \mid \lambda)P(\lambda) = \sum_v \binom{n}{k} e^{-kvt} \left(1 - e^{-vt}\right)^{n-k} \lambda e^{-\lambda v}$$

$$= \lambda \binom{n}{k} \sum_v e^{-kvt} \left(1 - e^{-vt}\right)^{n-k} e^{-\lambda v}. \tag{3.2}$$

Carrying out this computation allows the investigator to remove the parameter v from her computations. Appendix D reveals that the last line of expression (3.2) may be simplified to

$$P_k(t) = \binom{n}{k} \sum_{i=0}^{n-k} \binom{n-k}{i} (-1)^i \frac{\lambda}{(k+i)t + \lambda}. \tag{3.3}$$

Thus, the unconditional probability of the number of bird deaths is a function of the number of birds, k, the time t, and the parameter of the unconditional distribution of λ. While this distribution has no name, it is easy to manipulate since it is only a finite sum of fractions. Its shape for different values of t is illuminating (Figure 3.3).

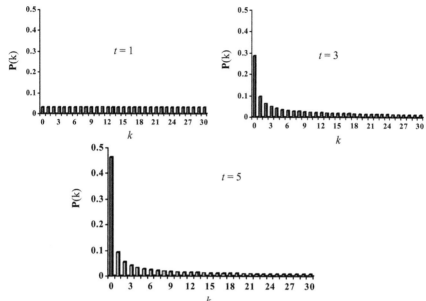

Figure 3.3. Compounding a binomial with an exponential $\lambda = 1$. The curves provide the distribution of the number of avian flu deaths in birds as a function of time.

It is instructive to compare the Figure 3.1 to Figure 3.3. The histograms of Figure 3.1 are what the investigator might have expected if she believed the unconditional distribution of the number of bird deaths followed a binomial distribution that was probabilistic in time (i.e., the probability of success was a function of time). However, these distributions were based on the survival parameter υ being constant. Figure 3.3 reveals the remarkable difference between the unconditional distribution of the number of birds deaths in the population, when the variability of the survival parameter is taken into account.

3.4 The Gamma Distribution and ER Arrivals
The gamma series of distributions, while interesting in their own right, have important applications in Bayesian biostatistics.

The gamma distribution is closely related to the exponential distribution, a distribution we introduced in Chapter Two. Recall that we developed the exponential distribution by considering the time until the first arrival from a Poisson process with parameter λ. The gamma distribution is simply the time until the rth arrival.[*] Its format is

---

[*] It can be shown mathematically that a gamma variable is the sum of r exponential variables each with parameter λ. This fits with our understanding of a gamma variable being the waiting time until the rth Poisson arrival, since this waiting time is merely the sum of the waiting times for each of the r arrivals, each one of which follows an exponential distribution with parameter λ.

$$f(x) = \frac{\lambda^r}{\Gamma(r)} x^{r-1} e^{-\lambda x}, \qquad\qquad (3.4)$$

where $\Gamma(r)$ is simply a function[*] that permits the sum (or integral) of this function to be one over all values of x, satisfying one of the major criteria of probability. The gamma function has two parameters: r (known as the scale parameter) and λ, the shape parameter. Its mean is λ/r, and variance λ/r^2. Different values for these parameters permit a wide variety of shapes for this commonly used probability distribution (Figure 3.4).

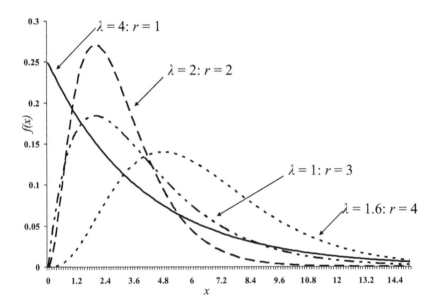

Figure 3.4. Different shapes available from the gamma distribution.

The gamma distribution's flexibility of shape will be particularly useful for us in our exploration of compounding now, as well as later, as we generate posterior distributions for biologic and health care related processes. The Bayesian is commonly faced with a parameter from a probability distribution that he or she believes has its own range of values. Assigning probabilities to these values requires them to have flexibility in the distribution choice. The gamma family of distribution, with its selection of two parameters λ and r is particularly rich, providing a wide range of shapes from which the worker may choose.

This distribution has an important application when compounded with the Poisson distribution. This famous process has been the object of much attention in

---

[*] $\Gamma(r)$ is simply known as the gamma function.

the computation and simulation world, e.g., [3] and has been directly applied to arrivals in emergency rooms as this next example illustrates.[*]

Example 3.2:
The growth of baby boomers will sharply increase the need for quality health care. However, as nurses move to the primary care, hospitals find that they cannot find enough nurses. Prospective nursing students are now commonly guided to enter other fields. The reasons are multitudinous, involving poor quality of work place due to increased patient loads and complaints about managed care. These influences are having a major effect just when many nurses themselves are retiring.[†]

A chronic shortage of nurses has left an emergency room critically low on this critical resource. While the deficiency does not impair the facility when patient flow is light, the shortage does have an impact when more than six patients are seen per hour. A biostatistician is asked to assess the arrival pattern of patients to this busy ER. Let X_t be the expected number of visits by time t. He is interested in the distribution of the number of patients seen in an hour, or X_1.

Recognizing that the arrival of patients to the ER meets the criteria of a Poisson process[‡] the worker examines the data, computing that, on average, there are 8 patient arrivals per hour. From this information, he graphs the distribution of the expected number of visits per hour (Figure 3.5).

This distribution has a strong central tendency, with the probability being highest around the mean arrival rate. From his assumption, he can compute the probability that there are six or more arrivals to the clinic per hour as

$$P[X_1 \geq 6] = \sum_{k=6}^{\infty} \frac{8^k}{k!} e^{-8} = 1 - \sum_{k=0}^{5} \frac{8^k}{k!} e^{-8} = 0.806, \tag{3.5}$$

indicating that the ER will be overburdened with patients approximately 80 percent of the time.

However, at the conclusion of this evaluation, he receives a histogram of the distribution of patients to the emergency room for the last week, revealing important deviations from the arrival pattern expected from the Poisson distribution (Figure 3.6).

---

[*] To the author's knowledge the application of the Poisson-Gamma compound distribution was first applied to emergency room visits by Dr. John. P. Young at The Johns Hopkins University, circa 1968.

[†] Taken from Facts about Nursing Shortage at www.nursesource.org/facts_shortage.html.

[‡] These criteria are independent arrivals with a constant arrival rate characterized by λ.

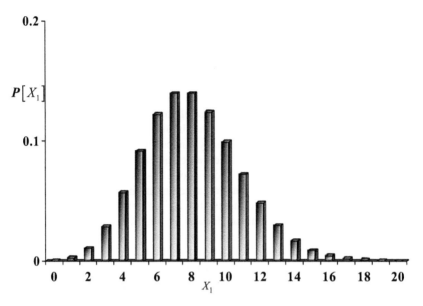

Figure 3.5. Distribution of the number of patients X_t in one hour assuming an underlying Poisson distribution with parameter $\lambda = 8$.

  The observed distribution has the same mean as the Poisson distribution, yet the probabilities assigned to different numbers of arrivals are remarkably different. The Poisson distribution has a greater tendency toward clustering around the mean, while the observed data demonstrate heavier tails. This is a critical difference, given the biostatistician is most interested in one of these "tail probabilities," i.e., $P[X_1 \geq 6]$. The difference between the observed and expected probability distribution is particularly vexing since, while the Poisson assumptions about patient arrivals are essentially valid, the Poisson distribution produces a poor fit. While the statistician is tempted to compute the desired probability from the distribution of the actual data, this estimate, based on the vicissitudes of the weekly data, can vary markedly from week to week.

  One approach to this dilemma is to consider possible variations, in the arrival rate λ itself. In fact, when the biostatisticians computes the distribution of the hourly arrival rate itself for different hours during the week, he observes that they do not remain at the value eight, but vary remarkably and asymmetrically (Figure 3.7).

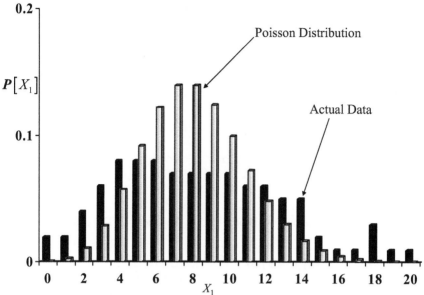

Figure 3.6. Comparison of the actual versus the observed distributions of patient arrivals to an ER. Both distributions have equivalent means, but the observed distribution has heavier tails.

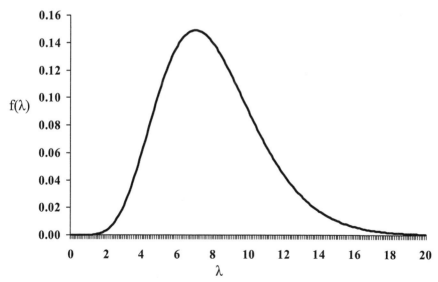

Figure 3.7. The marginal distribution of the patient arrival rates to an ER.. While the most common values of λ are relatively small, the distribution's skewness demonstrates the occurrence of high hourly arrivals, reflecting periods of intense ER activity.

It seems reasonable to use the gamma distribution to characterize the variability in the Poisson arrival rate where $\lambda = 0.5$ and $r = 8$. Thus, the worker recognizes that the $P[X_1 \geq 6]$ he computed from expression (3.5) was conditional on the value of $\lambda = 8$, and what he really needs is the unconditional distribution of X_1, the distribution of the variability of the arrival rate λ has been taken into account. Using the Law of Total Probability, he writes

$$P_k(t) = \sum_\lambda P_k(t \mid \lambda) P[\lambda]$$

$$= \sum_\lambda \frac{(\lambda t)^k}{k!} e^{-\lambda t} \frac{\alpha^r}{\Gamma(r)} \lambda^{r-1} e^{\alpha \lambda}. \qquad (3.6)$$

The simplification of this process is provided in Appendix E. The exact formula is

$$P[X_t = k] = \binom{k+r-1}{r-1} \left(\frac{\lambda}{\lambda+t}\right)^r \left(\frac{t}{\lambda+t}\right)^k. \qquad (3.7)$$

The unconditional distribution of X_1 follows a negative binomial distribution! The probability that there are k arrivals to the ER by time t, is the same as the probability that in a sequence of independent success-failure trials there are k failures before the rth success, where the probability of a success is $\lambda/(\lambda+t)$, and the probability of failure is $t/(\lambda+t)$. This is quite a remarkable result, generating an unconditional distribution for $P_k(1)$ that is easy to work with, namely,

$$P[X_t = k] = \binom{k+r-1}{r-1} \left(\frac{\lambda}{\lambda+1}\right)^r \left(\frac{1}{\lambda+1}\right)^k. \qquad (3.8)$$

Note that, as expected, the final result is not a function of λ, but instead a function of t (where in this case $t = 1$), and the parameters of the probability distribution of λ, i.e., α and r.

Going with the biostatistician's assumption that $\alpha = 1.0$ and $r = 8$ generates a negative binomial distribution with parameter $p = 0.5$, and $r = 8$ (Figure 3.8).

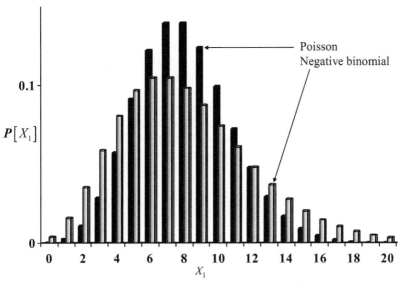

Figure 3.8. Comparison of the Poisson distribution $\lambda = 8$ and the negative binomial distribution for $p = 0.5$ and $r = 8$. Note the heavier tail of the negative binomial variable

The biostatistician now computes

$$P[X_1 \geq 6] = \sum_{k=6}^{\infty} \binom{k+r-1}{r-1} \left(\frac{\lambda}{\lambda+1}\right)^r \left(\frac{1}{\lambda+1}\right)^k$$

$$= \sum_{k=6}^{\infty} \binom{k+r-1}{r-1} (0.50)^r (0.50)^k$$

$$= 1 - \sum_{k=0}^{5} \binom{k+r-1}{r-1} (0.50)^r (0.50)^k$$

$$= 0.710.$$

a more accurate reflection of the strain on the emergency room.

■

3.4.1 Compound Gamma and Negative Binomial Distributions
One of the amazing findings about compounding distributions to obtain the marginal distribution of a variable is that the final solution can be very simple. One such case results from compounding a gamma distribution whose scale parameter follows a negative binomial distribution, as we will see in the following example.

Example 3.3: Storm Warnings

The North American hurricane season in general lasts from June 1 through November 1 of every year. However, the most powerful storms in the Gulf of Mexico are not seen until late August into September. This is primarily because huge storms require a vast reservoir of heat to sustain their energy, and it's not until late summer that the gulf is warm enough to maintain them. However, the Houston-Galveston metroplex, west of the Gulf has entered an unusual pattern in which they are struck by storms in June.

An environmental scientist is interested in assessing the time until this major metropolitan area is struck by one of these early storms. Beginning with a useful model, she believes that a gamma distribution may be a useful tool in making this prediction. If x is the time until a tropical storm arrives in weeks, she writes

$$f(x \mid n) = \frac{\alpha^n}{\Gamma(n)} x^{n-1} e^{\alpha x},$$
(3.9)

where n is a nonnegative integer. Thus according to this probability rule, the probability that the Houston-Galveston area is hit by a storm after time x is the area under this curve to the left of x (Figure 3.9).

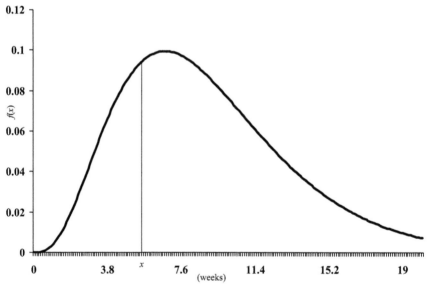

Figure 3.9. Modeled distribution of the probability of hurricane or tropical storm landfall in the Houston-Galveston metroplex where x is the number of weeks into the storm season. The probability that landfall occurs before time x is the area under the curve to the left of x, $P(x)$.

However, she believes that the pattern of storm strikes is changing, and actively explores the possibility that the parameter n from this distribution is not the same from year to year, but that it has its own probability distribution P_n. Assume P_n follows a negative binomial distribution with parameters r and p, i.e.,

$$P_n = \binom{n-1}{r-1} p^r (1-p)^{n-r}$$

for $n \geq r$. She is interested in the unconditional distribution of x, the probable time of a major tropical storm landfall, independent of the value of n. Using the Law of Total Probability, she writes

$$f(x) = \sum_n f(x \mid n) P_n$$

$$= \sum_{n=r}^{\infty} \frac{\alpha^n}{\Gamma(n)} x^{n-1} e^{-\alpha x} \binom{n-1}{r-1} p^r (1-p)^{n-r}. \qquad (3.10)$$

Appendix F demonstrates that expression (3.10) simplifies to a gamma distribution, i.e.

$$f(x) = \frac{[\alpha p]^r}{\Gamma(r)} x^{r-1} e^{-\alpha p x}. \qquad (3.11)$$

It is instructive to compare the conditional distribution of time to landfall, $f(x \mid n)$ with the unconditional distribution $f(x)$. Both are gamma distributions, but with different parameters. The conditional distribution has parameters α and n. However, since n has its own distribution, the unconditional distribution of time to storm time has parameters αp and r. Thus, the unconditional distribution draws its parameters from the conditional distribution of x and the marginal distribution of n.

In this example, the environmental scientist believes that $\alpha = 2.25$, $p = 0.5$, and $r = 4$, producing a marginal distribution of x with shape parameter $(2.25)(0.50) = 1.125$ and scale parameter $r = 4$ (Figure 3.10).

Thus, the marginal distribution of x suggests an earlier time for a major storm strike. For example, using the conditional distribution of x, the probability of a storm landfall in the first four weeks of the season is 0.105.[*] However, using the compound result, this probability is 0.475, over four times greater.

∎

Example 3.4: Substance Abuse Rehabilitation
As one example of compounding gamma distributions, we consider an example involving substance abuse.

---

[*] This probability is computed from Excel, using the built in gamma probability function.

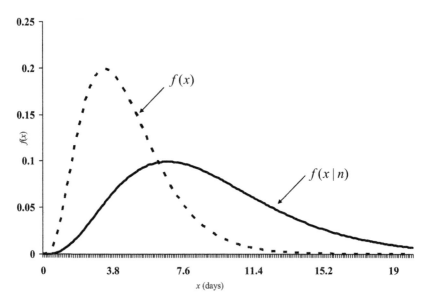

Figure 3.10. Comparison of conditional, $f(x|n)$, and marginal, $f(x)$, distribution of modeled time in days to tropical storm arrival. Each follows a gamma distribution.

Crystal methamphetamine, (known as crystal meth, "meth," or "crank") is an illegal derivative of methamphetamine. A member of the amphetamine class of drugs, it creates a temporary, false sense of increased energy in the user. People who ingest "meth" note increased physical strength accompanied by an euphoria of increased physical strength, mental focus, sharpened intellectual abilities, as well as enhanced sexual prowess and feelings of desirability. The precise pathophysiologic effects of the drug are increased heart rate and blood pressure, higher respiratory rate, and greater metabolic rate.

Over time, the user requires greater and greater drug quantities to attain the same "high," leading to the cravings that are the *sine qua non* of addiction. Chronic use of the drug generates prolonged fatigue, delusional thoughts, paranoid thought patterns, and permanent psychological damage. The effects on other organ systems are equally profound, leading to fatal kidney, liver, and heart failure.

Motivated by the rise in prevalence of methamphetamine use, counties have instituted and administered rehabilitation centers, which treat the patients' drug cravings. However, the addiction is as powerful as that of crack cocaine, making it a difficult condition to reverse.

Assume that several contiguous counties have developed their own rehabilitation facilities. Each uses a different set of counselors, employing various treatment strategies. However, all treatment centers experience a high rate of recidivism, and each tracks the time to methamphetamine reuse, which is the time from rehab discharge to the time the patient returns to abusing meth.

    In this example, assume that the time to reuse has been tracked and fol-lows a gamma distribution. However the distribution is different for each county's clinic; the scale parameter m is the same across clinics, but the shape parameter λ varies across clinics. Thus, if x is the time to reuse, then its probability function is

$$f(x) = \frac{\lambda_c^m}{\Gamma(m)} x^{m-1} e^{-\lambda_c x},$$

where λ_c refers to shape parameter from the cth rehabilitation center. The health care worker examines these gamma distributions from each of the counties overlaid on one another (Figure 3.11).

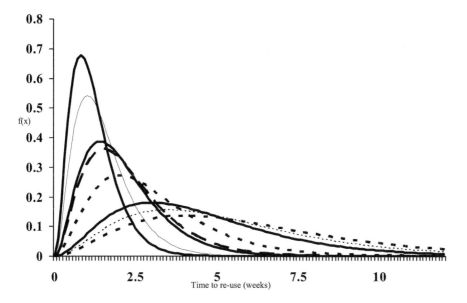

Figure 3.11 Hypothesized distribution of time to reuse of methamphetamine for eight different counties. The distributions are each gamma, but with a different shape parameter λ.

From Figure 3.11, each community has an early time of reuse for its patients, ac-knowledging the difficulty of treating this profound addiction. Several of the clinics are unable to postpone reuse beyond several days. Other centers can forestall re-cidivism to 2 to 4 weeks. However, each center is successful for a subgroup of their patients, postponing reuse for months.

    The health care worker is interested in determining the probability distri-bution of not just one clinic, but all clinics, with the view of extrapolating the re-sults to clinics that are not in this initial collection of rehabilitation centers. While he knows that the shape parameter is a continuous variable and could theoretically range from zero to infinity, he sees that the distributions have short average reuse times, which translate to smaller values of their shape parameters. He chooses to allow λ to have its own distribution. Let λ follow a gamma distribution, i.e.,

$$f(\lambda) = \frac{\alpha^r}{\Gamma(r)} \lambda^{r-1} e^{-\alpha\lambda} \qquad (3.12)$$

Thus, in this framework, each community "chooses" its shape parameter λ from the distribution expressed by equation (3.12), and then has drug reuse time produced from a gamma distribution with this shape parameter and scale parameter m.

The unconditional distribution follows from the application of the Law of Total Probability, which reveals

$$f(x) = \sum_{\lambda} f(x \mid \lambda) f(\lambda)$$

$$= \sum_{\lambda} \frac{\lambda^m}{\Gamma(m)} x^{m-1} e^{-\lambda x} \frac{\alpha^r}{\Gamma(r)} \lambda^{r-1} e^{-\alpha\lambda}. \qquad (3.13)$$

The mathematics reduce to the following unconditional distribution (Appendix G),

$$f(x) = \left[\frac{(r+1)r}{\alpha(r+m)} \right] \left(\frac{r+m}{r+1} \right) \left(\frac{\alpha}{\alpha+x} \right)^{r+1} \left(\frac{x}{\alpha+x} \right)^{m-1}. \qquad (3.14)$$

An initial inspection of this finding produced a disarmingly simple result. The first term, $\left[\dfrac{(r+1)r}{\alpha(r+m)} \right]$ is simply a constant, independent of the variable of interest, x.

The remainder of the expression is

$$\left(\frac{r+m}{r+1} \right) \left(\frac{\alpha}{\alpha+x} \right)^{r+1} \left(\frac{x}{\alpha+x} \right)^{m-1} \qquad (3.15)$$

a familiar, albeit somewhat disguised distribution. Assume a coin whose probability of a heads is $\alpha/(\alpha+x)$ is flipped $r + m$ times. Then the probability of $r + 1$ heads is provided by expression (3.15). It is a binomial distribution.

Note that we are not saying that the unconditional time to reuse follows a binomial distribution. The very nature of the continuous reuse variable makes this an impossibility. However, the unconditional distribution of this time is related to a binomial distribution. The variable of interest composes part of the probability of success, $p = \dfrac{\alpha}{\alpha + x}$. The shape of this distribution is a function of r and m (Figure 3.12).

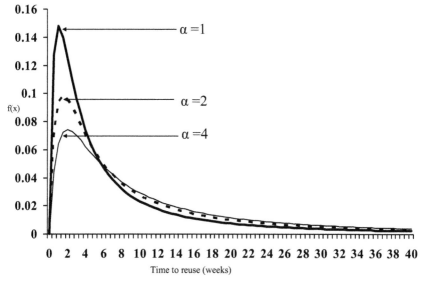

Figure 3.12. Example of compounding a gamma with a gamma distribution for predicting methamphetamine reuse time as a function of different values of α ($m = 2$, $r = 1$). Note the heavy skewness.

Note the extreme shift to the left for this distribution as a function of α, the scale distribution for the prior distribution of λ. It reflects the totality of the experience of the clinics demonstrating early reuse time for many of the patients. Note that the location of the most likely reuse times is not a function of the shape parameter of the distribution of λ itself. Regardless of the value of α, the most common reuse times are within 1 to 2 weeks of treatment termination. This news, the result of the ensemble experience for the established treatment centers with available data, is a sobering, but realistic assessment of the failure rates for contemporary rehabilitative therapy.

To continue this example, the assessment selected by the health care worker making this global assessment is provided (Figure 3.13). This figure demonstrates both the early recidivism rate, but also a fairly thick tail, supporting the concept that longer term success is possible with current therapy approaches.

3.6 The Normal Distribution

The most widely used probability distribution of the past 300 years, in fact, the one which is most "normally" or commonly used, is the "bell shaped curve" (Figure 3.14). After a brief review of its properties, we will implement this popular distribution in the compounding process.

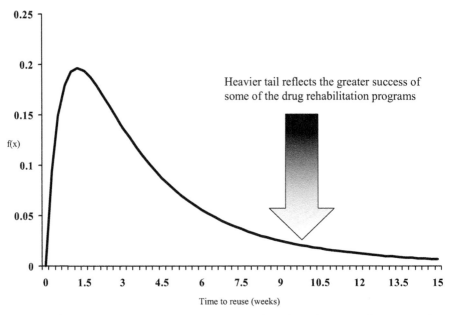

Figure 3.13. Unconditional distribution of time to methamphetamine reuse when community reuse times are relatively short ($m = 2$, $r = 1$, $\alpha = 5$).

3.6.1 Why Is the Normal Distribution Normally Used?

There are two main reasons why this distribution, formally known as the Gaussian distribution (named for Carl Frederick Gauss 1777–1855, Figure 3.15), is the most widely used probability distribution in applied statistics. The first is that there actually are processes (e.g., the movement of Brownian motion commonly used in the interim monitoring of clinical trials[4]) in which event probabilities of interest precisely follow this distribution, whose function is

$$f(x) = \frac{1}{\sqrt{2\pi}} e^{-\frac{x^2}{2}}. \tag{3.16}$$

The second and perhaps most important rationale for the common use of the normal distribution lies in the nature of events of interests. Frequently events whose probability we would like to find represent the combined action of many smaller events.

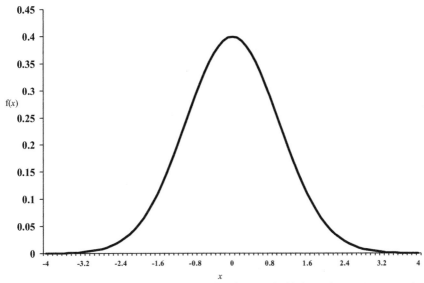

Figure 3.14. The standard normal distribution or "bell shaped curve" centered at zero with a standard deviation of one.

For example, suppose an epidemiologist is interested in the probability distribution of body temperature, a quantity whose mean we know to be 98.6 degrees Fahrenheit. However, body temperature itself is generated and maintained by a complex collection of actions, e.g., basal metabolic rate, activity, neural tone, and endocrine status. These in turn are composed of other influences. Thus, we might think of body temperature as the resultant of many different effects; many of these are positive, tending to increase body temperature, while many others are negative, reducing the temperature. Each individual influence is small, but it is the ensemble of these numerous, infinitesimal effects that produces the resultant body temperature.

In addition, it is the nature of these sums to assume more moderate than extreme values. This is because there are more ways to produce centrally located totals as demonstrated in the following example.

Example 3.5: Generating Central Tendency

Consider the behavior of a simple variable x that can only assume one of two possible values; $x = 0$ with probability 0.50, or $x = 1$ with probability 0.50. Certainly this variable demonstrates no inclination for central tendency (Figure 3.17, $n = 1$).

However, the situation changes at once when we add two of them. Let $y = x_1 + x_2$. An examination of the possible values of x_1 and x_2 reveals that y can have one of only three possible values.

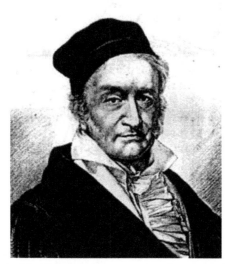

Figure 3.15. Portrait of Carl Frederick Gauss, one of the discoverers of the "normal" distribution, or the bell-shaped curve. From www-history.mcs.st-andrews.ac.uk/Indexes/G.html, School of Mathematics and Statistics, The University at St. Andrews, Scotland.

If $x_1 = 0$ and $x_2 = 0$ then $y = 0$
If $x_1 = 0$ and $x_2 = 1$ then $y = 1$
If $x_1 = 1$ and $x_2 = 0$ then $y = 1$
If $x_1 = 1$ and $x_2 = 1$ then $y = 2$

Each of these possibilities occurs with probability 0.25. Yet note that there are two events which produce the more moderate event of $y = 1$, and only one possible event that produces either of the extreme values of $y = 0$ or $y = 1$. Thus, since there are more combinations of (x_1, x_2) values that produce the moderate value of $y = 1$, the probability of this moderate value is greater (Figure 3.16) for $n = 2$.

The movement to central tendency increases as the number of variables in the sum increases. It is this movement that is captured in the central limit theorem, which states that sums of variables, suitably normalized, have probability distributions that can be nicely approximated by the normal distribution. Thus the veracity of the central limit theorem motivates the normal distribution's ubiquity.

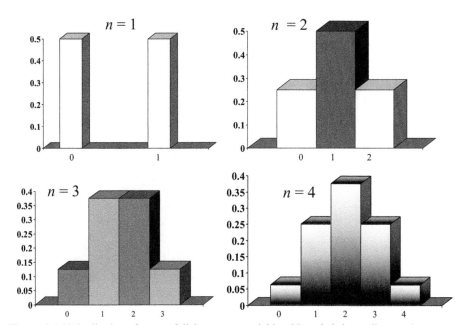

Figure 3.16 Distribution of sums of dichotomous variables. Note their immediate tendency to develop central tendency as more are combined.

3.6.2 Using the Normal Distribution
An important advantage in using the normal distribution is the relative ease of producing probabilities from it. Although the actual production of probabilities requires one to use a table (Appendix H), fortunately we need use only one table to produce probabilities for the many different normal distributions. This is due to the ease of transformation of normal random variables and the notion of symmetry.

3.6.3.1 Simplifying Transformations
The normal distribution is not just a single distribution, but instead represents an entire family of them. There are an infinite number of normal distributions, each one characterized by its unique mean μ and variance σ^2. The mean provides the location of the distribution, and the variance characterizes the dispersion of the variable around that mean (Figure 3.17).

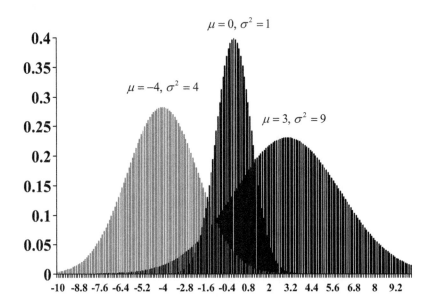

Figure 3.17. Different locations and dispersions of three normal distributions.

Figure 3.17 provides three illustrations of different members from the family of normal distributions, their locations and dispersal or "spread" governed by their means and variances of each. We refer to the normal distribution with mean μ and variance σ^2 as $N(\mu, \sigma^2)$.

      The fact that the location and the shape of a normally distributed variable is governed by its mean and variance suggests that the investigator must incorporate these two parameters into any computation of the probabilities using these distributions. Because there are an infinite number of combinations of these parameters, a first impression is that these computations can rapidly become unwieldy. Fortunately, this complexity is removed by the fact that each member of the family of normal distributions can be related or transformed to another normal distribution. This single normal distribution has a mean of zero and a variance of one, and is known as the *standard normal distribution*.

      Therefore, if X follows a normal distribution with mean μ and variance σ^2, then X can be transformed to a normally distributed variable with mean 0 and variance 1. Specifically, if X follows a normal distribution with mean μ and variance σ^2, then $(X-u)/\sigma$ follows a normal distribution with mean 0 and variance 1. This observation, in concert with the symmetry of the normal distribution about its mean permits us to compute all of the probabilities that we need from the normal distribution with relative ease.

Example 3.6

Assume blood glucose levels in a population of type II diabetic patients follow a normal distribution with mean $\mu = 189$ milligrams per deciliter (mg/dl) and variance $\sigma^2 = 100$. To compute the expected proportion of patients with blood sugar levels greater than 210 mg/dl, we simply calculate

$$P[X > 210] = P\left[\frac{X - 189}{10} > \frac{210 - 189}{10}\right] = P[Z > 2.1],$$

where the variable Z follows a $N(0,1)$ distribution. Appendix H does not provide the probability that $Z > 2.10$ directly. However, since the standard normal curve is symmetric about $Z = 0$, we compute $P[Z > 2.1] = P[Z < -2.1] = 0.018$, using Appendix H to compute this last probability. Thus, we would expect 1.8% of diabetic subjects to have a blood sugar greater than 210 mg/dl.

■

3.6.3. Compounding the Normal Distribution

One of most useful examples of compounding begins with the normal distribution. While the background mathematics that demonstrate this result are complicated (Appendix I), the result itself is straightforward and easy to use.

Assume that we have a variable that follows a normal distribution with mean θ and unknown variance σ^2. In this case, the variance is a known constant; however, θ itself follows a normal distribution, with known mean μ and known variance v^2. We are interested in the marginal distribution of the original variable x. The unconditional distribution of x is itself normally distributed, this time with mean μ and variance $\sigma^2 + v^2$.

In this case we have three occurrences of the normal distribution. The distribution of x given the parameter θ follows a normal distribution. The parameter θ itself follows a normal distribution. From these two assumptions, it follows that the unconditional distribution of x follows a normal distribution as well. We will repeatedly use this easily implemented finding.

Example 3.7

Patients in a phase II clinical study with elevations in diastolic blood pressure are administered a blood pressure reducing medication in liquid form. When provided the medication, they are expected to have a blood pressure reduction which is normally distributed with mean θ and variance $\sigma^2 = 36$. Any patient who had a blood pressure reduction that is not as large as 5 mm Hg, is considered a treatment failure. However, the bioavailability of the medication is in question, making the expected blood pressure reduction θ a variable. It is believed that θ is normally distributed with mean 10 and variance $v^2 = 9$. The investigator would like to know the proportion of treatment failures.

The solution is straightforward. The investigator understands, that, when in possession of the value of θ, the proportion of nonresponders is simply the probability that a variable following a normal distribution with mean θ and variance 10 is less than five. However, although she doesn't have the value of θ, she knows that it is also normally distributed with mean 10 and variance 9. Using the result of compounding normal distributions, she concludes that the unconditional distribution of the blood pressure reduction follows a normal distribution with mean 10 and variance $36 + 9 = 45$. She therefore computes the proportion of nonresponders as

$$P[X < 5] = P\left[\frac{X-5}{\sqrt{45}} > \frac{10-5}{\sqrt{45}}\right] = P[Z < 0.745] = 0.773.$$

By this criteria, most patients are nonresponders.

This compounding result reveals that the distribution of x and θ are both normal, and both have the same mean. However, the variances are quite different (Figure 3.18).

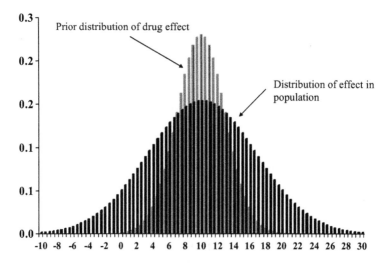

Figure 3.18. Distribution of blood pressure reducing effect. The effect of the drug in the population is less predictable than the effect of the drug based on its "prior" distribution.

Problems

1.   From Example 3.1, the probability of k deaths in n birds with the Avian flu was derived to be

$$P_k(t) = \binom{n}{k} \sum_{i=0}^{n-k} \binom{n-k}{i} (-1)^i \frac{\lambda}{(k+i)t+\lambda}. \tag{3.17}$$

Using equation (3.17) where $\lambda = 1.5$, compute each of the following probabilities.

    a. P[out of twenty birds, there are less than 10 deaths in 1 week]
    b. P[out of twenty birds, there are less than 10 deaths in 2 weeks]
    c. P[out of twenty birds, there are less than 10 deaths in 3 weeks]

2.   Assume the time to motor vehicle accident at a dangerous intersection follows a Poisson distribution with shape parameter $\lambda = 3$ accidents per week. Compute the probability there will be six or more accidents in two weeks.

3.   Now assume that the λ follows a gamma distribution with shape parameter $\alpha = 3$, and scale parameter $m = 2$. Find the unconditional distribution of the number of accidents in two weeks, and compute the probability that there will be six or more accidents in two weeks based on this new distribution. Compute and compare the means and variances of each of these two distributions.

4.   The yearly frequency of supreme court nominees follows a Poisson distribution [5]. A political scientist watches the inauguration of a new U.S. president and is interested in computing the probability distribution of the number of supreme court seats that will be vacant over the next four years. Compute the probability distribution of the number of supreme court vacancies using the Poisson distribution with parameter $\lambda = 0.37$.

5.   Assume now that the parameter λ follows a gamma distribution with shape parameter $\alpha = 3$ and scale parameter $r = 9$. Compute the distribution of the number of vacancies on the supreme court using this distribution.

6.   An epidemiologist carefully observes the outbreak of a new measles epidemic. She expects the incubation period (time to the first onset of symptoms) in days to follow a gamma distribution with scale parameter 2. However, its scale parameter also follows a negative binomial distribution

$$P_n = \binom{n-1}{r-1} p^r (1-p)^{n-r}$$

$r = 2$ and $p = 0.60$. Compute the probability that the incubation period is greater than three days, using the unconditional distribution of the incubation duration.

7.   An outpatient clinic for an orthopedics department has patients waiting to
      see physicians. The waiting time for patients follows an exponential distribu-
      tion. However, the parameter λ follows a gamma distribution with shape pa-
      rameter $\alpha = 2$ and scale parameter $r = 4$. Find the unconditional distribution
      of the waiting time.

8.   The duration of commencement speaker's addresses follow a gamma distri-
      bution, where the shape parameter $\alpha = 30$. Assume the scale parameter fol-
      lows a negative binomial distribution with $p = 0.2$, and $r = 8$. Compute the
      probability that a commencement address lasts more than 30 minutes.

9.   The radius of a cloud of toxin at time t follows a normal distribution with
      mean μt and variance $\sigma^2 = 500t$. Assume that the mean μ is not constant, but
      follows a normal distribution with mean $300t$ and variance $500t$. Compute
      the unconditional probability that the radius is greater than 500 for $t = 1$.

References

1.   Hill B. (1953). Observation and experiment. *New England Journal of Medicine*
     248:995–1001.
2.   Moyé L.A., Kapadia A.S. (2000). *Difference Equations in Public Health
     Applications*. New York. Marcel Dekker/Taylor and Francis. Chapter 11.
3.   Wang M.L., Houshmand A.A. (1999). Health care Simulation: A case study at
     a local clinic. *Proceedings of the 1999 Winter Simulation Conference*.
4.   Moyé L.A. (2005). *Statistical Monitoring of Clinical Trials. Fundamentals for
     Investigators*. New York. Springer-Verlag.
5 . Callen E., Leidecker H. (1971). A mean life on the Supreme Court. *American
     Bar Association Journal* **57**:1188–1192.

4
Completing Yo r First Bayesian Comp tations

4.1 Compounding and Bayes Procedures

Our review of basic probability and new found familiarity with the Law of Total Probability now permits us to extend the work of the previous chapter to complete our first Bayesian computations.

Both Bayesians and frequentists recognize the importance of the parameters of probability distributions. In fact, we cannot compute probabilities of some of the most basic events using these distributions without knowledge of them. In fact, Bayesians almost always, while frequentists sometimes, refer to the probability distribution of the event x as $P[x \mid \theta]$, or $f(x \mid \theta)$, explicitly denoting the relationship between the probability distribution of x and the parameter on which use of that distribution is based. However, we commonly do not know the value of the relevant parameter, signified in this discussion by θ. Frequentists estimate θ as though it had one and only one value in the population. However, to the Bayesian, the parameter θ has intrinsic variability of its own. Bayesians capture this useful information about the location of θ in the prior distribution, denoted as $P[\theta]$, or $\pi(\theta)$.

Identifying this information has two useful purposes. The first is that it permits a worker to identify the unconditional probability distribution of x, by carrying out a weighed sum of the values of the parameter of θ. This is what the Law of Total Probability permits, i.e.,

$$P[x] = \sum_{\theta} P[x \mid \theta] P[\theta]. \qquad (4.1)$$

This equality allows us to compute the unconditional distribution of x from its conditional distribution, i.e., converting $P[x \mid \theta]$ to $P[x]$, a conversion known as compounding.

However, useful as the compounding process is,[*] it is only an intermediate point in the Bayes computation. The Bayesian is not so interested in starting with

---

[*] Examples are provided in Chapters Two and Three.

$P[x \mid \theta]$ and going on to compute $P[x]$; the Bayesian wants to move from $P[x \mid \theta]$ to $P[\theta \mid x]$. This is the process of "inversion" of the probability, i.e., reversing the conditions of the probability computation, first stated by Bayes and Laplace. Recall from Chapter One that Bayes Theorem provides the inversion formula, simply stating

$$P[\theta \mid x] = \frac{P[\theta \cap x]}{P[x]} = \frac{P[x \mid \theta] P[\theta]}{\sum_{\theta} P[x \mid \theta] P[\theta]}, \tag{4.2}$$

or, when working with continuous distributions

$$\pi(\theta \mid x) = \frac{f(x \cap \theta)}{f(x)} = \frac{f(x \mid \theta) \pi(\theta)}{\sum_{\theta} f(x \mid \theta) \pi(\theta)}. \tag{4.3}$$

The denominators in the right-hand sides of each of these expressions are precisely the results from the Law of Total Probability. Thus, in order to complete the inversion process, we simply need to carry out a final division. This process of compounding followed by division generates the posterior distribution of θ.

　　　　The purpose of this chapter is to gain some basic experience with obtaining posterior probability distributions. We will start with the most simple cases, then allow the examples to increase in complexity and realism.

4.2 Introduction to a Simple Bayes Procedure.
Our first example identifying a Bayes procedure utilizes a discrete conditional distribution and discrete prior distribution. The procedure we establish here is that used in most cases of posterior distribution identification. After identifying the conditional distribution, either $P[x \mid \theta]$ or $f(x \mid \theta)$, and the prior distribution of θ, $\pi(\theta)$, we use the law of total probability to obtain the unconditional distribution of x, and then carry out the division to obtain the posterior distribution $\pi(\theta \mid x)$.

Example 4.1
An orthopedic clinic is staffed by one of two physicians, Dr. Diane Two and Dr. Peter Three. The number of nurses assisting Dr. Two is either one or two; the probability that she has one nurse assisting her is $1/2$, and with probability $1/2$ she has two nurses assisting her. Dr. Three requires the help of either 1, 2, or 3 nurses, each with probability $1/3$.

　　　　If x is the number of nurses in the clinic then we can easily identify the probability distribution of x if we know which of the two doctors is staffing the clinic. Let's assume that $\theta = 2$ means that Dr. Two is seeing patients, and $\theta = 3$ identifies Dr. Three as the staff doctor at the clinic. Then, remembering our notation from Chapter 1,

$$P[x \mid \theta = 2] = \frac{1}{2}1_{x=1} + \frac{1}{2}1_{x=2}$$

$$P[x \mid \theta = 3] = \frac{1}{3}1_{x=1} + \frac{1}{3}1_{x=2} + \frac{1}{3}1_{x=3}. \tag{4.4}$$

Thus, we can compute the probability distribution of the number of clinic nurses, by simply knowing whether Dr. Two or Dr. Three is the staff physician that day. We may more succinctly write this distribution as

$$P[x \mid \theta] = \frac{1}{\theta} \sum_{i=1}^{\theta} 1_{x=i}. \tag{4.5}$$

Suppose that on any given day, the probability that Dr. Two is seeing patients is ⅔, and Dr. Three is at the clinic for ⅓ of the time. Recall that the value of θ denotes the doctor at the clinic, so we may also write.

$$P[\theta] = \frac{2}{3}1_{\theta=2} + \frac{1}{3}1_{\theta=3}. \tag{4.6}$$

Based only on information about doctor availability, if someone asks, "How likely is it that Dr. Two was in the clinic today?" our answer can only be that this doctor's probability of being in the clinic is ⅔. There is no other condition or known event that occur in the clinic that permits us to adjust this estimate one way or the other. However, if we were told, "There were 2 nurses in clinic today. Now, what is the probability that Dr. Two is the physician seeing patients?" a Bayes procedure provides the answer.

The answer to this question requires us to carry out the classic inversion process of Bayes and Laplace. We know $P[\theta]$. We must obtain $P[\theta \mid x]$. To do this we must invert $P[x \mid \theta]$ to $P[\theta \mid x]$.

Bayes Theorem states

$$P[\theta \mid x] = \frac{P[\theta \cap x]}{P[x]} = \frac{P[x \mid \theta]P[\theta]}{\sum_{\theta} P[x \mid \theta]P[\theta]}. \tag{4.7}$$

From the conditions of the problem, we know that

$$P[\theta \cap x] = P[x \mid \theta]P[\theta] = \frac{1}{\theta} \sum_{i=1}^{\theta} 1_{x=i} \left[\frac{2}{3}1_{\theta=2} + \frac{1}{3}1_{\theta=3} \right].$$

Thus we can write the posterior distribution as

$$P[\theta \mid x] = \frac{\dfrac{1}{\theta}\displaystyle\sum_{i=1}^{\theta} 1_{x=i} \left[\dfrac{2}{3}1_{\theta=2} + \dfrac{1}{3}1_{\theta=3}\right]}{\displaystyle\sum_{\theta}\dfrac{1}{\theta}\displaystyle\sum_{i=1}^{\theta} 1_{x=i} \left[\dfrac{2}{3}1_{\theta=2} + \dfrac{1}{3}1_{\theta=3}\right]}. \tag{4.8}$$

We should pause for a moment to examine the numerator and denominator of this expression. The denominator is a quantity that we have familiarity computing from the previous two chapter. We recognize it as a function only of the data point x. However, the numerator is a function not just of x but also of θ. Thus, the posterior distribution is a function of θ, exactly what it must be in order to compute the probability of a value of θ.

The numerator allows us to compute the joint values of θ and x, and requires that we know each of these values. For example, if we wanted to know the probability that Dr. Two was in the clinic along with two nurses, then $x = 2$ and $\theta = 2$ and we would write

$$P[x = 2 \cap \theta = 2] = \frac{1}{\theta}\sum_{i=1}^{\theta} 1_{x=i} \left[\frac{2}{3}1_{\theta=2} + \frac{1}{3}1_{\theta=3}\right].$$

Since one of the conditions of the problem is that $\theta = 2$, any term involving the indicator function $1_{\theta=3}$ becomes zero. We continue, writing

$$P[x = 2 \cap \theta = 2] = \frac{1}{\theta}\sum_{i=1}^{\theta} 1_{x=i} \left[\frac{2}{3}1_{\theta=2} + \frac{1}{3}1_{\theta=3}\right] = \left(\frac{2}{3}\right)\left(\frac{1}{2}\right)\sum_{i=1}^{2} 1_{x=2}$$

$$= \left(\frac{2}{3}\right)\left(\frac{1}{2}\right) = \frac{1}{3}.$$

The denominator of the posterior distribution is simply the sum of these probabilities over the only two values of θ, i.e., 2 and 3, and is easy to simplify

$$\sum_{\theta}\frac{1}{\theta}\sum_{i=1}^{\theta} 1_{x=i} \left[\frac{2}{3}1_{\theta=2} + \frac{1}{3}1_{\theta=3}\right]$$

$$= \frac{1}{2}(1_{x=1} + 1_{x=2})\frac{2}{3} + \frac{1}{3}(1_{x=1} + 1_{x=2} + 1_{x=3})\frac{1}{3}$$

$$= \left(\frac{2}{6} + \frac{1}{9}\right)1_{x=1} + \left(\frac{2}{6} + \frac{1}{9}\right)1_{x=2} + \frac{1}{9}1_{x=3}$$

$$= \frac{4}{9}1_{x=1} + \frac{4}{9}1_{x=2} + \frac{1}{9}1_{x=3}. \tag{4.9}$$

This is the marginal distribution of the number of nurses.[*] We substitute this result into equation (4.8) to write

$$P[\theta \mid x] = \frac{\dfrac{1}{\theta}\sum_{x=i}^{\theta} 1_{i=1}\left[\dfrac{2}{3}1_{\theta=2} + \dfrac{1}{3}1_{\theta=3}\right]}{\dfrac{4}{9}1_{x=1} + \dfrac{4}{9}1_{x=2} + \dfrac{1}{9}1_{x=3}}. \tag{4.10}$$

Let's compare this formula's result with our intuition. Recall that only Dr. Three works with three nurses. Therefore, the posterior distribution should reveal that $P[\theta = 3 \mid x = 3] = 1$. From formula (4.10), we find that

$$P[\theta = 3 \mid x = 3] = \frac{\left(\dfrac{1}{3}\right)1_{x=3}\left(\dfrac{1}{3}\right)}{\left(\dfrac{1}{9}\right)1_{x=3}} = \frac{\dfrac{1}{9}}{\dfrac{1}{9}} = 1,$$

confirming our understanding of the problem.

We now have the formula we need to update the prior probabilities of the availability of physicians. For example, we know that the prior probability that Dr. Two is in the clinic is ⅔. However, what if we now know that there are two nurses in the clinic? We can therefore update the probability of Dr. Two's presence by using equation (4.10) to calculate

$$P[\theta = 2 \mid x = 2] = \frac{\left(\dfrac{1}{2}\right)1_{x=2}\left(\dfrac{2}{3}\right)}{\left(\dfrac{4}{9}\right)1_{x=2}} = \frac{\dfrac{2}{6}}{\dfrac{4}{9}} = \frac{3}{4},$$

and we see that the posterior probability has updated this probability from ⅔ to ¾.

4.3. Including a Continuous Conditional Distribution

Recall that there are four components from which a Bayes posterior distribution is constructed. The first is the prior distribution, or the distribution of the parameter of interest that is not based on the current data x. The second distribution is the distribution of x given the parameter θ. This is known as the conditional distribution since it is (of course) conditional on the value of the parameter θ. The third distribution is the marginal distribution of x, and the fourth is the posterior distribution of θ given x.

---

[*] Note that the sum of the probabilities for all possible values of the number of nurses is $4/9 + 4/9 + 4/9 = 1$, exactly the sum that a proper probability distribution should have.

In the previous example of our first complete Bayes procedure we examined the posterior distribution resulting from a combination of very simple distributions for the prior distribution of θ and the conditional distribution of x given θ. In this next example, we will incorporate a well recognized distribution introduced in Chapter Two, using it to help consider the possible likely values of its parameter.

Example 4.2: Hepatitis Sera Production

A strain of monkeys has been carefully selected to test their ability to produce a protective serum against a new strain of hepatitis. Hepatitis is a viral infection that targets the liver. In its most culminant form, the virus destroys the billions of hepatocytes that compose the structure of the liver, shredding the huge organ. With only a critically weakened, dysfunctional liver to rely on, the organism cannot detoxify many of the compounds that are by-products of both digestion and metabolism. The results are cataclysmic. In rare cases, convulsions ensue three to four days after infection, followed by coma. Without a liver transplant, the organism dies in less than a week after the initial infection.

A small number of primates known to be resistant to the hepatitis virus are set aside for infection with the virus in an attempt to generate optimal quantities of antiserum. Although the monkeys will each survive their infections, no one knows how likely it is that they will produce adequate levels of antiserum. Let the probability of adequate antiserum production be reflected by the parameter θ. In this simple example, the scientists believe that θ is equal to either 0.10, 0.65, or 0.90.

Ten monkeys are infected and observed for adequate antiserum production. Let x be the number of monkeys that produce adequate antiserum. Since θ is assumed to be constant from primate to primate, and each monkey's ability to produce adequate antiserum production is independent of any other primate's capability, then observations in these primates are really a sequence of Bernoulli trials. Therefore, if the investigators knew the value of θ, they could compute the distribution of the number of monkeys that will produce adequate antiserum as

$$P[x = k \mid \theta] = \binom{10}{k} \theta^k (1-\theta)^{10-k}, \qquad (4.11)$$

where $x = 0, 1, 2, 3,..., 10$. From a frequentist perspective, a good estimator of θ is the proportion of monkeys who produce adequate antiserum.

The experiment is carried out, and all ten primates are infected. Seven of the ten monkeys are observed to produce adequate antiserum, and the scientists carry out a quick computation, producing an estimate of θ of $\frac{7}{10} = 0.70$. A cursory examination of the initial candidate choices for θ suggests that the value $\theta = 0.65$ is the most likely, since, of the three candidate values, 0.65 is closest to the observed estimate of 0.70. The frequentist concludes that of the three prior values of θ, $\theta = 0.65$ is most likely the correct one.

However, to a Bayesian, this is an incomplete examination. While the possible values of θ have been provided, there was no probability assessment of the likelihood of these values. This missing component reduces the impact of the prior values of θ on the final solution.

For example, suppose the investigators believed not just that there were only three possible values of θ, but that there is a 45% chance that the probability of adequate antiserum production is 0.10, a 5% chance that this probability is 0.65, and a 50% chance that this probability of adequate antiserum production is 0.90. We have now converted the catalog of possible values of θ to a prior distribution for θ, written in our standard notation as

$$\pi(\theta) = 0.451_{\theta=0.10} + 0.051_{\theta=0.65} + 0.501_{\theta=0.90}. \tag{4.12}$$

Note that the function of this prior distribution is to assign probability to possible values of θ. The frequentist, flummoxed by this step, wonders on what basis this probability is assigned. However, to the Bayesian, probability is subjective, not just based on relative frequency; it is perfectly appropriate to let it reflect the degree of truth the investigators feel is captured by each of the three estimates.

Using a Bayesian formulation, we write the binomial distribution as the conditional distribution of x given θ, $f(x|\theta)$, and proceed with our standard Bayesian formulation.

$$\pi(\theta|x) = \frac{f(x|\theta)\pi(\theta)}{\sum_\theta f(x|\theta)\pi(\theta)}, \tag{4.13}$$

which in case of these investigators, becomes

$$\pi(\theta|x=k) = \frac{\binom{10}{k}\theta^k (1-\theta)^{10-k} \left(0.451_{\theta=0.10} + 0.051_{\theta=0.65} + 0.501_{\theta=0.90}\right)}{\sum_\theta \binom{10}{k}\theta^k (1-\theta)^{10-k} \left(0.451_{\theta=0.10} + 0.051_{\theta=0.65} + 0.501_{\theta=0.90}\right)}$$

$$= \frac{0.45\binom{10}{k}\theta^k (1-\theta)^{10-k} 1_{\theta=0.10} + 0.05\binom{10}{k}\theta^k (1-\theta)^{10-k} 1_{\theta=0.65} + 0.50\binom{10}{k}\theta^k (1-\theta)^{10-k} 1_{\theta=0.90}}{\sum_\theta 0.45\binom{10}{k}\theta^k (1-\theta)^{10-k} 1_{\theta=0.10} + 0.05\binom{10}{k}\theta^k (1-\theta)^{10-k} 1_{\theta=0.65} + 0.50\binom{10}{k}\theta^k (1-\theta)^{10-k} 1_{\theta=0.90}}.$$

While this may appear formidable it is actually quite easy to evaluate. The denominator (as always) is simply an example of compounding. We only need to sum over the three possible values for θ to calculate

$$\sum_{\theta} 0.45 \binom{10}{k} \theta^k (1-\theta)^{10-k} \mathbf{1}_{\theta=0.10} + 0.05 \binom{10}{k} \theta^k (1-\theta)^{10-k} \mathbf{1}_{\theta=0.65} + 0.50 \binom{10}{k} \theta^k (1-\theta)^{10-k} \mathbf{1}_{\theta=0.90}$$

$$= 0.45 \binom{10}{k} (0.10)^k (0.90)^{10-k} + 0.05 \binom{10}{k} (0.65)^k (0.35)^{10-k} + 0.50 \binom{10}{k} (0.90)^k (0.10)^{10-k}.$$

Placing this result in the denominator of (4.13), we may now write the posterior distribution as

$$\pi(\theta \mid x=k) = \frac{0.45 \binom{10}{k} \theta^k (1-\theta)^{10-k} \mathbf{1}_{\theta=0.10} + 0.05 \binom{10}{k} \theta^k (1-\theta)^{10-k} \mathbf{1}_{\theta=0.65} + 0.50 \binom{10}{k} \theta^k (1-\theta)^{10-k} \mathbf{1}_{\theta=0.90}}{0.45 \binom{10}{k} (0.10)^k (0.90)^{10-k} + 0.05 \binom{10}{k} (0.65)^k (0.35)^{10-k} + 0.50 \binom{10}{k} (0.90)^k (0.10)^{10-k}}.$$

Recall that the investigators found seven of ten primates produced adequate antiserum, allowing us to compute

$$\pi(\theta \mid x=7) = \frac{0.45 \binom{10}{7} \theta^7 (1-\theta)^3 \mathbf{1}_{\theta=0.10} + 0.05 \binom{10}{7} \theta^7 (1-\theta)^3 \mathbf{1}_{\theta=0.65} + 0.50 \binom{10}{7} \theta^7 (1-\theta)^3 \mathbf{1}_{\theta=0.90}}{0.45 \binom{10}{7} (0.10)^7 (0.90)^3 + 0.05 \binom{10}{7} (0.65)^7 (0.35)^3 + 0.50 \binom{10}{7} (0.90)^7 (0.10)^3}.$$

The denominator is merely a constant, easily computed to be 0.0413. We are now ready to evaluate the probabilities of different values of θ.

$$P[\theta = 0.10 \mid x = 7] \quad = \pi(\theta = 0.10 \mid x = 7) \quad = \quad \frac{0.45 \binom{10}{7} (0.10)^7 (0.90)^3}{0.0413} \quad = \quad 0.00009$$

$$P[\theta = 0.65 \mid x = 7] \quad = \pi(\theta = 0.65 \mid x = 7) \quad = \quad \frac{0.05 \binom{10}{7} (0.65)^7 (0.35)^3}{0.0413} \quad = \quad 0.305$$

$$P[\theta = 0.90 \mid x = 7] \quad = \pi(\theta = 0.90 \mid x = 7) \quad = \quad \frac{0.50 \binom{10}{7} (0.90)^7 (0.10)^3}{0.0413} \quad = \quad 0.695.$$

Note that the most probable value of θ by this calculation is not 0.65, but 0.90, a different selection from that of the "frequentist" investigators.

The difference in the solution requires a closer examination. The data from the experiment generated 7 successes in 10 trials, suggesting that a reasonable estimate from this one research effort was $\frac{7}{10} = 0.70$, an estimate that of the three choices, was closest to 0.65, supporting the idea that the best estimate of θ was 0.65. However, the Bayesian procedure came to a different conclusion, suggesting that the value of 0.90 was the most likely; this solution was more than three times as likely as the estimate of 0.65, and many times more likely than the value of 0.10. What has happened here? Where is the disconnect?

The answer is provided in a single word — prior. The prior distribution for θ, i.e., $\pi(\theta) = 0.451_{\theta=0.10} + 0.051_{\theta=0.65} + 0.501_{\theta=0.90}$, places most of the prior belief about the value of θ on the extremes, 0.10 and 0.90, with minimal prior belief placed on the value of 0.65. Thus, the Bayes procedure took the data provided by the experiment, and integrated it with the information provided in the prior. It was the prior information that forced the Bayes assessment to focus not on 0.65, but 0.90. This solution demonstrates the strong link that Bayesian analyses can forge between the prior information and the posterior distribution of θ.

As another illustration, suppose the prior distribution for θ from this example had placed equal weight on each of the three possible values for, θ i.e.,

$$\pi(\theta) = 0.3331_{\theta=0.10} + 0.3341_{\theta=0.65} + 0.3341_{\theta=0.90}. \qquad (4.14)$$

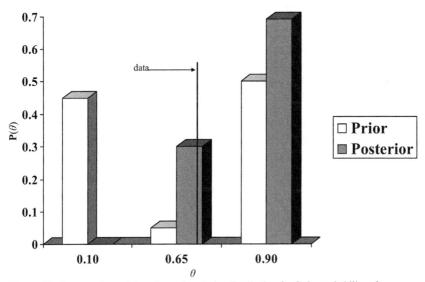

Figure 4.1. A comparison of the prior and posterior distribution for θ, the probability of adequate antiserum production from a collection of monkeys. Note that the prior distribution, in combination with the observed data, suggests a larger value of θ then the data do when considered alone.

This prior places no preference on each of the three candidate values of θ. Then, the posterior probabilities for the values of θ based on $x = 7$ can be computed from equation (4.13) for this new prior, showing $P[\theta = 0.10 \mid x = 7] = 0.000028$, $P[\theta = 0.65 \mid x = 7] = 0.815$, and $P[\theta = 0.90 \mid x = 7] = 0.185$. This set of posterior probabilities aligns nicely with the investigators first conclusion that the most likely value of θ is 0.65.

∎

This example reveals the power that the prior distribution can have on the Bayes process to shape the posterior distribution. While this embeds great flexibility in the Bayesian approach, it also requires investigators to carefully consider their prior distribution, since its use must be successfully defended to the medical and biostatistical communities. As we will see in Chapter Five, from the frequentist's perspective, the influence of the prior distribution is one of the greatest weaknesses of the Bayes perspective.

4.4. Working with Continuous Conditional Distributions

In this example of a Bayes procedure, we will use a continuous conditional distribution and a simple, dichotomous prior distribution. Again, the process is as before. Compute the joint distribution as the product of the conditional distribution and the prior distribution of the parameter, find the marginal distribution by compounding, and then carry out the division to find the posterior distribution of the parameter of interest.

Example 4.3: Astrocytomas

Primary brain cancers are called astrocytomas. These astrocytomas are graded from the mildest (stage 1) to the most dangerous (stage 4). Stage 4 astrocytomas, otherwise known as *gliobastoma multiforme*, are locally invasive, producing a rapidly deteriorating clinical course.

An investigator understands that the average survival time of a patient with gliobastoma multiforme is twenty weeks, and believes she has identified a therapy that will prolong this short survival time. She wishes to use a Bayes procedure to assist in the evaluation of her data.

This investigator denotes the time until death (in weeks) for her patients by t. She expects that this time follows an exponential distribution with parameter θ, i.e., $f(t) = \theta e^{-\theta t}$.[*] If her therapy has no effect, then she believes the value of $\theta = 0.05$. However, if the therapy is effective, the survival duration will be prolonged to 36 weeks, consistent with $\theta = 0.028$.[†] So she is interested in assessing the evidence based on the data from one patient for these two alternative values for θ. The investigator can do this through an evaluation of the posterior distribution of θ given the patient's survival time t.

Let's first solve this problem in general. The conditional distribution of t given θ is the exponential distribution, $f(t \mid \theta) = \theta e^{-\theta t}$. To construct the prior distribution, the investigator recognizes that the parameter θ can be one of only two

---

[*] This distribution was introduced and discussed in Chapter Two.
[†] Since the average value of t in weeks is θ^{-1}, the new estimate of θ is assumed to be $1/36 = 0.028$.

possible values. Let's identify them as θ_1 or θ_2. She lets $\theta = \theta_1$ with probability p, and $\theta = \theta_2$ with probability $1 - p$. Thus, in this general case, we write

$$\pi(\theta) = p\mathbf{1}_{\theta = \theta_1} + (1-p)\mathbf{1}_{\theta = \theta_2}. \tag{4.15}$$

We now have the ingredients we need to identify the posterior distribution of θ. Given the patient's survival time t, we wish to compute the posterior probability distribution of θ, $\pi(\theta \mid t)$.

Begin by using our general formula for computing the posterior distribution, i.e.,

$$\pi(\theta \mid t) = \frac{f(t \mid \theta)\pi(\theta)}{\sum_\theta f(t \mid \theta)\pi(\theta)}, \tag{4.16}$$

And substituting the probability distributions for this problem in involving brain cancer survival, we can write

$$\pi(\theta \mid t) = \frac{\theta e^{-\theta t}\left(p\mathbf{1}_{\theta=\theta_1} + (1-p)\mathbf{1}_{\theta=\theta_2}\right)}{\sum_\theta \theta e^{-\theta t}\left(p\mathbf{1}_{\theta=\theta_1} + (1-p)\mathbf{1}_{\theta=\theta_2}\right)}. \tag{4.17}$$

This is an easy posterior probability function to work with. Its denominator quickly simplifies to $p\theta_1 e^{-\theta_1 t} + (1-p)\theta_2 e^{-\theta_2 t}$, and the posterior distribution becomes

$$\pi(\theta \mid t) = \frac{\theta e^{-\theta t}\left(p\mathbf{1}_{\theta=\theta_1} + (1-p)\mathbf{1}_{\theta=\theta_2}\right)}{p\theta_1 e^{-\theta_1 t} + (1-p)\theta_2 e^{-\theta_2 t}}$$

$$= \frac{p\theta e^{-\theta t}\mathbf{1}_{\theta=\theta_1} + (1-p)\theta e^{-\theta t}\mathbf{1}_{\theta=\theta_2}}{p\theta_1 e^{-\theta_1 t} + (1-p)\theta_2 e^{-\theta_2 t}}.$$

The posterior probabilities for θ_1 and θ_2 are

$$P[\theta = \theta_1 \mid t] = \frac{p\theta_1 e^{-\theta_1 t}}{p\theta_1 e^{-\theta_1 t} + (1-p)\theta_2 e^{-\theta_2 t}}$$

$$\tag{4.18}$$

$$P[\theta = \theta_2 \mid t] = \frac{(1-p)\theta_2 e^{-\theta_2 t}}{p\theta_1 e^{-\theta_1 t} + (1-p)\theta_2 e^{-\theta_2 t}}.$$

With the general solution in hand, we can find the specific values of these probabilities based on the data of this problem. The two possible values of θ are $\theta_1 = $

0.05, and $\theta_2 = 0.028$, corresponding to a mean survival time of 20 weeks and 36 weeks, respectively. Let's also assume that $p = 0.50$, reflecting the investigator's lack of preference for either of these two prior values of θ. Equally weighting the candidate values of θ in the prior distribution is the hallmark of a *non-preferential prior distribution*. We will have much more to say about these in a later chapter.

Using these values, the posterior probability statements become

$$P[\theta = 0.05 \mid t] = \frac{(0.5)(0.05)e^{-0.05t}}{(0.5)(0.05)e^{-0.05t} + (0.5)(0.028)e^{-0.028t}}$$

(4.19)

$$P[\theta = 0.028 \mid t] = \frac{(0.5)(0.028)e^{-0.028t}}{(0.5)(0.05)e^{-0.05t} + (0.5)(0.028)e^{-0.028t}}.$$

Based on our understanding of this problem, we would expect that a shorter survival time favors the value of $\theta = 0.05$ as this value is associated with the shorted average survival time. The longer the patient's survival, the more support the data provides for the value of θ associated with longer survivals (Figure 4.2).

Figure 4.2 confirms our intuition. Confining our attention to the scenario for $p = 0.50$ (non-preferential), we see that as the survival time of patients increase, the probability that the average survival time is short (i.e., that $\theta = 0.05$) decreases. Also larger values of t also provide some support $\theta = 0.05$. Note that for a survival of sixty weeks, the posterior probability $P[\theta_1 = 0.05 \mid t = 60]$ remains above 0.20.

However, to the Bayesian, there is another important component of this problem — the value of p. The non-preferential solution reflected equal weight of evidence supporting the two candidate values of θ. However, what if the medical community was skeptical of claims that the average patient survival with glioblastoma multiforme was greater than twenty weeks? They might choose values of p as high as 0.75, or even 0.90, also reflected in Figure 4.2. In these cases, the posterior probability $P[\theta_1 = 0.05 \mid t]$ is larger for all survival times, requiring an extremely long survival time to overturn the conventional belief that $\theta = 0.05$.

This last paragraph is reminiscent of statistical hypothesis testing. However, there are important differences that emerge at once. In the standard frequentist approach, the investigator sets replaces her intuition that $\theta = 0.028$ with the "null" hypothesis that $\theta = 0.05$, i.e., the idea that they don't believe but must embrace for a time until they reject it. She then gathers data and asks how likely is the data, given the null hypothesis that $\theta = 0.05$. If the "data are not likely" she then rejects the null hypothesis.

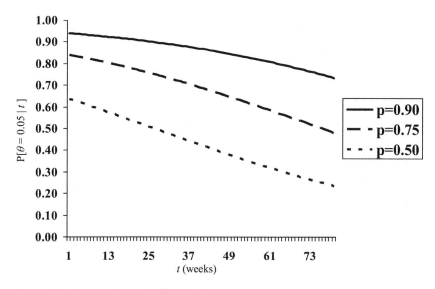

Figure 4.2. The posterior probability that the average survival is 20 weeks in patients with grade 4 astrocytoma as a function of survival time t, and the prior probability, p.

However, the Bayesian's reasoning is more direct. She believes that $\theta = 0.028$, and places some probability on this degree of belief. She then updates her assessment of the probability based on the data. For example, her prior belief may be $P[\theta = 0.028] = 0.10$. However, if she observes the patient has survived 40 weeks, her posterior assessment, using equation (4.19) is updated from 0.10 to $P[\theta = 0.028 \mid t = 40] = 0.870$, a substantial increase. ∎

4.5. Continuous Conditional and Prior Distributions

In this example, we extend our repertoire of computing posterior distributions by working with continuous prior and continuous normal distributions. The example demonstrates a popular illustration, further cementing the importance of this popular distribution, and introducing the concept of conjugate priors.

Example 4.4: Testing for Diabetes Mellitus

Diabetes mellitus is a disease of abnormal glucose metabolism, whose long-term consequences are heart attacks, strokes, kidney disease, blindness, and amputation. There are two forms of diabetes mellitus.[*] Type I, typically beginning in childhood is an uncommon autoimmune disease where the body's immune system attacks the insulin producing cells of the pancreas. Type II diabetes is a disease where the body

---

[*] Another form of diabetes is diabetes insipidus, which is an endocrine disorder that leads to electrolyte disorders.

is resistant to the insulin it produces, and both blood insulin levels and blood glucose levels are higher than normal. Associated with obesity, type II diabetes mellitus is increasing in prevalence; currently 21 million Americans are afflicted with the disorder.

A diabetologist is interested in assessing the insulin level of his patient, which in this case, typically hovers around 8 milli-international units per milliliter (mIU/ml). Levels greater than 13 are associated with insulin resistance. The diabetologist needs to know if his patient's insulin level is greater than 13 mIU/ml.

A sample of the patient's blood is drawn and sent to a local laboratory, known for its high standards. Rather than assess only the one sample, they divide the blood specimen into four aliquots, running the insulin assessment on each of these. They then return the average insulin level from these for aliquots to the physician. In this case, the lab results for the patient are 13.5 mIU/ml. What should this physician conclude?

Commonly, the physician will decide that the insulin level is now in the abnormal range, and then follow this assessment with a cascade of clinical judgments and recommendations. However, a Bayesian approach suggests a different decision process.

From the Bayesian perspective, the investigator is interested in an accurate depiction of the patient's insulin level, but he understands that there is more than one source of variability. The first of course is the variability of the lab measurement. Even though the process of taking a mean value of four measurements reduces the variability of the insulin assessment, this substantial variability remains. Let θ be the blood insulin level. Assume that it follows a normal distribution with mean μ and variance v^2. The laboratory attempts to assess θ through a collection of n measurements. We let $x_1, x_2, x_3,..., x_n$ be these n measurements of blood insulin levels. The diabetologist is interested in a measure of the location of θ. Specifically, he is interested in whether the patient's insulin level is greater than 13.

However, there is a second source of variability, the insulin level itself. This physician recognizes that his patient's insulin level is not a fixed constant, but is itself constantly varying due to changes in the patients glucose level, activity level, and extent of disease. Thus, the diabetologist must estimate a parameter that is constantly changing. In the absence of data, he would estimate the value of θ as μ. However, how can he combine this knowledge with the results of the laboratory test? A Bayesian might describe this problem as identifying the posterior distribution of θ given the data.

In the presence of n laboratory assessments, let's assume that x_i follows a normal distribution with mean θ and variance σ^2. We know that if $x_1, x_2, x_3,..., x_n$, which represent the results of each of the individual tests are independent and have the same normal distribution, then $\bar{x}_n = \dfrac{1}{n}\sum_{i=1}^{n} x_i$ is itself normally distribution with mean θ and variance σ^2/n. This is the conditional distribution of $\bar{x}_n$ given θ, or $f(\bar{x}_n | \theta)$. Thus, the answer to this physician's question resides in an examination of the posterior distribution of θ given $\bar{x}_n$ has been observed.

To compute the posterior distribution for θ, we proceed as before, writing

$$\pi\left(\theta \mid \overline{x}_n\right) = \frac{f\left(\overline{x}_n \mid \theta\right) \pi\left(\theta\right)}{\sum_{\theta} f\left(\overline{x}_n \mid \theta\right) \pi\left(\theta\right)}. \tag{4.20}$$

However, recall that we have already identified the denominator of the expression on the right side of equation (4.20); it is a normal distribution with mean μ and variance $\sigma^2/n + \upsilon^2$. It only remains to find the quotient of equation (4.20), a computation that is fully developed in Appendix I. These computations reveal that the posterior distribution is normal, with mean μ_p and variance v_p, where

$$u_p = \frac{\upsilon^2}{\upsilon^2 + \sigma^2} \overline{x}_n + \frac{\sigma^2}{\upsilon^2 + \sigma^2} \mu ;$$

$$\tag{4.21}$$

$$v_p^2 = \frac{\upsilon^2 \sigma^2}{\upsilon^2 + \sigma^2}.$$

In this case a "normal" prior, when combined with a "normal" conditional distribution, produces a "normal" posterior distribution. A distribution that simultaneously appears as the prior, conditional, and posterior distribution is known as a *conjugate family of distributions*. Though they have some weaknesses, conjugate distributions are commonly used because the results are easy to work with, and it is easy to compare the prior and posterior information.

In this particular example involving diabetes mellitus, a comparison of the means, variances of the prior, conditional and posterior distribution is illuminating (Table 4.1).

Table 4.1. Mean and variance of insulin levels in conjugate. normal Bayes computation

		Distribution	
	Prior	Conditional	Posterior
Mean	8.00	13.50	11.52
Sigma	1.00	0.75	0.60
Variance	1.00	0.56	0.36

The mean insulin level from the prior distribution is 8 mIU/ml, a level within the normal range of 0 to 13. The lab test reveals that the insulin level is abnormal. However, the mean of the posterior normal distribution is 11.52, still in the normal range (Figure 4.2)! Although the test result is positive, the mean of the posterior Bayes distribution remains below 13 mIU/ml (Figure 4.3).

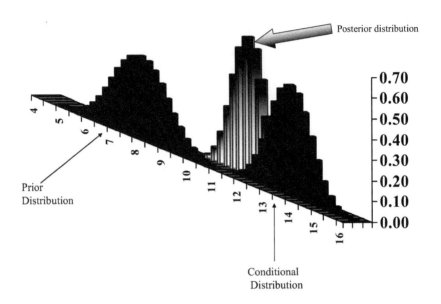

Posterior distribution

0.70
0.60
0.50
0.40
0.30
0.20
0.10
0.00

Prior
Distribution

Conditional
Distribution

Figure 4.3. Distribution of insulin levels in the conjugate normal setting.

Figure 4.3 provides the prior distribution of θ, the insulin level, the conditional distribution, and the posterior distribution. Note that the posterior distribution is centered between the prior and conditional distributions. The prior distribution of θ has exerted its influence on the location of the posterior distribution, pulling its mean into the range of normal insulin levels.

This influence is a direct consequence of equation (4.21), that demonstrates that the mean of the posterior distribution is a weighed average of the mean of the prior and conditional distributions. The weights are the variances. Thus, the relative magnitude of the prior and conditional distribution variances determine the location of the mean of the posterior distribution.

As an illustration of this effect, assume that the laboratory was less precise, and produced a larger variance. In this case, we would expect a smaller posterior mean, reflecting the heavier influence of the relatively more precise prior distribution of the mean insulin level (Table 4.2).

Table 4.2. Mean and variance of insulin levels in conjugate normal Bayes computation: Less precise lab data.

		Distribution	
	Prior	Conditional	Posterior
Mean	8.00	13.50	9.10
Sigma	1.00	2.00	0.89
Variance	1.00	4.00	0.80

Table 4.2 demonstrates the effect of increasing the variance of the conditional distribution on the posterior distribution mean and variance. The mean is now lower, closer to the mean of the prior distribution (Figure 4.4).

An examination of the distribution reveals the anticipated effect; the posterior distribution is closer to the prior distribution than that produced by the laboratory. The location of the posterior mean must be between the mean of the prior and the conditional distribution. It will be centered exactly between the two means when the variances are equal, i.e., when the prior information is as precise as the information provided by the data.

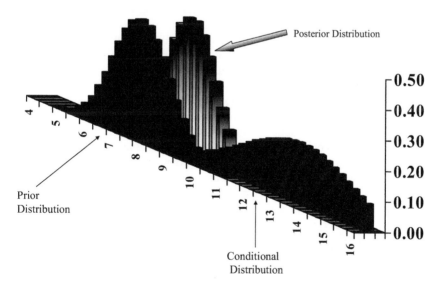

Figure 4.4. Distribution of insulin levels in the conjugate normal setting. The imprecision of the lab data has produced a conditional distribution with a larger variance, pushing the posterior distribution closer to the prior distribution.

■

Example 4.5: Clinical Trial Compliance

As a final example, consider the problem of estimating the degree to which patients take their assigned medicine in clinical trials, commonly known as patient compliance. The issue of compliance is critical. Several studies, e.g. the Lipid Research Clinics [1] designed to examine the effect of a medication on a clinically important intervention, have had that attempt undermined by the patients unwillingness to stay on their therapy for the duration of the study. Some of the reasons why patients may choose not to remain on study medication are undesirable side effects associated with the therapy, patient disenchantment with the study, and "pill-sharing," or the practice of a patient sharing their medication with their family members can decrease patient compliance with the study drug.

The vitiating impact of poor study compliance on a clinical research effort requires that the study investigators work to first attain and then maintain a high compliance level; this in turn requires that they have accurate measures of patient compliance. Taking pill counts (i.e., computing the proportion of pills not ingested when the patient returns to clinic with their bottle of unused medication) and direct patient interrogatories, while helpful, are not definitive.* Investigators are best informed about patient compliance by assessing measures that are objective, e.g., serum or urine levels that are directly impacted by the active agent.

Consider a clinical trial that will assess the effect of a compound designed to increase the level of high density lipoproteins (HDL) and thereby improve patient survival in patients at risk of having a heart attack. In this study, patients are randomly allocated to one of two treatment arms; active therapy or placebo therapy. All patients receive medication in the form of a pill to be taken once per day. Patients who are randomized to the control group will receive placebo therapy for their HDL levels. The levels of these patients are anticipated to remain the same, and they will therefore experience the population mortality rate. Patients who are randomized to the active therapy are expected to experience an increase in HDL levels which is believed will have a favorable effect on mortality.

The investigators believe that measuring the patients HDL levels would be the best measure of compliance in the study. In this example, the investigators focus on the compliance of patients in the active group. If these patients take their active medication, then the investigators anticipate in the first three months of the study these patients will experience an increase in their HDL levels by μ milligrams per deciliter (mg/dl), where μ is a known constant with a standard deviation of σ, also known. However, the effect that any given patient experiences is modulated by their compliance θ, which is unknown.

The investigators define compliance θ as the proportion of the assigned medication that a patient actually takes. Thus $0 \leq \theta \leq 1$, and the HDL increase that a given patient experiences with is $\theta\mu$. For example, if the investigators expect a 15 mg/dl increase in HDL levels if the patient is fully compliant, but the patient is

---

* For example, patients can discard unused medication, or, in an attempt to please their physician, simply not tell the truth about their pill taking behavior.

75% compliant with their therapy, then that patient will experience a $(0.75)(15$ mg/dl) = 11.25 mg/dl increase in HDL level.

The investigators' goal is to estimate the patient's compliance based on their change in HDL. Specifically, they wish to know whether the likelihood that a patient is compliant with therapy is less than 80%. These patients will be targeted for special attention by the investigations in an attempt to improve their compliance with therapy.

This question can be easily formulated from a Bayesian perspective. We will assume that a patient's compliance θ follows a uniform distribution on the [0,1] interval. Thus, in the absence of any information about the patient's change in HDL level, the investigator has no idea of what the patient's compliance level is. We say that $\pi(\theta) = 1_{\theta \in [0,1]}$.

Assume that the HDL increase that the patient experiences, x, when their compliance is known is normally distributed with mean $\mu\theta$, and variance σ^2. It remains for the investigators to identify the posterior distribution of θ given the value of their HDL increase. We write

$$\pi(\theta \mid x) = \frac{f(x \mid \theta)\pi(\theta)}{\sum_\theta f(x \mid \theta)\pi(\theta)} = \frac{\frac{1}{\sqrt{2\pi\sigma^2}} e^{-\frac{1}{2\sigma^2}(x-\mu\theta)^2} 1_{\theta \in [0,1]}}{\int_\theta \frac{1}{\sqrt{2\pi\sigma^2}} e^{-\frac{1}{2\sigma^2}(x-\mu\theta)^2} 1_{\theta \in [0,1]}}. \tag{4.22}$$

From Appendix J, this can be written as

$$\pi(\theta \mid x) = \frac{\frac{1}{\sqrt{2\pi\sigma^2}} e^{-\frac{1}{2\sigma^2}(x-\mu\theta)^2} 1_{\theta \in [0,1]}}{\frac{1}{\mu}\left[\Phi\left(\frac{\mu-x}{\sigma}\right) - \Phi\left(\frac{-x}{\sigma}\right) \right]} \tag{4.23}$$

where $\Phi(x)$ is the cumulative distribution function of the standard normal distribution function evaluated at x. The probability that a patient is noncompliant with the therapy based on the change in their HDL level is

$$P[0 \le \theta \le c] = \frac{\left[\Phi\left(\frac{c\mu-x}{\sigma}\right) - \Phi\left(\frac{-x}{\sigma}\right) \right]}{\left[\Phi\left(\frac{\mu-x}{\sigma}\right) - \Phi\left(\frac{-x}{\sigma}\right) \right]}. \tag{4.24}$$

We can easily evaluate expression (4.24). For $c = 0$, we expect $P[0 \le \theta \le c]$ to equal zero, which is what the formula confirms. For $c = 1$, $P[0 \le \theta \le c] = 1$, again confirming our intuition.

As an example of the use of formula (4.24), assume that the expected change in HDL levels in this study for patients in the active group is 5 mg/dl with a standard deviation of 2 mg/dl. The patient is observed to have a 3 mg/dl increase in HDL level. The investigators can compute the likelihood the patient was less than 80% compliant using formula (4.24)

$$P[0 \le \theta \le c] = \frac{\left[\Phi\left(\frac{c\mu - x}{\sigma} \right) - \Phi\left(\frac{-x}{\sigma} \right) \right]}{\left[\Phi\left(\frac{\mu - x}{\sigma} \right) - \Phi\left(\frac{-x}{\sigma} \right) \right]}:$$

$$P[0 \le \theta \le 0.80] = \frac{\left[\Phi\left(\frac{(0.80)(5.0) - 3.0}{2.0} \right) - \Phi\left(\frac{-3.0}{2.0} \right) \right]}{\left[\Phi\left(\frac{5.0 - 3.0}{2.0} \right) - \Phi\left(\frac{-3.0}{2.0} \right) \right]}$$

$$= \frac{\Phi(0.50) - \Phi(-1.50)}{\Phi(1) - \Phi(-1.50)} = \frac{0.691 - 0.067}{0.841 - 0.067} = 0.806,$$

revealing that this patient who has experienced only a 3 mg/dl increase in HDL has an 81% probability of being noncompliant with therapy. One can easily compute the relationship between the probability of noncompliance and the change in HDL (Figure 4.5).

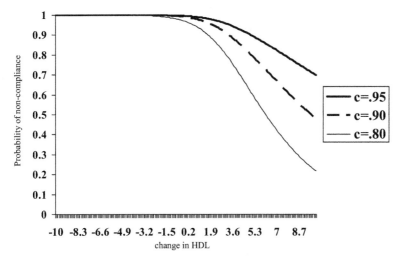

Figure 4.5. Probability that a patient's compliance is less than c as a function of the change in HDL level in six months; $\sigma = 2$ mg/dl.

Figure 4.5 reveals that for decrease or small increases in HDL, the probability of noncompliance is high. However, for further increases in HDL, the probability of noncompliance decreases. Figure 4.5 also demonstrates that if the definition of noncompliance increases to 90% or 95%, the likelihood of noncompliance also increases, an expected result since more stringent definitions of compliance require greater increases in HDL to meet the compliance definition.

However, the utility of this evaluation is sensitive to the value of σ, with larger values of the standard deviation increasing the likelihood of a noncompliance assessment (Figure 4.6). The increased variance in the HDL measurement leads the posterior distribution to require even larger increases in HDL levels before it reduces the likelihood that the patient is noncompliant.

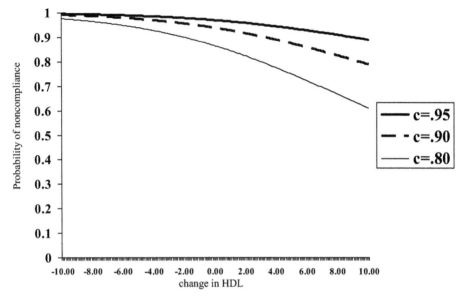

Figure 4.6. Probability that compliances is less than c as a function of the change in HDL level in six months; $\sigma = 5$ mg/dl.

■

This chapter has provided our first computations for posterior distributions. The process thus far has been straightforward, requiring a compounding procedure followed by a division. However, the implications of the result are critical for biostatistics, and are the subject of the next chapter.

Problems

1   A patient is taking two medications, an antihypertensive or an anti-inflammatory drug but refuses to take both each day, taking either one or the other on any particular day. Each has a similar spectrum of side effects. For the first medication (an antihypertensive) a patient has a 33% chance of having headaches, a 10% chance of having nausea, a 17% chance of dizziness, and a 40% chance of having no adverse effects at all. For the anti-inflammatory medication, the patient has a 30% chance of nausea, 30% chance of a headache, 10% chance of dizziness, and a 30% probability of no adverse effects. Since the patient is likely to have adverse effects with the antihypertensive agent, he takes it three out of four days randomly, taking the anti-inflammatory agent on one in four days. The patient calls the doctor's office, complaining of a headache. He can't remember which medication he took this morning.

        a.   Compute the posterior probability of medication type given the occurrence of adverse events.

       b.   What is the probability that it was the antihypertensive?

2   Rocky Mountain spotted fever and Tsutsugumushi's fever are both ill-nesses produced by ricketsia. Rocky Mountain spotted fever, produced by a bite from the tick *Dermasanter androsoni* begins with a rash that starts centrally and spreads locally, while the rash associated with Tsutsugu-mushi's fever (produced from a chigger bite) begins peripherally, and moves centrally. In the U.S., a patient is 100 times as likely to have Rocky Mountain spotted fever than Tsutsugumushi's fever, while in Japan, a pa-tient is 50 times more likely to have the latter rather than the former. The time to rash follows an exponential distribution in each case, with a mean time to fever of five days for Rocky Mountain spotted fever and twelve days for Tsutsugamchi's fever.

       a.   Compute the posterior distribution of the occurrence of the dis-ease (either Rocky Mountain spotted fever of Tsutsugamcuchi's fever) given the time of fever onset.

       b.   What is the probability that a patient located in China has Tsutsugumushi's fever given their fever occurs on day 8?

       c.   What is the probability that a patient located in the U.S. has Rocky Mountain spotted fever given the fever occurs on day 8?

3   Patients can have mid back or lower back injuries. Sixty percent of pa-tients who arrive at the clinic have low back injuries. Sixty percent of pa-tients with low back injuries have primary difficulty bending forward, while 30% have trouble with hyperextension of the back and 10% have primary difficulty bending from side to side. For patients with mid back injuries, 40% have difficulty bending from side to side, while 30% have difficulty with hyperextension, and 30% have difficulty bending over.

       a.   Find the posterior probability distribution of the location of back injury given the primary motion difficulty.

       b.   A patient arrives complaining of back pain. On exam she is found to have primary difficulty bending from side to side. What is the probability this patient has a mid back injury.

4   An emergency room physician would like to differentiate between the presentation of acute appendicitis versus ruptured ectopic pregnancy in young women by using the white blood cell count. He observes that in young women patients with acute appendicitis, the white count is normally distributed with mean 15,000 white blood cells per cubic centimeter (wbc cc^{-1}) and standard deviation of 3,500. However, in women with ectopic pregnancies, the mean wbc count is 18,000 wbc cc^{-1} and the standard de-viation is 2,000. In his community, women are two times as likely to pre-sent with a ruptured appendix than with an ectopic pregnancy.

       a.   Compute the posterior probability that a women has an ectopic pregnancy given her wbc count.

b. A young woman presents with a wbc count of 21,250. What is the probability that she has a ruptured ectopic pregnancy based solely on this information.

5   The common cold is currently affecting a local community. This season, there are two variants; an adenovirus, and a rhinovirus. The adenoviral infection is three times as common as that due to the rhinovirus. However, the symptom complexes are somewhat different. The adenovirus infection produces a fever that lasts no more than 48 hours, while the rhinovirus induced fever lasts no more than 72 hours. Assume that the fevers are uniformly distributed on these intervals. A patient has a fever lasting 48 hours.

a. Find the posterior distribution of the type of infection given the duration of the fever.

b. What is the probability that the patient has the rhinovirus infection?

6   *Klebsiella pneumonia* is a gram negative bacterium that commonly resides in the gastrointestinal tract. Although it is relatively harmless when confined to the large colon, Klebsiella can cause disease when introduced to other organ systems, most notably pneumonia. Affecting primarily people with underlying chronic disease with an immunosuppressive component e.g., alcoholism, cancer, or diabetes, the mortality rate from this infection is high. A laboratory works to isolate a particular strain of the *Klebsiella pneumonia*, by obtaining its velocity coefficient k, e.g., the constant that describes the rate of growth of the organism during its exponential phase $y_t = y_0 e^{kt}$, where if y_t is the number of organisms at time t. Let $\theta = 1, 2, 3, 4$, identify the strain of *Klebsiella*. The laboratory's history of identifying strains of this particular bacteria is well-known to its workers (Table 4.3). If the strain of the organism is known, then its velocity coefficient is normally distributed with a mean value as provided in Table 4.3 and variance of 3.

Table 4.3 Prior distribution of *Klebsiella pneumomia* presence.

θ	Strain	$P[\theta]$	Mean velocity coefficient
1	6557A	0.02	5
2	8704	0.46	7.5
3	6557C	0.24	2
4	6466D	0.28	8.9

For a particular infected patient, a specimen of *Klebsiella pneumonia* is obtained and its mean velocity coefficient is found to be 3.

    a.   Find the posterior probability of Klebsiella strain given the velocity coefficient.

    b.   What is the probability that this patient is infected with strain 6557C.

7   An automobile accident on a nearby superhighway brings four patients, one with blood type A, the other three with blood type B to the local emergency room. with severe blood loss. Quickly depleting its blood supplies, the hospital puts out a call to local citizens to donate blood. Local citizens are screened for each of the needed blood types. The probability of a match for type A is 0.10, while the probability of a match for the patients with type B is 0.20. One patient is needed to complete the match for each of the accident victims. Upon the eighth screened patient, the lab technicians shouts triumphantly, "We have completed the matches for one of the patients!"

    a.   Find the posterior distribution of the blood type given the number of screened patients to meet a patient's blood supply need.

    b.   What is the probability that match was for blood type A?

8   Patients with schizophrenia commonly complain of bizarre ideations (e.g., that they have new organs implanted by an intelligence agency); the frequency between these can be reduced with modern antipsychotic therapy. A patient is either taking no medications, one medication, or two medications to control these manifestations of their disease. The time to the next bizarre ideation follows a gamma distribution, where

$$f(t) = \frac{\alpha^r}{\Gamma(r)} t^{r-1} e^{-\alpha t}.$$

For this example, the psychiatrist estimates α by $\hat{\alpha}$, and r by $\hat{r}$, using $\hat{\alpha} = \frac{\bar{x}^2}{s^2}$, and $\hat{r} = \frac{\bar{x}}{s^2}$ where $\bar{x}$ and s^2 are the mean and variances of the time to bizarre ideations. If a patient is not taking his drug, then the mean time to bizarre ideation is 0.9 days with a variance of 1. If the patient is taking one of his medications, then the mean time to bizarre ideation is eight days with a standard deviation of four days. If the patient is taking both of his medications, then the mean time to bizarre ideation is 30 days with a standard deviation of 8 days. The likelihood that a patient is taking no medication is 0.25, taking one medication is 0.57, and taking both medications is 0.23.

    a.   Compute the posterior probability that a patient is taking one medication, given the time to bizarre ideation.

b. Given the patient did not experience a bizarre ideation for 17 days, compute the probability that the patient is not taking both of his medications.

9   There are two types of commonly occurring food poisoning in a community, one produced by *Staphylococcus aureus*, the second caused by *Clostridium perfringens*. Each infection generates intense diarrhea requiring fluid replacement. The time from food ingestion to the onset of symptoms follows a negative exponential distribution, with the mean time to *Staphylococcus aureus* induced symptoms being six hours, while the mean time to diarrhea induced by *Clostridium perfringens* is nine hours. In a community where the prevalence of *Staphylococcus*-induced food poisoning is five times that due to *Clostridium*, the members of a picnic group arrive at the emergency room each complaining of intense diarrhea beginning ten hours after the outdoor meal.

  c. What is the posterior distribution of the type of infection, given the duration of time between food ingestion and diarrhea?

  d. What is the probability that the picnic group is suffering from Clostridium induced disease?

10 After an intense urban flood during one of the hottest summers on record, several survivors experienced an acute illness beginning with painful muscles and joints, swelling and bleeding from the mouth and nose. Ten days later, many are dead. Investigation reveals that the cause is a viral agent that causes hemorrhagic fevers. There are two suspected viral agents, V_1 and V_2. The probability of death within ten days of the first symptoms from agent V_1 is 0.25. The probability of death within ten days of the appearance of symptoms following infection by the second virus is 0.95. Specialists believe that the less lethal V_1 is fifty times more likely than V_2 to be the cause of the illness. You contact a health care worker on the scene, who tells you that of 40 patients infected with the virus, 39 are dead within ten days of the infection.

  a. Compute the posterior probability distribution of the viral agent given the proportion of patients who have died with ten days of symptom onset.

  b. Compute the probability that the more lethal agent V_2 is the cause of this outbreak.

Reference

1. The LRC Investigators (1984). The lipid research clinics coronary primary prevention trial results. *Journal of the American Medical Association* **251**: 351–374.

5

When Worlds Collide

5.1 Introduction

One can fill volumes with the intellectual conflicts between Bayesians and frequentists. The prologue of this book provides a brief overview of these discussions, the referenced articles and textbooks describing the combative exchanges between each camp's zealots.

However, newcomers to Bayes procedures are easily disoriented by the traditional arguments posed by each camp. Several claims have been swept away by modern technology or ground down by recent experience. Other contentions have been offered from a general perspective, ignoring the unique position of biostatistics and its connection to clinical medicine. It is therefore difficult for a novice studying these historical tracts to identify the contemporary distinguishing features between the two camps.

Following the hypothetical example of Pratt [1], this chapter compares the frequentist and Bayesian perspectives using a fictitious conversation between a neurologist, a frequentist statistician, and a Bayesian. The interaction of these discussants delineates the modern fault lines between these two opposing camps.

She knew what was coming. Anxious to postpone the battle for just a moment longer, she stood quietly at the back of the audiorium, its empty seats soon to be filled with investigators. *Your investigators*, she thought. Allowing her eyes to follow the long, sloping aisle as it descended, she saw two men on the stage, caught in the bright light flooding down from the ceiling. Sighing, Celia Manseur, M.D., walked down toward the stage to join them.

Leon Thomas, tall and thin, wearing his trademark white vest sat comfortably on the edge of the table, one leg resting of the floor, the other swinging back and forth. Leaning his head with its full mane of gray hair back, he laughed gently at a comment made by his counterpart, Jeremy Stone. Standing several feet from Leon, Jeremy stood, feet spread apart, arms loosely crossed over his tieless shirt and blue blazer, shaking his head in amusement.

Having fun, are we boys? she thought. *We'll see how long that lasts.* "Sorry I'm late," she said, climbing the steps to the stage to join them. "Sounds like you're getting along just fine without me."

"Of course we are" Jeremy answered, ambling over to shake Celia's hand. "Especially when we're not discussing anything important."

"Nice to see you as always, Celia," Leon called from the other side of the table, "although I'm surprised that you wanted to get together just two hours before the steering committee meeting. You must have a million things to do before this first major planning session. What's this all about?"

"Right to the point as always, Leon. I wanted the three of us to meet because I received these two statistical analysis plans from each of you, and—"

"Is there anything wrong with them?" Jeremy interrupted.

"That's the problem," she replied, pulling them out of her valise, and tossing them onto the smooth table where they slid for a few feet before stopping. "I just don't know."

"I asked you both to submit reports laying out the design of this clinical trial and—"

"Please. Let's all sit down here," Leon said.

"Thanks. You know the importance of this study. It's the first major trial since the use of aspirin to study the effect of a new medication that we believe will actually prevent strokes."

"Yes," Jeremy said. "There are over 600,000 strokes in the United States each year alone. Dramatically reducing that burden has tremendous public health implications. But the intervention you'll be studying has serious adverse effects. The final risk-benefit assessment will be critical. Whatever the results, Celia, your study's impact will be profound."

"Well, I think my group did a decent job with the stat analysis component," Leon said. "It's a straightforward evaluation. The annual stroke event rate of patients in the control group of the study will be about 10%, producing a two-year cumulative event rate of 19%. Based on Celia's estimation," Leon continued, nodding to her, "the active therapy will produce a 20% reduction in the event rate. This means that patients who are randomized to the active group will have 80% of the strokes that will occur in the control group."

"Yes," Celia said. "You computed that the sample size for this study, assuming a two-side type I error rate of 0.05 and 90% power, would be 4,118 people. So, 2059 recruited to each of the study's two treatment arms and followed for two years is what you think we need to answer the scientific question."

"That's exactly right," Leon replied. "The analysis of the trial will be equally uncomplicated, following well-accepted procedures. I can't imagine what the problem is Celia. It's pretty straightforward."

"Yes, Leon, it's a well considered plan. Yet, Jeremy," she continued, nodding to the other statistician, "has another perspective."

"I understand what Leon has generated," Jeremy began." As always, it's well written, but in my view, it contains some cumbersome reasoning. Plus, it's more expensive than necessary. We can do just as good a study with fewer patients."

"Uh oh," Leon said, wrinkling his nose at a fictitious aroma. "Isn't that a Bayes scent I smell?"

"Sweet, isn't it."

"All kidding aside, Jeremy, these Bayes arguments, however fashionable, would just be a distraction from the results of a major clinical experiment. We want the point of the study to be the stroke results, not some new-fangled statistical analysis."

"Sure, Bayes procedures are innovative, but the approach isn't new." Jeremy got up and slowly walked around the table. "In fact, it's been available for longer than the frequentist 'hypothesis testing' point of view. The Bayesian perspective is clear and simple. Celia, as a scientist and practicing physician, you'll understand its basic appeal. We start with a scientific idea that you believe. In this case, it would be that this new method of stroke prevention reduces the stroke rate. You then collect relevant data, learning how the data influence your early belief. Your initial evaluation of the hypothesis' truth either increases or decreases based on the data. It's quite natural."

"Many good workers are skeptical of that approach, as you know, Jeremy."

"That's a real shame, Leon," Jeremy replied, stopping behind his friend, and putting his hands gently on Leon's shoulders, "because what I've described is the scientific method. Are you saying you and other frequentists have taken a stand against this fundamental principle?"

"OK, OK, Jeremy," Leon said, waving his hand and smiling in mock surrender. "Finish making your point."

"Bayes procedures parallel the scientific method nicely. As scientists, in fact, as humans, we formulate ideas. We believe things. Bayesians demand that we place prior probabilities on those beliefs. Those are what make up 'the prior'. The data that we subsequently collect update these prior probabilities."

"I follow that," Celia said, "but the scientific method has been around for four or five hundred years. If Bayes procedures follow it so closely, then why are they just coming onto the scene now?"

"They've been waiting for the right tools, Celia," Jeremy said, taking a seat across from the neurologist. "The Bayesian concept started in the eighteenth century. In fact, it was commonly used for over 130 years. However, the problems they tried to solve were too tough. Exceeded their computational ability. Sixty years ago, they were beyond anyone's ability to solve them. Modern day computing's changed that."

"Well, how complicated are they?"

"Not too bad, really. Complex enough to need a computer, but not so complex that we can't solve them. Celia, I freely admit that Bayesian computations can be complicated," Jeremy continued, holding his open hands out in front of him. "But complicated computations, in and of themselves, are no reason to avoid a solid approach to a hard problem. Frequentist calculations are also complex. You know what logistic regression is, right?"

"Yes," Celia responded.

"And you know how to interpret the regression coefficients, odds ratios, confidence intervals, p-values, all that stuff, right?"

"Sure. We commonly write papers using these measurements."

"Great. How do you compute the information matrix?"

"What?" she asked. "What kind of question is that? Why are you asking me?"

"I'm asking if you can carry out the necessary linear algebra to derive and compute Fisher's information matrix. After all, it's an important background calculation that must be completed to get the odds ratios and the other quantities you said you used. Can you fill in the elements of the information matrix?"

"Of course not. I don't need to do that to get my work done."

"Exactly my point, Celia. It's a background computation that's both necessary and complicated, but it's not one you yourself do. You merely interpret the end result, right? That's precisely how the Bayes background calculations work. You can't condemn Bayes work because it's complicated. We do a lot of complicated things in science. This is just one more."

"I get it."

"Jeremy," Leon interrupted. "You're completely missing the point. I'm not rejecting Bayes procedures merely because they're complicated. I reject them here because they're unfamiliar to the clinical community. They're alien. Foreign. No one knows how to react to them, or to interpret them. Frankly, I'm sorry to say, the medical community just doesn't trust them."

"I don't know about the medical community, but you sure don't. I'm not surprised. The way to gain trust is to start with simple problems, gain some insight from that initial work, and then use that insight to help solve more complicated problems."

"You mean," Leon asked, "we should get more experience. 'Learn as we go?'"

"Sums it up nicely."

"Well, you may be right, but this is neither the time nor the experiment for that We're getting ready to begin a huge project here, Jeremy. The sponsor's spending millions of dollars on this research product. We just can't hand that colossal investment of money, time, and resources over to an untested procedure, hoping to learn a little something about it. There's too much at stake for that."

"It's not untested, and in any event, if we follow your proposal, we are handing the same resources to a poorly formulated concept."

"How so?"

"Bear with me." Turning to Celia, Jeremy asked, "Before you could get funding for this trial we're here to discuss today, there was a phase II clinical trial that was carried out first, right?"

"Sure. We executed a much smaller study in the same types of patients we plan to evaluate in this larger study." *Finally,* she thought to herself. *Here's a question that I know how to answer*

"What was the effect size?"

"It showed an 18% reduction in strokes."

"Was it positive?"

"We got a good result — 'p' of 0.16."

"Ah ... reporting study results as p-values. I guess we can thank Leon and his frequentist friends for that. OK. Oh point one six. That's greater than 0.05, right?"

"Yesssss...," Celia replied, letting her voice trail off.

"So the study was negative, right?

"No. You can't say that. It was a pilot study. I— "

"But the p-value was greater than 0.05, and it had to be less than 0.05 to be positive.

"Yes, but it wasn't powered—"

"Well, how could you design a huge, expensive phase III study on the foundation of a negative phase II result?"

"Because we didn't expect the p-value to be less than 0.05, Jeremy. Like I said, the phase II study wasn't powered for efficacy."

"Then why not skip all of the mumbo-jumbo about 'p less than 0.05' if you didn't really expect it? Just say in the beginning of the Phase II trial that you expect the effect size to be about 15−20% and the p-value between 0.10 and 0.30."

"I … I don't know. And I have to say, I've wondered that myself."

"I'm pushing you to make a point," Jeremy replied, smiling gently. "Leon told us Bayesian ideas were alien. I'm simply saying that frequentist ideas, while familiar, make no sense. It seems silly to have an unrealistic expectation from a Phase II study. Why expect it to be positive at the 0.05 level when you know that's pretty near impossible. All that happens is that in the end, you backtrack to a more appropriate argument when you see the data, right? Why not design the study more reasonably to begin with?"

"The answer is that you are stuck with the frequentist traditional interpretation of p-values," Jeremy continued. "The medical community has accepted the false message that 'p-values had better be less than 0.05 before the study is considered positive.' As you pointed out, the p-value paradigm didn't make any sense for you in your phase II study. But you were compelled to use it anyway. One of my colleagues says, next to nuclear weapons, p-values are the worst invention of the 20th century.

"Fortunately," Jeremy concluded, "you chose to interpret your phase II effort reasonably. Bayesians want more reasonable designs as well. We don't have p-values."

"Well," Celia asked, "what do you use in their place?"

"Posterior probabilities. These probabilities are the result of updating prior probabilities with relevant data."

"A process that is no better than the prior probabilities on which they are based, Celia," Leon inserted. "Don't be fooled. When Jeremy describes this prior probability, what he's really saying is 'guesswork.' Can I get a word or two in here please?"

"Sure."

"So," Leon said, "this posterior distribution is based on prior information, right? Tell me, Jeremy, what prior information would you use for this stroke study?"

"We have some useful preliminary stroke rate estimates for both the control and the treatment group."

"Great. What probability will you place on this 'information'?"

"That depends on how strongly the neurologists believe the information."

"Believe? You're allowing their belief in the therapy to affect the study's results? You have to be kidding. Don't they know?"

"No," Jeremy replied. "We have to choose a prior probability, based on what the literature says, how the community perceives the effect, how the investigators react to different effect sizes —"

"Oh I get it – you guess"

"An educated guess."

"But a guess nevertheless. And, since the posterior distribution is based on the prior distribution, then guessing wrong about the prior means the posterior distribution will also be wrong. That's true too isn't it?

"Yes, Leon, that's a possibility, but you frequentists run the same risk."

"Not by guessing about a prior or posterior distribution"

"I disagree," Jeremy replied. "Say that you're designing a clinical trial. How do you choose the effect size? From prior information. The same as we Bayesians do. And what happens if you get it wrong? Suppose that you design a clinical trial to detect a 60 percent reduction in the control group event rate. Now you don't really know that the effect size will be 60 percent. You just 'arrive' at it, using it to compute the required sample size.

"Now," Jeremy continued, "suppose when you carry out the study, you don't find a 60 percent reduction, but instead, discover a much more modest effect size — say, 30 percent. Because you 'guessed wrong' about the effect size, the observed 30 percent reduction is not large enough to fall into the critical region, but it's nevertheless clinically significant. So, while the clinical investigators believe the discovered effect size is clinically relevant, the 30 percent reduction is not statistically significant. Your wrong 'guess' about the effect size has ruined the chance of the study to show that a clinically significant effect is actually statistically significant. Frequentists can make good or bad initial estimates, just like Bayesians."

"First of all, Jeremy," Leon responded, "the effect size chosen would have been based on the minimal clinical difference, not guesswork, second—"

"It's still an estimate that you make in the absence of firm knowledge."

"Well," Leon asked, "if we frequentists are not so different than you Bayesians, then why do you reject the entire frequentist argument out of hand?"

"Because frequentists act like they actually know the values of control group event rates and effect sizes when they don't. They therefore confuse investigators, regulators, and certainly the medical community."

"Well, what prior probability would you put on these effect size 'guesses' of yours, Jeremy?" Leon inquired.

"We would choose a reasonable value."

"And that value is?"

"In this problem, since the neurologists are quite uncertain about the effect size, we would use a non-preferential prior."

"Whoa" Celia exclaimed. "What's that?"

"It's a distribution that does not put more weight on one prior estimate than another. All prior estimates of the effect size are treated the same. So, there's no preference."

"Ah yes," Leon replied with a huge smile. "This is the part I love Bayesians argue about the important contribution of choosing a prior distribution. They tell us how 'flexible' it makes their approach to the problem. How 'adaptable' the procedures are. How 'honest' the process is But, when their time comes, and they are asked to commit, Bayesians, throw all of that flexibility and adaptability right out the window by choosing a non-preferential prior. Kind of like prior *non*-information. It's really laughable."

"Unlike frequentists, a Bayesian doesn't pretend to have information when no information is available," Jeremy responded. "All I'm saying is that some problems have more prior information than others. When we have it, we utilize it with an appropriately weighted prior. When we don't, then we don't and we use a non-preferential prior. The point is, Leon, one doesn't have to retreat to the frequentist approach just because of the absence of prior information. The Bayesian procedures are useful when prior information is either plentiful or absent."

"Weighted?" Leon asked. "Well, when you have prior information, how exactly do you decide what weight to place on it?

"The weights are based on the beliefs of the neurologists."

"What you really mean is that, you assign probabilities, right?"

"Yes, we listen to the clinicians, study the literature, speak to the experts in the field, and then attach a probability."

"So, you make it up."

"It's based on the relative strengths of the beliefs of the scientists."

"Like I said, Jeremy — you make it up. That's a critical difference between you and me. You're content to make the probability up. I need to measure it. To me, probability is corporeal, while to the Bayesian, it's ethereal."

"I'm not following this," Celia said.

"To me, probability is concrete, Celia. Here's an example. You give a coin to a Bayesian and ask, 'Is the coin fair?' He replies, 'What do *you* think?' and then makes up a probability based on your belief. He then flips the coin 100 times and combines the result with your assessment. That's not what I do."

"What do you do?"

"I simply snatch the coin from you and flip it The only information I need is the result of the tosses. Jeremy needs your subjective assessment, your beliefs and your feelings about the coin. Your feelings are between you and him. If you want an answer, just give me the coin, let me toss it, and I'll tell you"

"And, Leon, if every toss cost you a $1,000, you would be foolish not to use prior information to help reduce the number of tosses," Jeremy interjected.

Probability makes its greatest contribution when anchored to reality, Celia," Leon responded.

"Yes," Jeremy replied, "but the perception of reality is subjective—"

"Oh no you don't, Jeremy," Leon answered. This is not a philosophy class. Here's the difficulty. Celia, right now you are in the midst of designing a large clinical trial that will study thousands of patients. You will direct the expenditure of hundreds of thousands of man hours of effort, and millions of dollars, to do what? Evaluate the effectiveness of a new stroke therapy, or to put a new statistical procedure based on a belief system to the test?"

"And with that argument as a drumbeat," Jeremy interrupted, "clinical trial methodology marches backwards. Leon, the entire concept of randomization was new 70 years ago. Innovative. Threatening to the status quo. However, because it was well considered and used cautiously, the use of randomization in clinical trials has risen to the pinnacle in clinical research methodology. In fact, randomization helped to define the clinical trial. Wasn't that a chance worth taking? Or do you disagree with any innovation?"

"Yes, it was," the frequentist conceded. "However, it developed slowly over time, allowing investigators and regulators to become familiar with it."

"A process which precisely describes the evolution of Bayes procedures," Jeremy interjected. "They have been studied for decades. With each passing year, workers become more comfortable with them, computing tools advance, and the correct use of prior information improves."

"But your reliance on prior information is a critical weakness in clinical trials," Leon replied. "The frequentist approach, the perspective that accepts probability only as relative frequency, is comprehensible, well established, and works. Even Bradford Hill, who was a premier epidemiologist and very skeptical of the frequentist approach to statistics, did not argue for the Bayes approach. This eloquent scientist, who convinced skeptical doctors to accept the concept of randomization and the use of blinding in clinical studies, knew better than to get them involved in Bayes procedures. And—"

"If memory serves, he didn't argue for your *p*-values either."

"And it's no surprise why," Leon continued, focusing again on Celia. "Bayesian procedures are too subjective. They deliberately mix subjective, sometimes even capricious, shifting impressions with objective data. Constructing a clinical trial using Bayes procedures is like building a mansion on sand. It won't take long before the entire edifice, no matter how elegant, crumbles. Clinical trials must be evidence-based, Celia. That's what the frequentist requires. We take one fact-based step at a time. We don't even let you start with what you believe. You must start with what you don't believe.

"We insist," Leon continued, "that you begin with what is established, not what you want, or hope, or dream will be true. You start with what is accepted, because that is the closest community approximation to the truth. That's the null hypothesis. In order to take the next step forward, you must build a fact-based case. We require that the scientist affirmatively and clearly disprove the current community standard. When you have rejected this standard, you have set a new standard. The next scientist cannot just assume what he or she believes is true, they must prove that the new standard that you helped to create is wrong."

"Setting my other concerns aside for the moment," Jeremy interjected, "what you have described is a wasteful process if there is good prior information that you ignore."

"Well, Jeremy, if there's that much prior information that informs the process so completely, then why bother with the experiment at all? But, of course we all know the sad answer to that question don't we? We execute the experiment because there really isn't good prior information. There is only prior belief. Bayesians embrace these soft prior beliefs while frequentists reject them. Frequentists in biostatistics understand the many blind alleys false prior beliefs lead to.

"My goodness, Celia," Leon said, leaning across the table to engage the neurologist, "look at how many times prior beliefs have been wrong in the past. Did you know that, for 1500 years, physicians believed that the presence of pus in a wound was a good sign? They carried out medical procedures that would increase the likelihood that pus would be generated. Why? Because their belief was based on an erroneous statement in an early Roman medical text."

"People weren't doing any real evaluations of what they did then," Celia said.

"And what would Bayesians have done in a clinical trial designed to test whether producing pus was good?" Leon speculated, leaning back in his chair. "They would have searched the literature to gauge current opinion, eh Jeremy? They would have spoken to experts and learned that the overwhelming consensus of opinion was that pus was beneficial, right? These strong but false beliefs about the benefit of pus would have been the foundation of their prior 'information' that would have been built into the research effort, making it even tougher to demonstrate the worthlessness of pus-producing therapies."

"And, Leon, your null hypothesis would have been that pus was good as well, right?" Jeremy inquired. "After all, that idea was the state of the science at the time, and the null hypothesis assumes the state of the science is true."

"You've hit the nail right on the head, Jeremy. That would most definitely have been our null hypothesis. But the final mathematical formula we frequentists use to estimate the effect size of the therapy would *not* have included that belief. The effect size estimate would be based on only the data. The data would speak for itself, and not be muzzled by the misleading prior information."

"Well, I guess that's a fine history lesson," Celia said, checking her watch, "but we need to get back to the issue at hand."

"My point is simply this," Leon asserted. "The time-tested frequentist approach makes you uncomfortable as a physician precisely because it does an admirable job of protecting you from your weakness, Celia."

"Oh really? And exactly what weakness is that?"

"Your need to believe that the therapy you are studying is going to work"

"I don't see how in the world you can think that's a weakness," Celia said.

"I in no way mean to offend you. You are a dedicated scientist. If you weren't I wouldn't work with you. Clearly you are a devoted physician and specialist, but you are also human. You care about the patients that you see, with a compassion that is uniquely yours and amplified by the oath you took. As a neurologist, you know what strokes can do to people — you see the ravaging effects of this disease every day. The early deaths. Its crippling effects in survivors. Strong people reduced to helplessness. Dynamic personalities enfeebled. You're part of that, Celia. You work with it day after day, and you want to do something about it. You just don't look for a cure, you ache for one I'm not criticizing you for this. We nonphysicians rely on your drive to make anything and everything to improve our lives. I don't fault you for it. In fact, I honor you.

"So," Leon continued, "when you as an investigator learn of a potential new treatment that promises safe, effective prevention of strokes, you can't help but give it the benefit of the doubt because you've seen so much pain and suffering produced by the current, inadequate standard of care. It's only human to believe the new therapy can make a difference. But, unfortunately, this human feeling can be misleading."

"That's the practice of medicine," Celia said.

"Now, look what the research process does to your belief, Celia. As a clinical scientist, you want to work with this potentially new therapy, study its potential, and hopefully develop it into a useful tool in the war against strokes. But first you must build support for this new therapy, convincing others that your therapy is useful. So you speak with other investigators about this therapy, email them, meet with them, debate and argue with them, eventually persuading several that what is now known as 'your approach' is a promising one. You defend your point of view with conviction. You must persuade other believers with different beliefs. How can you possibly get them to align with you without first being a believer yourself? You must believe in the therapy you advocate.

"And when you have persuaded your team of researchers, you must begin a quest for funding. You go to private companies, philanthropic organizations, granting agencies. Each of these funding sources is deluged with other ideas, protocols and requests such as yours. They want their resources to have the greatest effect, to do the most good. So, everything else being equal, who are they going to fund, investigators who fervently believe in an idea, or scientists who blandly state 'we don't really know what the result will be, so we want to simply make an objective assessment'?

"Look at your situation now, Celia. In about forty minutes you're going to present this protocol to a room full of investigators and nurses who want to prevent strokes. They are connected to each other and to you by the conviction that this intervention has a good chance of preventing strokes. You are believers in this therapy."

"And exactly what's the problem with that?" Jeremy asked.

"The problem is that, while in the beginning you may have been objective, the nature of the process converts you to a true believer by the time you get to actually carrying out the science. Remember that fervent, well-intentioned beliefs are commonly wrong in medicine. The role of the frequentist statistician, Celia, is to protect you from your strong convictions about the effects of an untested therapy. Since you don't know if your belief is right or wrong, why rely on it in a study designed to test it?"

"I can't speak about other fields," Leon added, "but in medicine, subjective probability is just allowing nonevidence based opinions, which can no longer get in the front door, to sneak in the back one. And you don't have to look far to find clinical trial examples that have overturned commonly held 'beliefs.' The CAST investigators didn't see how the use of new antiarrhythmic therapy could make people with dangerous heart rhythms worse. But that's exactly what the medicines did. All of the prior information suggested these medicines would save lives. Yet, the medicines killed people.

"Many surgeons believed osteoarthritic knees would benefit from a procedure that cleaned out the joint space of its loose, dysfunctional cartilage remnants. The prior information said this would be the most beneficial. It wasn't."

"Well, we have to have beliefs in the practice of medicine, Leon," Celia said.

"Why?"

"Because without them, we would be indecisive. How could we advocate therapy to patients if we didn't?"

"And that's the trap," Leon replied. "Your beliefs and 'priors' get you clinicians into trouble because you can't separate out the good ones from the bad ones. You don't have prior information, you have prior suspicions."

"Bayesians say that you should accept these prior suspicions, allowing them to alter the result. Frequentists say 'Prove it' To frequentists there is no middle ground. You either know something or you don't"

"No pale pastels, eh, Leon?" Jeremy inserted. "I understand your enthusiasm for frequentist-based clinical trials, but keep in mind that the very trials you just described were the ones that produced the misleading results. In fact, they do it so often that some divisions of the FDA require two well-designed and well-conducted clinical trials to show that an intervention is effective. Not one, but two."

"That's right, Jeremy," Leon responded instantly. "So why make the situation worse, by weakening the clinical trial corpus with a Bayes injection?"

"Because, we don't have the luxury of your presumption. There is always middle ground. The time for your simplistic approach to prior information is over. It served a useful role for a short time, but now, its over. It's time for it to leave the stage."

"Speaking of leaving the stage, Celia" Leon said, "how much more time do we have?"

"The meeting starts in a half hour," Celia replied, checking her watch. "We have some time left."

"Clinical investigation," Jeremy began, "was a mess in the 1930s and 40s. Articles contained 10% data, 90% belief. The new introduction of frequentist-based statistical analyses changed that, by providing a clear, solid structure to the design and analysis of clinical research. It was the right thing at the right time. But now," Jeremy continued, "its time is over. Leon, frequentists have done a good service for the medical community for several decades. A very short time in the history of science, but it was an important contribution nevertheless. Things were out of balance, and your presence helped to balance them. Frequentists reacted understandably to the bad use of prior information sixty years ago. That was a good lesson to learn."

"Well," Leon said "at least we can agree on something today. I thought you were going to say that we learned the wrong lesson from this experience."

"No. You learned the right lesson too well. You say the medical community hasn't grown up, Leon. You'd better take another look around. It's a whole new set of numbers This community whose insight you disparaged has pioneered some remarkable research."

"With clear catastrophes."

"Catastrophes that we have learned from. Just like catastrophes in economics, in space travel, in meteorological prediction. Yet despite the setbacks — setbacks that, by the way, occurred on the frequentists' watch — we have advanced. Many sophisticated clinical investigations that are under way now were beyond the wildest dreams of the established clinical scientists 60 years ago. We now carry out multi-armed clinical trials. Merged phase II / phase III clinical trials. Trials with complex statistical monitoring rules. Trials within trials, that include prospectively declared, adequately powered subgroup analyses.

"Yet despite these advances in methodology and philosophy, Leon, you would deny clinical investigators the right to take the next step they have earned. You're like an overprotective parent, who won't let his or her son move from the children's clothing section up to the young men's section, because you're comfortable with where they are and don't want to run the risk of change. Well Leon, like it or not, change is here. You can play an important role in this evolution of thought, smoothing the transition, but, whether you're active or not, the transformation is under way. The time is now."

"Using untested prior information to fuel future studies is a destructive force, Jeremy"

"Just because bad automobile drivers cause accidents doesn't stop you from driving, Leon. Just where would science be if it followed your philosophy of 'once bad — always bad.' Should innovative surgeons choose not to inform the community of new procedures just because they fear the presence of a few inferior surgeons will harm patients with this new tool? Should Celia cease her investigation because she knows some doctor at some point will misuse it? Leon, if it would have been left to you, the modern world would have given up on the idea of flight because they knew at some point that an airplane would eventually crash. You argue that we shouldn't grow because growth is dangerous. But, we have to grow anyway. The use of prior information can be watched, monitored, and controlled. We need flexibility in its use. Bayesians provide that flexibility."

"So do frequentists," Leon responded.

"Really? You mean, like the 'flexibility' that says a p-value must be less than 0.05 in all research endeavors? Here we are, 80 years later, still trying to dig out from the results of Fisher's manure experiment."

"I don't understand," Celia interjected. "Manure experiment?"

"Yes, the father of frequentist statistics carried out an agricultural experiment evaluating the effects of manure. The 0.05 level came from that."

Celia shook her head in amazement.

"Leon and his frequentist friends foisted Fisher's 0.05 proclamation on us all," Jeremy continued. "They watched it happen. Heavens They helped it happen, by writing manuscripts that showed investigators how to carry out procedures that would lower the p-value, rather than how to carry out better investigation."

"Listen— " Leon responded.

Jeremy held his hand up. "I don't want to fight. I'm just acknowledging as I'm sure that you would, that the p-value selection of 0.05 was never meant to be rooted in stone. We are stuck with oh-five not because of frequentist flexibility but because of your hyper-rigidity. Many frequentists contend that this criterion should be thoughtfully reconsidered. And you are right to do so. But it requires good, clear, prospective thinking, and that's what Bayesians argue for," Jeremy continued. "Sadly, disciplined thought will be rejected by bad researchers. They will always be with us. But nevertheless the field of clinical investigation must advance. With self-control and with clear thought, but it must make progress. The technology is here, and the research community is ready. So, what are you waiting for?"

"Celia," Leon responded, "the clinical community is not ready for these hypermodern arguments. We're not just talking about mathematics here; we're talking about the fate of patients at risk of having strokes. Keep in mind that Bayes procedures have been around for 200 years. They never got much traction. They are untested assessments — runaway mathematics. Even though your clinical therapy payload may be valuable, the Bayes engine is not for you. It'll never get off the ground in medicine.

"Think very, very carefully before you take the fateful Bayes step, Celia," Leon continued. "It will attract criticism like large magnets attract iron bars. The issue won't be the effects of your treatment — it will be the mathematics that you used to measure your therapy's effects. The only way your treatment will be accepted as beneficial is if its benefit is confirmed by a time tested, accepted, standard, frequentist procedure, a confirmation procedure that will add weeks to the study and thousands of dollars to the overall bill. And, heaven help you if the Bayesian result is in one direction, and the frequentist evaluation in the other Your study will die a futile, suffocating death in the quicksand of controversy.

"Well, Celia?" Leon inquired. "Do you want to be an established neurologist, or a renegade?"

"What he's really asking," Jeremy said, "is do you want to be handcuffed to the past, or use modern tools that provide the flexibility you need. Sure, we use prior information. When it's solid, we incorporate it. We'd be silly not to use reliable information when it's readily available. However, it's the Bayesian who makes decisions based on the observed data. I bet you never heard of the likelihood principle, Celia?"

"One more new thing this morning, I guess."

"The likelihood principle states that only relevant data useful to answering your scientific question is the data that's been collected. Other observations that have not been observed are irrelevant. Does that make sense to you?"

"Yes," Celia responded. "Seems like it's hardly worth bothering about. Why draw conclusions from data you don't have?"

"Actually. It's kind of self-evident, isn't it. Why make a decision based on data you didn't observe? You don't buy a car based on cars that you didn't examine. You don't choose a job based on jobs you don't apply for, or never heard of, so why make decisions based on data that we didn't observe?"

"Seems silly to do that."

"Well, don't just tell me," Jeremy said. "Tell my friend, Leon. That's what he does. Frequentists violate this principle all the time."

"How does statistics do that?" the neurologist answered.

Taking his glasses off to clean them, Jeremy began. "Frequentist significance testing, is based on the rejection or acceptance of the null hypo—"

"You mean rejection or nonrejection of the null hypothesis, don't you?" Leon interrupted.

"Listen to him, Celia. Do you honestly want to turn your clinical experiment over to this kind of statistical double talk?"

She merely shrugged her shoulders.

"It used to be that you didn't have a choice. Now, you do. Anyway, according to the frequentist, you don't accept the null — you just can't reject it. That kind of syntax may make sense to a frequentist, but it hasn't, doesn't, and won't make sense to the practicing community. Research is difficult enough without having to jump through the semantic hoops the frequentists have created. Working with the frequentist perspective is like bumbling through a hall of mirrors. One positive result is a type I error, but another's not — that one's real. Another result appears to be negative, but they say 'No, it's not really negative — it's simply a type II error.' They have created a confusing maze based on reverse thinking. It's time the research community left the amusement park."

"You mean, left the frying pan, and leaped into the fire, don't you" Leon added.

"No, but I need to get back to the likelihood principle. To the frequentist, the same data, using different underlying distributions, can produce different results. That's a violation of the likelihood principle. Here's an example. Let's say you measure blood pressure with a digital meter. Make sense to use a normal distribution for these pressures?"

"I guess so," Celia responded.

"That's not a trick question, Celia. Tricks live in Leon's bag, not mine. Using an electronic meter, you compute the DBP's of all of your patients. Each patient has a diastolic blood pressure less than 100, and you easily calculate the mean of these pressures. Later, you learn that the meter you used to measure DBP wouldn't work if the DBP was greater than 100. Does that fact change how you compute the mean?"

"No," Celia answered.

"Why not?" Jeremy asked.

"Well, because no blood pressures occurred in the range where the meter was broken."

"It would change Leon's calculation. He'd say you couldn't use a normal distribution; you'd have to truncate it."

"Even though the DBPs were never in the range where the meter was broken? You can't be serious, Leon" Celia asked.

Nodding, Leon responded, "Jeremy's absolutely right. That's exactly what I'd do."

"Well, let's all be very sure to understand what we just heard. The distribution that Leon would use to describe your data was selected not by the data, but by the process that produced the data. Data that you didn't observe affected the distribution Leon was going to use. This, Celia, is a clear violation of the likelihood principle. Do you want to commit your multimillion dollar trial to that kind of philosophy?"

"Jeremy. It amazes me how you continue to miss this fundamental point. We are interested in generalizing results. If Celia only cared about the blood pressures of the people whose DBP she took, then of course she would be right to ignore the defect in the meter. However, in statistics we focus on the thousands, or tens of thousands, or millions of patients whose DBP we did not measure. We want to generalize. And in that larger group will be found subjects with DBPs greater than 100. That's why the distribution must be truncated."

"So, both approaches are reasonable—"

"Depending on the point of the exercise, Celia. It is the goal of the study that begets the methodology, and the methodology, not the data, determine the analysis plan. Sure we have rules that we go by. Clinical investigation would be lost without them. We rely on them, and so do you, Celia. What you just heard from Jeremy is exactly why you shouldn't use the procedures he advocates. He has, in one fell swoop, just abandoned the two-tailed test."

"What?" Celia asked. "How'd he do that?"

"Two-tailed testing ensures that there is adequate protection for the finding that a therapeutic intervention may produce harm," Leon explained. "At the beginning of the study, the investigator creates a critical region so that the null hypothesis is rejected for hazard as well as for benefit. Commonly, this means dividing the type I error in two, placing half in the hazard side of the distribution and half on the benefit side. However, at the study's conclusion, the test statistic can only fall on one side of the distribution — it can't be in both. Doctors commonly look at this and ask 'Why, when we now know what side of the distribution the test statistic is on, must we bother with the type I error allocated in the other tail?' But statisticians have successfully argued that since they said prospectively that they would divide the type I error in two, investigators should follow through on their original plan. Bayesians argue that since the data do not identify harm, than regardless of what you determined up front, you can put all of your type I error on the benefit side."

"Right" Jeremy said. "Even when the investigation is over, and the test statistic falls clearly in the benefit side revealing that no harm has been done, you frequentist still argue that, since you were concerned about harm in the beginning, you must be concerned about harm in the end, even though there was no evidence of harm. You're shackled by a well meaning, but false *a priori* belief, Leon. If *that's* not being misled by *a priori* belief, than nothing is

"But actually," Jeremy added, smiling at his friend, "we don't have type I error in the Bayesian paradigm, right? All we have is the likelihood that the scientific hypothesis is true. The conclusions are much easier to understand. The intervening computations can be more complex, I admit, but the conclusions make more sense."

"We'd better sum this up now," Celia responded, noting that investigators were beginning to file into the auditorium. "Leon?"

"Sure. Doctors have reported on the treatments they have used for hundreds of years. Many of those assessments are worthless because they were degraded by either poor observation or built-in biases. For centuries, it was anathema for physicians to test some of their own most valued treatments. That's why Celia's predecessors bled patients for so long. And, when they did try to collect data, they didn't understand how their point of view affected the results of their work.

"When clinical trials appeared in England in the 1940s, clinicians were this methodology's strongest opponents. Many doctors hated the idea of blinding, and rejected the concept of randomization. It's not hard to understand why. Who among us would want their loved ones to have their treatment option selected by a doctor flipping a coin? I know that's simplistic, but that's the view they took.

"Clinical trials have transformed clinical investigation from the subjective to the objective. While the technology has advanced, the thinking of medical researchers has *evolved*. They understand the importance of objective measures. When they use therapy based on belief and not objective data, disaster strikes, e.g., the harmful effects of hormonal replacement therapy in post-menopausal women. Medicine, at long last, is finally striding to a future with big steps because it actually, finally, is testing the beliefs on which therapy was founded. Your immediate predecessors, Celia, were no longer content to rely on history or tradition to educate you. They demanded data — data that was objectively obtained with clear, consistent rules, and objectively analyzed according to national, and more recent, international standards.

"And now, after all of this effort and perseverance, along come the Bayesians. They say that you can incorporate prior information into your answer. You can rely on your untested intuition because it's your intuition. Be honest, Celia, doesn't that approach strike a sympathetic chord in you?"

"I must admit that it does."

"Then that's a chord that you must murder Obliterate it. Despite what Bayesians say, the influence of prior experience is one of contamination, not liberation. Maybe we'll be ready for it soon, but only when we have good, clear ways to measure and accurately assess prior information. That's not now. Trying to use this novel tool today is like a 17th century man trying to fly. He's two hundred years too early, and he's going to get hurt."

"But what about using prior information that's available?" Celia inquired.

"Come on now That's nothing more than intellectual seduction. Bayesians wrap this notion of prior distribution in elegant mathematics, but it's the same dark assertion that has pulled at the shadowed corners of investigator's minds for centuries namely, 'Your belief is correct, self-evident, and needn't be completely tested.' Now, in all fairness to Jeremy, that may not be the message that he and his fell Bayesians mean to transmit, but I assure you, that's the answer that doctors receive.

"And, by the way, Celia, where were these Bayesians when frequentists were patiently instructing clinical investigators these past sixty years. Bayesians were nowhere to be found when frequentists were educating clinical investigators about research discipline. They were AWOL when frequentists argued repeatedly that clinical research methodology should be structured, that research questions should be stated objectively, that null findings be as easily interpretable as positive ones, and that doctors must be concerned about the possibility of harm even when they 'believe' that no harm will occur. Bayesians were curiously absent for the five decades that these arguments raged furiously.

"And now, just when the investigator community finally understands the problem that stems from relying on their own untested assumptions, along come the Bayesians who have the temerity to suggest that 'Well, after all, prior information is a good thing.' It's just the same old argument, that is, providing mathematical justification for physicians to toss away their research discipline and once again embrace their old, first love — prior belief That's great in religion, Jeremy, but it poisonous to science. What you're doing to clinical scientists is akin to giving a 10 year old a handgun, and then saying, 'Now, be careful.' They just can't be careful enough because they're not ready."

"But Leon," Celia responded, "it's undeniable that these procedures are increasing in popularity."

"Have you ever been to the beach, Celia?" Leon asked.

"Well, sure, what does that —"

"Just because the tide is high, doesn't mean it will always be so. It always recedes. It may shape the landscape a little, but the waters always withdraw."

Turning to Jeremy, Celia asked, "Any final words?"

"Only this," Jeremy asserted. "Frequentist thinking is doomed to the ash heap of history for the simple reason that it denies the one persistent, common trait of humans. We learn by updating our prior experience. If it won't die today, then it will die tomorrow, or the next day." But it's on the way out. We've grown beyond it."

Investigators were now streaming into the room. Celia thanked each of her friends, coming away from the discussion with much more knowledge, but the same level of confusion. As she walked to the podium to prepare for her first address as Principal Investigator, the same uneasiness that had prompted her to meet with the statisticians remained, and as the audience of scientists looked to her for leadership, she wondered, *Is my problem a Bayes problem or not?*

Reference

1. Pratt J.W. (1962). Discussion of A. Birnbaum's "On the foundations of statistical inference." *Journal of the American Statistical Association* **57**:269–326.

Chapter 6
Developing Prior Probability

6.1 Introduction

Disconnecting probability from relative frequency both adds to and subtracts from the persuasive power of Bayes' evaluations in biostatistics. The dividend from this uncoupling is the resilience of Bayes procedures. Separated from the hard and fast rule that all probability measurements must have their root in a relative frequency determination,[*] the Bayesian is free to develop probability on something else. These alternative sources commonly rely on a complicated orchestration of knowledge, training, experience, and expertise that can be debated but, in the end, are difficult to either reject out of hand or completely embrace. Bayesians must quantify these beliefs in order to include them in their calculations, but the subjective impressions themselves need not be the result of an observed experiment.

The obvious trouble with the use of subjective probability is that it can be false. Even when based on the opinions of experts and thought leaders, subjective impressions are commonly wrong impressions. Thus, while the admonition "have a true opinion and be certain of it" is the goal of the clinical Bayesian, in medicine it is much easier to be certain of an opinion than to have that opinion be true.

However, this dilemma, once acknowledged, is not insurmountable. Diligent prior probability construction can incorporate substantial flexibility, and the plasticity of the underlying mathematics allows the investigator to incorporate both strong belief and substantial uncertainty within the construction of their prior distribution. After this has been achieved, the sensitivity of the final result to changes in the prior distribution can provide a sense of stability to the final solution.

6.2 Prior Knowledge and Subjective Belief

Despite the knowledge explosion in disease and its treatment in the 20th century, the unexpected result remains a stubbornly common occurrence in medicine and clinical research. Our inability to dependably forecast a treatment effect in a clinical research effort forces the investigator to rely on a combination of impression, experience, and insight. This permits the investigator to plug the gap between an incomplete prior knowledge base that suggests many possible actions, on the one hand, and the execution of one single, incisive action on the other. This hole is filled by the essence of the decision maker herself, who must call on her expertise

---

[*] The relative frequency argument states that the probability of an event must be based on a mathematical calculation. This computation is the proportion of outcomes that generate that event. Thus, $P[A] = \dfrac{\text{total number of outcomes that produce } A}{\text{total number of outcomes}}$.

and intuition in order to choose from among the many candidate actions (Figure 6.1).

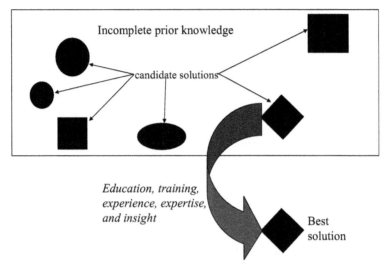

Figure 6.1. Incomplete prior information can only offer several candidate courses of action. The final selection is based on characteristics of the clinicians and investigators.

The second year medical student who must obtain a history on a deaf-mute patient, and the third year student who is vomited upon by a patient while conducting an examination are both rapidly immersed in making clinical determinations in the face of partial knowledge. By the time they have become the expert surgeon in the operating suite and the accomplished emergency room physician, they are experts at making decisions in the face of incomplete information.

Yet, while clinicians develop this talent, sharpen it, and in the best of circumstances wield it with breathtaking effectiveness, the Bayesian is challenged to incorporate this prior knowledge into their decision process. This incorporation consists of 1) separating prior knowledge from prior belief, and 2) placing this prior knowledge within a mathematical metric.

We will define prior belief as the mix of fact-based knowledge with subjective impressions. Acting on prior belief and its important subjective component is unavoidable in clinical medicine simply because we are required to treat diseases that we incompletely understand. Physicians rapidly develop guidelines for treating patients because patients and their desperate families need their help, and doctors have an oath-bound obligation to provide it.

For example, over twenty million patients in the United States have type II diabetes mellitus. Its consequences are devastating, and practitioners are reminded that each day, patients have heart attacks and strokes because of it, suffer amputations and blindness due to it, and experience renal disease because of it. Treatment is urgently required.

In this setting, consider the contemporary range of answers to the question "Does tight control of blood sugar elevations in patients with type II diabetes reduce the occurrence of the disease's consequences?" Many health care workers answer an immediate affirmative with no hesitation, pointing to 1) the underlying theory of the disease, 2) the findings about this relationship in patients with type I diabetes mellitus, and 3) their own clinical impressions. Others examine new revelations about the pathophysiology of the disease, the absence of good data in type II diabetes mellitus, the adverse event profiles of the medications used to treat type II diabetes, in combination with their own experiences to conclude that tight control of blood glucose levels is not worth the risks of the medicines used to achieve it. Thought leaders on either side of the issue passionately debate it; they believe they know. However, in the absence of definitive information, no one knows.* And while our knowledge about this critical issue is obtained from both scientific experimentation and by deduction, we are chastened by Albert Einstein, who reminds us that "Nature does not educate us beyond our own experiences."

While prior belief can be "certain," prior information is frequently incomplete, and, although we desire a degree of belief of "1" in all true propositions, and "0" in all false propositions, this lofty standard rises above what is achievable in science [1]. Our health care research tools remain rudimentary. One useful device that we researchers use on our quest is the measuring rod of consistency. The observation that a set of different experiments, carried out by different investigators, in different patients, using different study designs produce similar results, bolsters our belief in the truth of these results. In this circumstance, our prior belief is smoothly updated and refined through the cascade of consistency.

Yet even consistency can be a difficult track record to sustain. The suggestion that the anticholinesterase inhibitor vesnarione was first helpful [2] and then harmful [3] in patients with congestive heart failure (CHF) flummoxed the cardiology community, wreaking havoc with its "priors." It is difficult to create a consensus on prior information when different experiments purporting to study the same problem produce conclusions that are mirror images of each other.

The situation is complicated by funding restraints that require researchers to present plans for "reasonable" hypotheses when the definition of reasonable is caught firmly in the grasp of incomplete and sometimes unreliable prior information. Thus, researchers commonly cannot study hypotheses that may be true simply because their truth is judged unlikely by the funding source.

Thus, in medicine, the Bayesian must be especially cautious when using prior information. Since this source is irretrievably bound up with prior, subjective belief whose validity can rarely be investigated, its use requires caution and vigilance. One such precaution is the use of the counterintuitive prior.

6.3 The Counterintuitive Prior

There are two main sources for prior probabilities. One is the consensus among medical experts. The second is literature based. Commonly these two sources are

---

* ACCORD is a multimillion dollar, National Heart Lung and Blood Institute sponsored clinical trial to address this very question.

combined to construct prior probability. The underlying idea is that consistency, when combined with clear observation and careful reasoning, has the power to reveal the truth.

However, in medicine, we need to understand the misleading role false prior information can play. Thus, our discussions will incorporate the reality that we, despite our best efforts, do not have good foreknowledge of the value of the parameter. A useful way to begin constructing prior probabilities is therefore to divide the distribution between what we believe we know, and what we must acknowledge that we don't know.

Example 6.1: Hospitalization in Heart Failure

An investigator wishes to determine the probability of hospitalization for patients with CHF or a weakening of the heart's ability to function effectively. Heart attacks, chronic hypertension, and diabetes mellitus are just three of the many causes of this condition. With progressive loss of pumping capacity, the heart's ability to provide blood to the major organ systems deteriorates and the patient progressively weakens. The lungs are particularly affected as they fill with fluid, blocking the body's ability to exchange carbon dioxide for oxygen. Without medication, the patient will ultimately die from multiple organ failure.

The investigator believes that in his patient population, the likelihood that patients with CHF who are followed for one year will be hospitalized is 0.28. However, being unsure, he places positive probability uniformly between 0.20 and 0.35, writing the prior distribution as $\pi(\theta) = \frac{1}{0.15} \mathbf{1}_{\theta \in [0.20, 0.35]}$.

However, while reflecting some of the investigator's uncertainty about the location of the one year hospitalization rate, this prior probability distribution does not fully reflect the degree of uncertainty of the location of θ. We must differentiate between what the investigator believes he knows from the truth. Thus, while he thinks that θ lies in the [0.20, 0.35] interval, in fact, it could be anywhere between [0, 1]. Even in the face of this investigator's beliefs, this "counterintuitive" possibility must be admitted, and should be included in the prior distribution as well. An alternative prior distribution would be

$$\pi(\theta) = p \frac{1}{0.15} \mathbf{1}_{\theta \in [0.20, 0.35]} + (1-p) \mathbf{1}_{\theta \in [0,1]}, \tag{6.1}$$

for $0 \le p \le 1$. This formulation permits emphasis on the values of θ which the investigator has pinpointed, but also reflects the event (however unlikely it is in the investigator's eyes) that he might be wrong. The appearance of the distribution for alternative values of p reveals the different possible levels of influence of this "counterintuitive" component of the prior distribution (Figure 6.2).

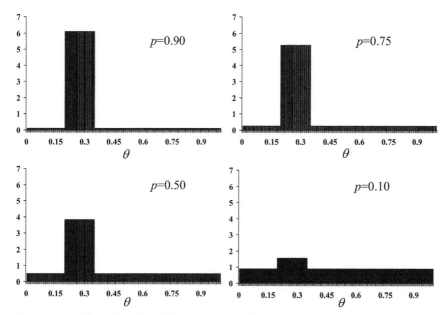

Figure 6.2. Effect of weight of the "counterintuitive" component of the prior distribution.

Figure 6.2 demonstrates the influence of the counterintuitive component on the prior distribution of the one year cumulative incidence rate of hospitalization for CHF. For large values of p, this counterintuitive segment of the prior distribution is minimal. However, decreasing values of p reduce the prior weight that is placed on the relatively tight region of θ in which the investigator believes the value of θ resides, strengthening the greater role of the counterintuitive portion of the prior, and its effect on the posterior distribution of θ.

In order to compute the posterior distribution of θ, we can rewrite $\pi(\theta)$ as

$$\pi(\theta) = \left(1 + 5.667p\right)\mathbf{1}_{0.20 \leq \theta \leq 0.35} + \left(1-p\right)\mathbf{1}_{0 \leq \theta \leq 0.20} + \left(1-p\right)\mathbf{1}_{0.35 \leq \theta \leq 1} \qquad (6.2)$$

If, in the coming year, the investigator learns that of his 80 patients with CHF x of them have been have been hospitalized, based on our work in Chapter Four, he can write

$$\pi(\theta \mid x) = \frac{P[x \mid \theta]\pi(\theta)}{\sum_{\theta} P[x \mid \theta]\pi(\theta)}$$

$$= \frac{\binom{80}{x}\theta^x (1-\theta)^{n-x}\left[\left(1 + 5.667p\right)\mathbf{1}_{0.20 \leq \theta \leq 0.35} + \left(1-p\right)\mathbf{1}_{0 \leq \theta \leq 0.20} + \left(1-p\right)\mathbf{1}_{0.35 \leq \theta \leq 1}\right]}{\binom{80}{x}\left[\left(1 + 5.667p\right)\int_{0.20}^{0.35}\theta^x (1-\theta)^{n-x}\,d\theta + \left(1-p\right)\int_{0}^{0.20}\theta^x (1-\theta)^{n-x}\,d\theta + \left(1-p\right)\int_{0.35}^{1}\theta^x (1-\theta)^{n-x}\,d\theta\right]} \qquad (6.3)$$

a formulation that can be assessed with the help of Appendix B.

The value of the parameter p equation (6.3) measures the influence of the non-informative, or counterintuitive assessment of the location of θ, small values of p reflecting relatively low confidence in the investigator's initial beliefs (Figure 6.3).

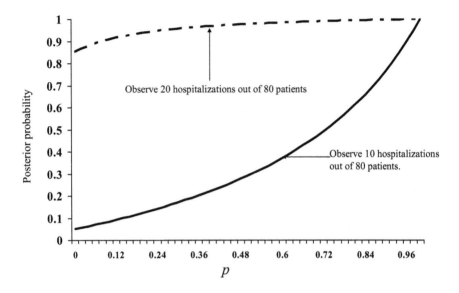

Figure 6.3. The posterior probability that the one year hospitalization rate is between 0.20 and 0.35 as a function of the prior distribution. Note the influence of a non-informative prior in the presence of unexpected results.

Figure 6.3 demonstrates the role of informed prior information on the posterior probability that $0.20 \le \theta \le 0.35$, which was the investigator's intuition. When 20 of 80 patients with CHF are hospitalized, this rate of 25% is consistent with the investigators initial belief and produces a high posterior probability for the event that $0.20 \le \theta \le 0.35$. This posterior probability remains high for even low values of p, (i.e., values of p that emphasize the counterintuitive component of the prior distribution that θ is not in this range). Clearly, observing 20 hospitalizations in 80 patients observed for one year generate high posterior probabilities of the investigator's belief that $0.20 \le \theta \le 0.35$, irrespective of the role of counterintuitive prior information.

However, the circumstances are altered when the data are less consistent with the specific intuition of the investigator. In the case where only 10 of 80 patients with CHF are hospitalized, the observed event rate is substantially less than what the investigator expected. Large values of p suggest that the posterior probability that $0.20 \le \theta \le 0.35$ continues to be high, a result not supported by the data. For example choosing $p = 0.99$ generates $P[0.20 \le \theta \le 0.35 \mid \bar{x} = 0.10] = 0.90$, demonstrating the ability of a prior distribution to overwhelm the data obtained from the conditional distribution.

However, a more circumspect value of $p = 0.50$, signifying that there is only 50% confidence in the investigator's initial assumption, produces a posterior probability of $P[0.20 \leq \theta \leq 0.35 \mid \bar{x} = 0.10] = 0.29$, a more modest and reasonable assessment. Thus, medium values of p, serving to moderate the investigator's prior belief, protect the posterior distribution from the unanticipated event.

A critical value in these calculations is p. As it increases from zero to one, the investigator's prior belief plays a greater role in the prior distribution, limiting the support for counterintuitive findings. Thus, before any there can be any general acceptance of a posterior result, there must be clear elaboration of the sensitivity of the posterior findings to the fundamental assumptions in the prior distribution.

Sensitivity analyses comprises this evaluation. If there were absolute, unshakable confidence in the prior distribution, such an evaluation would be unnecessary since deviations from the prior knowledge would be unjustified. However, in biostatistics, prior information is most always disputed, with different perspectives providing different weight to beliefs about the location of θ.

The sensitivity of the posterior probability is best demonstrated when the observed data fall near the boundary of the region of interest. For example, if 29 hospitalizations occur in 80 patients, the observed rate of 0.363 falls just above the upper boundary of the region of interest, $0.20 \leq \theta \leq 0.35$. Is the finding supportive of the investigator's intuition? It depends on how strongly the investigator's belief is reflected in the prior distribution, i.e., how large is the value of p (Figure 6.4)?

Of course, an alternative way to review this is to compute the posterior probability not just of one region of θ but alternative regions of θ as well (Figure 6.5).

Figure 6.5 depicts the wide range of values of the posterior probability that the one-year hospitalization rate lies between 0.20 and 0.35. There are two important implications of this curve. The first is that the investigator must choose the prior probability with great care. The scientist is in the best possible position when they have chosen the prior probability p prospectively before the research is completed. This early choice protects the investigator from the criticism that they have allowed the data (which has already provided an appropriate contribution to the posterior solution through the conditional distribution) to inappropriately select the prior probability as well. Thus a useful tact is to first settle on an *a priori* value of p, consistent with both their intuition and the need to reflect the possibility of a counterintuitive finding.

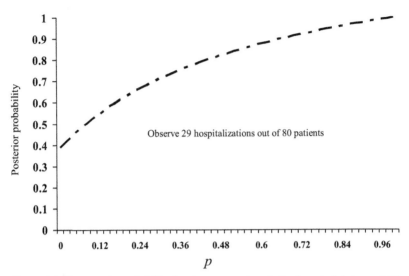

Figure 6.4. The posterior probability that the one-year hospitalization rate is between 0.20 and 0.35 as a function of the prior distribution when the observed data suggest the event rate is 36%. In this case, the posterior probability is quite sensitive to the role of counterintuitive prior information.

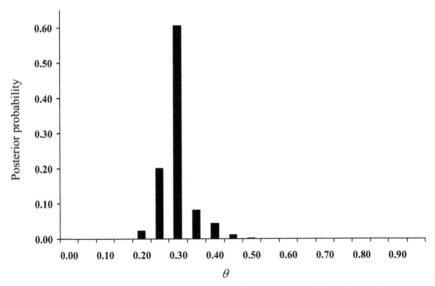

Figure 6.5. Posterior probability distribution for θ when p, the probability of the nonintuitive prior, is 0.50.

A second implication is for the audience receiving the result. While this informed community may accept the underlying methodology and the form of the posterior distribution, its members may disagree with the investigator over the value of p in the prior distribution. Bayes procedures invite this flexibility by inviting the consumer to replace the investigator's prior distribution with their own. This allows each audience member to produce their own posterior distribution and solution to the research question from the same research. Thus, one research endeavor, well designed and executed can generate a host of posterior distributions, each of which serves the need of the consumer group.

For the rest of the chapter, we will continue to provide counterweight to the investigator's *a priori* beliefs by incorporating a counterintuitive component to the prior information.

6.4. Prior Information from Different Investigators

The construction of prior probabilities commonly begins with the consultation of several experts, who based on their knowledge and expertise, have an understanding of the likely location of the parameter of interest. However, while these joint discussions can be useful and sometimes generate spectacular new ideas, its product, like that of the belief system of a single investigator, must be treated with caution.

Two useful approaches to take when constructing prior distributions from multiple experts are to either 1) allow them to reach consensus among themselves or 2) maintain the independent assessments of their opinions.

The consensus approach permits their interaction to alter their personal assessments of the parameter's location. At the conclusion of the conversation, the investigators have each arrived at a perspective on the prior distribution that is different than their original one.

The independence approach does not permit the experts to modify their opinions based on the assessment of other experts who are being contemporaneously solicited. It instead gathers the perspectives of each of the investigators and then simply multiplies the prior probabilities together to produce a new prior probability. Consider the following example.

Example 6.2: Hurricane Prediction

The arrival of the twin devastating hurricanes Katrina and Rita in August–September 2005 capped a tropical storm season of unprecedented ferocity. During this singular year, there were 28 named storms, 15 hurricanes, and 4 category five storms, each of these record setting numbers typifying the unanticipated fury of this unusual season (Figure 6.6).[*]

---

[*] There were so many storms, that the National Hurricane Center, exhausting its predetermined list of storm names, resorted to the Greek alphabet, requiring the letters alpha, beta, gamma, delta, epsilon, and zeta before the 2005 season mercifully ended.

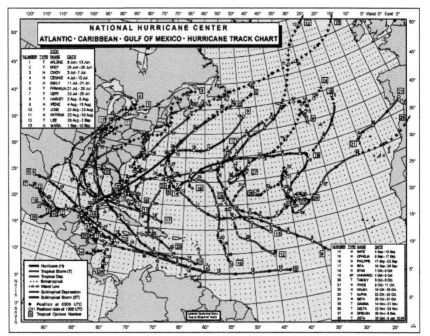

Figure 6.6. Official tracks of the named tropical storms in 2005. Reproduced from the National Hurricane Center.

Meteorologists commonly presage the tropical storm season (which arrives the first day of June) with a prediction of the expected number of tropical storms and hurricanes, using these predictions to convey the urgency of adequate preparations for the East and Gulf Coasts of the United States.

Assume we have three experts who provide their sense of the number of hurricanes expected in an upcoming hurricane season. The three meteorologists, M_1, M_2, and M_3, when queried, have estimated the expected number of named tropical storms along with the probability of that estimate (Table 6.1). Each meteorologist provides a probability distribution of the number of storms. For example, meteorologist M_1 believes the probability that there will be exactly eleven named storms in the upcoming tropical storm season with probability 0.023, while M_2 assigns only 0.002 probability to this event, and M_3 believes the probability of exactly eleven named storms is 0.114. The task before the statistician is to synthesize this information into a uniform assessment of the probability distribution of the number of anticipated named topical storms. The prediction of meteorologist M_3 is the most dire, suggesting the possibility that there may be as many as twenty named storms in the upcoming year (Figure 6.7).

Table 6.1 Storm Predictions of Three Meterologists (M₁, M₂, and M₃)

Number of named storms	Meterologist Assessment			Consensus	Independence
	M₁	M₂	M₃		
1	0.015	0.073	0.000	0.006	0.000
2	0.045	0.147	0.002	0.022	0.004
3	0.089	0.195	0.008	0.052	0.033
4	0.134	0.195	0.019	0.091	0.124
5	0.161	0.156	0.038	0.128	0.237
6	0.161	0.104	0.063	0.149	0.264
7	0.138	0.060	0.090	0.149	0.185
8	0.103	0.030	0.113	0.130	0.087
9	0.069	0.023	0.125	0.101	0.050
10	0.041	0.013	0.125	0.071	0.017
11	0.023	0.002	0.114	0.045	0.001
12	0.011	0.001	0.095	0.026	0.000
13	0.006	0.000	0.073	0.014	0.000
14	0.003	0.000	0.052	0.007	0.000
15	0.001	0.000	0.035	0.003	0.000
16	0.000	0.000	0.022	0.001	0.000
17	0.000	0.000	0.013	0.001	0.000
18	0.000	0.000	0.007	0.000	0.000
19	0.000	0.000	0.005	0.000	0.000
20	0.000	0.000	0.002	0.000	0.000

The consensus approach encourages the meteorologists to assemble and discuss their beliefs. These discussions encourage them to share not just their conclusions but the basis for these results, each expert offering the others the opportunity to alter their perspectives, while allowing their own to be available for recalibration (Table 6.1, consensus column).

An alternative approach permits the statistician to develop a summary prior distribution based on the three scientists' responses. Let p_{ij} be the prediction of the ith meteorologist for j storms. Then the independence assessment n_j may be computed as

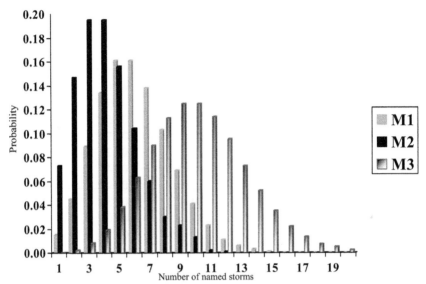

Figure 6.7. Independent predictions of the number of named storms by three meteorologists M_1, M_2, and M_3.

$$n_j = \frac{p_{1j}p_{2j}p_{3j}}{\sum\limits_{j=1}^{20} p_{1j}p_{2j}p_{3j}}, \qquad (6.4)$$

where the quantity in the denominator, $\sum\limits_{j=1}^{20} p_{1j}p_{2j}p_{3j}$, assures that the probabilities sum to one. A comparison of the consensus and independent assessment reveals the difference in the two distributions; in this case, the consensus assessment is skewed to a larger number of named storms (Figure 6.8).

6.5 Meta-Analysis and Prior Distributions

Commonly the basis of an expert's opinion is the result of a collection of studies. Each expert studies the results of the different, sometimes disparate results, and then carries out an assessment. This evaluation is an internal synthesis of the data, in which they review the effect of distinctive study designs, patient populations, patient follow-up duration, and statistical analyses on the results. This internal, mental synthesis produces a final data-based result that the expert believes is justified.

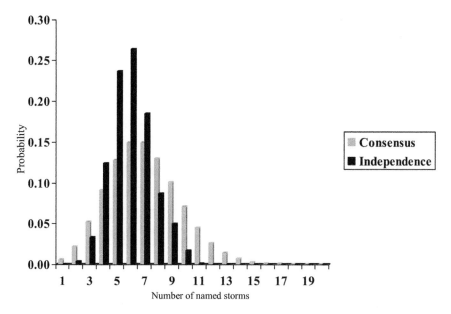

Figure 6.8. Comparison of a consensus versus an independent assessment of the opinions of three meteorologists. Note that the consensus predictions are skewed to the right.

There are circumstances in which researchers attempt to carry out this synthesis mathematically, a result commonly known as meta-analyses. *Meta-analyses* are the collection of processes that generate the combined results from several different independent studies designed to address the same scientific question. The literature contains useful discussions of the strengths and weaknesses of meta-analyses [4]. The controversies they can produce are commonly focused on the studies included in the analyses, e.g., when an analysis of corticosteroid use for brain injury [5] was believed to be flawed based on the exclusion of an influential study that demonstrated a benefit [6].

Example 6.3: HMG-CoA Reductase Inhibitors (the "statins")

In this example, we will build a prior distribution from the meta-analytic results in involving HMG-CoA reductase inhibition. Colloquially referred to as "the statins," the agents have proven to be an effective agent in the reduction of low density lipo-protein cholesterol (LDL-C). However the translation of this cholesterol lowering effect to reductions in mortality remained to be proven. Three studies were carried out to assess this effect in patients without a history of atherosclerotic disease (WOSCOPS) [7], or patients with a history of this disease (secondary prevention) in the United States (CARE) [8], and Australia (LIPID) [9].

At the inception of these studies, plans commenced for a meta-analysis of the results of the studies combining the effects of therapy on the cumulative total mortality rate [10]. These prospective plans permitted the investigators to build similar infrastructure into the three trials. They tested the same dose of medication, and used the same definitions for endpoints. The results of the meta-analysis produced an overall therapy effect of 20% reduction in the total mortality rate attributed to pravastatin [11] (Figure 6.9).

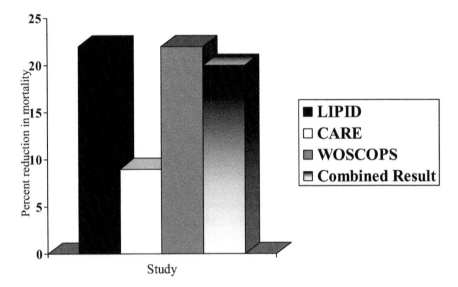

Figure 6.9. Percent reduction in total mortality for three cholesterol reducing clinical trials. The last bar represents the combined result.

The combined estimate of the percent reduction in mortality is 20%. However, in order to consider the possible inaccuracy in this result, we include a counterintuitive component in the prior. In this case, allow θ to follow a normal distribution with mean of 0.20 and standard deviation equal to the standard deviation of the estimate, 0.038. However, although this spreads the possible values of the effectiveness of the medication well above and below the meta-analytic estimate, it does so symmetrically. This symmetric extension can lead to an overestimation of the percent reduction of mortality, overestimating the effectiveness of the intervention. To reduce this consequence of the non-intuitive prior, we assume that the distribution is "asymmetrically" normal. For values of the efficacy θ that are less than 0.20, we place a normal distribution with a mean of 0.20. For greater values of efficacy, we assume a normal distribution that is scaled to reduce the probability of these larger values. The prior distribution is

$$\pi(\theta) = 2p \frac{1}{\sqrt{2\pi(0.038)^2}} e^{-\frac{1}{2}\left(\frac{\theta-0.20}{0.038}\right)^2} \mathbf{1}_{\theta \leq 0.20} + 2(1-p) \frac{1}{\sqrt{2\pi(0.038)^2}} e^{-\frac{1}{2}\left(\frac{\theta-0.20}{0.038}\right)^2} \mathbf{1}_{\theta > 0.20}.$$

for $0 \leq p \leq 1$. (Figure 6.10).

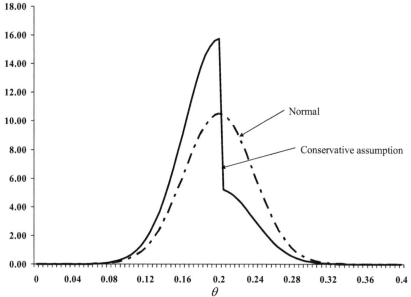

Figure 6.10. Alternative priors for "statin" induced reduction in mortality based on a symmetric (liberal) and asymmetric (conservative) assumption. The asymmetric prior distribution reduces the emphasis on overestimates of efficacy ($p = 0.75$).

This mixture deemphasizes larger values of θ, a reasonable conservative assumption when assessing the effectiveness of a therapy.

6.6 Priors and Clinical Trials

We have provided two examples in this chapter of what we have characterized as a *counterintuitive prior*. A counterintuitive prior probability distribution is a distribution that places prior probability on possible values of the parameter that the investigators believe will not actually occur. This may initially appear to be a contradiction to the Bayesian spirit since one of the motivations of Bayes analysis is to implement reports and advice that is reliable, i.e., prior "information," not "disinformation." However, the background information available to clinical researchers and biostatisticians can be tenuous, and in some cases, the best information has proven to be inaccurate.

Clinical trialists understand both the importance and frequent unreliability of prior information; in these circumstances, it can be impossible to separate prior information from prior belief, and here, prior belief is frequently wrong. The twin complexities of disease-occurrence prediction, and treatment efficacy prediction generates a volatile brew of strongly held but inaccurate impressions. In order to combat the counterproductive effect of using strongly held prior information in clinical trial methodology, we must balance this ineluctable tendency with a reflection of the suspected imprecision of that information. This procedure is necessary not only when prior information is incomplete but when there is a strong likelihood that the prior information is wrong.

In clinical trials which assess the effect of a therapy on a dichotomous endpoint (e.g., total mortality), two critical assessments in the trial's design are the control group event rate (e.g., the overall mortality rate in the control group) and the magnitude of the effect of therapy. Each of these prospective evaluations is critical for identifying the number of patients needed in the study and ultimately the human, financial, and material resources needed for the study's execution. Understanding the importance of these assessments, clinical investigators work hard to precisely determine these parameters. However, clinical experience demonstrates that despite these sometimes Herculean efforts, underlying event rates cannot be assessed accurately.

6.6.1 Difficulties in Estimating the Underlying Event Rate
Predicting the event rate of patients in the control group of a clinical trial may seem a straightforward task at first. After all, much of the world's relevant medical literature is available to investigators, and many of these contributions focus on the natural history of the disease process.

However, these contemporary literature and experienced-based assessments cannot consider all of the pertinent factors that determine the clinical events of patients with the disease in question. The clinical event rate is commonly linked to the prevalence of risk factors for the event. For example the occurrence of heart attacks is greater in patient populations with hypertension, *ceteris paribus*. If patients are to be recruited from a population of patients with a different constellation of risk factors than the populations reviewed in the literature, then the literature based event rates may be of reduced relevance.

This set of circumstances can be created by the medical community as it strives to reduce risk factor levels in vulnerable populations. The consequences of this worthy effort increases the inaccuracy of the event rate predictions. For example, the heart attack rate has progressively declined over the past three decades due to the introduction of both population based risk avoidance strategies in concert with lipid reduction and anticoagulation therapies, e.g., aspirin. The occurrence of smaller event rates had to be anticipated in trials that followed patients who were for the first time being exposed to these therapies; however, there was little contemporary literature on which to base reliable estimates.

The Survival and Ventricular Enlargement Study (SAVE) was a clinical trial designed in 1986 to assess the effect of the angiotensin converting enzyme inhibitor (ACE-i) captopril on the total mortality rate of patients who had left ventricular dysfunction [12]. Initial estimates of the cumulative placebo group mortality rate were 24%. However, the investigator believed that patients in SAVE would experience a smaller event rate because of the availability of improved therapy for heart failure. They therefore reduced their estimate of the cumulative mortality rate in the control group from 24% to 20%, producing a conservative estimate for this critical estimate. However, at the conclusion of the trial, the cumulative control group event rate was 23%. The investigators had adjusted in the right direction, but it was impossible for them to precisely foresee the actual value of the control group cumulative mortality rate[*]

The difficulties with estimating the control group event rate translate at once to problems with constructing a prior probability distribution for the control group event rate. Traditional sample size computations assume the control group event rate is known with certainty; however, acknowledgement that this rate is not known *a priori* doesn't help one identify the rate. Thus, any prior distribution for the control group rate must reflect the uncertainty of the scientists' best expectations.

6.6.2 Difficulties in Estimating a Study Intervention's Effectiveness

Predicting the magnitude of the therapy effect in a clinical trial is both essential and difficult. The *primum movens* of a study is to clearly and precisely generate this measure of the therapy's effect. However, sample size computations and the financial underpinnings of the trial require that this effect's magnitude be predicted before the study begins, a prediction that is fraught with difficulty. We can't deduce the result of an important experiment — we must execute it to know the effect.

The difficulty with predicting the efficacy of a clinical trial is that it is bound up with the investigators hopes and beliefs about the effect of therapy. Typically there is great controversy that surrounds its estimation. In the current climate of resource constraints, conducting a clinical trial is infeasible if the medical community believes the therapy will have no effect. It is equally impractical when the medical community accepts the effect of the therapy before the trial begins.[†] Trialists find it easiest to carry out clinical trials when there is no consensus in the medical community about the effect of therapy. Yet it is in precisely these circumstances that arriving at a consensus for the prior information is at its most difficult.

In addition, clinical trials can provide profound surprises, stupefying the prior beliefs of the experts. Two examples of the order shattering surprises that these trials can deliver are UKPDS and CAST. In these examples, relying on the prior information available and not providing some room for an unexpected result would have badly served the investigators.

6.6.2.1 UKPDS

The United Kingdom Prospective Diabetes Study (UKPDS) was a multicenter, prospective, randomized, intervention trial of 5102 patients with newly diagnosed type 2 (non-insulin-dependent) diabetes mellitus from 23 centers in England, Northern Ireland, and Scotland. The corpus of research has produced over fifty publications

---

[*] In fact the inability to reliably predict the control group event rate in a clinical trial has generated a new adaptation of the traditional design in which the investigators prospectively agree to continue the study not until a prespecified number of patients have been followed for a predetermined duration of time, but instead to follow them until a predetermined number of clinical events have occurred. This permits the investigators the freedom to adapt their trial to any perturbation in the control group event rate, diminishing the need for a precise and accurate estimate of this rate prospectively.

[†] This was a problem in the CAST clinical trial, which will be discussed later in this section.

dealing with different aspects of the study. Here, we will focus on the magnitude of effect.

This study was designed to evaluate the impact of improved blood glucose control on the complications of diabetes mellitus with particular emphasis placed on reductions in morbidity and mortality [13]. The endpoint that the UKPDS investigators chose was quite complex, since diabetes mellitus increases the 1) cumulative total mortality rate, 2) fatal and nonfatal myocardial infarction rate, 3) fatal and nonfatal stroke rate, 5) the rate of end state renal disease, 5) the prevalence of blindness, and 6) the prevalence of non-traumatic amputations. A complete description of the endpoint and the analysis plan is available [14].

When the UKPDS was started in 1977, the investigators believed that the improved blood glucose control might reduce the incidence of diabetes-related complications by 40% [15]. However, in 1987, after the trial had begun, an interim review of the data revealed that is was very unlikely that a 40% reduction in the cumulative incidence of the endpoints would be seen. The investigators announced that they were now interested in detecting at least a 20% reduction in the incidence of the combined endpoint, for which they had adequate power [16, Table 6]. Later, as the trial progressed, the investigators determined that a 15% reduction in the occurrence of the composite endpoints was more realistic.

However, the final UKPDS results reported in 1998 [17], were even less dramatic; 12% reduction in the cumulative incidence rate of any diabetes-related complication (95% CI 1% to 21%; $p = 0.029$). Thus the investigators were not able to reliable assess the magnitude of therapy effect at the study's inception, but even during the execution of the study, when their assessment was informed by the data that they were collecting, they remained unable to accurately predict it. Precise information for the effect was available, but this precise information was not accurate.

6.6.2.2 CAST
The "arrhythmia suppression" theory demonstrates the difficulties that occur when effect magnitude is based on strong but incorrect physician belief [18].[*]

Heart arrhythmias can be dangerous, and, in the middle of the 20th century, many cardiologists believed relatively minor heart irregularities e.g., premature ventricular contractions (PVCs) could spawn major life threatening arrhythmias. A new generation of medications (e.g., ecanide, flecanide, and moritzacine) that produced fewer side effects than the traditional antiarrhythmic agents were developed. Early studies, frequently carried out without a control group, suggested that this therapy might be beneficial. Ultimately, belief in the therapy was so strong, that the drugs were approved by the Food and Drug Administration (FDA) without a supporting pivotal clinical trial to support.

When a clinical trial to examine the effect of these therapies was finally executed, its investigators quickly learned that they faced an uphill fight for recruitment of patients into the trial. The practicing clinical community, having been persuaded by the leading cardiology opinion leaders and the FDA's approval of the

---

[*] Much of the discussion is taken from Thomas Moore's book entitled *Deadly Medicine*.

drugs, already believed the drugs were effective in suppressing dangerous heart arrhythmias and prolonging life. Why, they asked, were they now being asked to allow their patients to participate in a study in which there was a good chance that their patients' life sustaining medication would be substituted with a neutral placebo? The investigators, many of whom believed in the therapies' benefits, struggled for an effective riposte.

The trial investigators themselves were so convinced of the therapies' benefits that they insisted on a one-sided trial design. Thus, the trial would not be stopped if the therapy showed clear statistical evidence of harm. Thomas Moore in *Deadly Medicine* states (pages 203–204),

> "The CAST investigator ... wanted a structure that eliminated the possibility of ever proving that the drugs were harmful, even by accident. If the drugs were in fact harmful, convincing proof would not occur because the trial would be halted when the chances of proving benefit had become too remote."

The clinical community and investigators all believed that this therapy, so desperately needed for the treatment of serious arrhythmias, would be positive.

However, an interim analysis of the study results in the control group revealed that among 725 patients randomized to placebo there were 22 deaths. However, in the active group out of 730 patients randomized to the active therapy, 56 died. In a trial whose motivation was questioned by a clinical community who believed its question had already been answered in the positive, all could see that active therapy was almost three times as likely to kill patients as placebo. In this one-sided experiment the p-value was 0.0003, in the "other tail" [19].

The investigators reacted to these devastating findings with stupefaction. They had placed their "prior" all on the benefit side of the distribution, yet the final results resided exclusively in the "harm tail." Their *a priori assessment* of efficacy was completely wrong, and while the cardiology research community was shaken by the findings, the heart of the clinical community was broken by the realization that medications they believed to be beneficial were in fact killing patients.

There were many lessons the medical research community could learn from CAST. One of them was the inadvisability of relying on strong expert opinion about an effect size. The more strongly held the opinion, the greater the need for skepticism.

6.6.2.3 Wavering Prior Opinions

Expert belief should have a basis in fact. It is certainly appropriate, perhaps even critical that the facts be distilled through the filter of the expert's knowledge, training, experience, and expertise. However, its foundation must be rooted in fact. Clinical trials are candidates for this foundation. However, the facts from clinical trials must be more than mere descriptors of the findings in the sample; they must extend from the finding to the population at large. When the clinical trial results are themselves untrustworthy, the prior information (whose basis is in their unreliable results) become equally worthless.

Consider the collection of ELITE trials and its impact on knowledge about the use of therapy for CHF. The use of ACE-i therapy increased dramatically as a treatment for CHF in the 1980s. However, these medications were association with important, and sometimes, use-limiting adverse events e.g., hypotension, chronic cough, and angioedema. Angiotensin II type I receptor blockers (ARBs) were developed with the expectation that these agents would be safer than the original ACE-i's while continuing to confer a survival benefit for patients with CHF.

The Evaluation of Losartan in the Elderly Study (ELITE) I [20] was designed to directly compare the relative safety of angiotensin II type I receptor blockers to that of ACE-i's inhibitors. The prior belief was not that ARBs would provide longevity benefit, but that instead they would simply confer a safety advantage; in this case the safety advantage was improved renal function. Thus, one could imagine a "prior" that was neutral for a mortality effect, but focused on the ARBs to more successfully maintain patient renal function.

This double-blind study randomized 722 patients and followed them in a double-blind fashion for 48 weeks. Just prior to the end of the study, an additional endpoint was added. This measure was the composite endpoint of death and/or admission for heart failure. At the conclusion of ELITE I, the investigators determined that the increase in serum creatinine was the same in the two treatment arms (10.5% in each group; risk reduction 2%; 95% CI: -51 to 36; $p = 0.63$). However, they also discovered that 17 deaths occurred in the losartan group and 32 deaths in the captopril group, a finding equivalent to a risk reduction of 46% (95% CI 5 to 69; $p = 0.035$).

This surprising finding led to a substantial adjustment in the prior information about the effects of losartan. According to the authors, "This study demonstrated that losartan reduced mortality compared with captopril; whether the apparent mortality advantage for losartan over captopril holds true for other ACE inhibitors requires further study." Others even went so far as to attempt to explain the mechanism for the reduction in sudden death observed in ELITE 1 [21,22]. The "posterior" sense from ELITE was that there was no improved kidney protection for the drug, but that losartan could prolong the lives of patients who would have taken standard ACE-i therapy.

This new posterior information was used as the prior information for ELITE II [23], which, to the investigators' credit, was executed to confirm the superiority of losartan over captopril in improving survival in patients with heart failure. The primary endpoint in ELITE II was total mortality, requiring that twice as many patients as recruited in ELITE I be followed for twice as long.

At the conclusion of ELITE II, the cumulative all-cause mortality rate was not significantly different between the losartan and captopril groups (280 deaths in the losartan group versus 250 deaths in the captopril group, 17.7% versus 15.9%; hazard ratio 1.13 (95% CI: 0.95 to 1.35, $p = 0.16$). In fact, there was a trend to excess mortality in the losartan group. Thus, losartan did not confer a mortality benefit in the elderly with CHF when compared to captopril as suggested by ELITE I, and the prior information, would once again need to be radically altered. In the face of ELITE II, the investigators conceded, "More likely, the superiority of losartan to captopril in reducing mortality, mainly due to decreasing sudden cardiac death seen in ELITE, should be taken as a chance finding."

6.6.2.4 Conclusions on Nonintuitive Priors

Prior information is commonly central to the posterior result of the Bayesian analysis. The absence of an appreciation for the counterintuitive research finding can produce misleading results. Consider the following example.

An investigator is interested in determining the probability of abscess formation in patients with HIV infection. This rate θ he firmly believes lies between 0 and $1/2$, although he confesses he has no idea where in this range it resides. He therefore selects as his prior $\pi(\theta) = 21_{0 \le \theta \le \frac{1}{2}}$. Out of n patients with HIV infection, he believes the number of patients with abscesses x, follows a binomial distribution, i.e., $P[x = k \mid \theta] = \binom{n}{k} \theta^k (1-\theta)^{n-k}$. Following our development from Chapter Four, we can write the posterior distribution of θ (the abscess rate) given k (the number of patients with abscesses) as

$$\pi(\theta \mid x = k) = \frac{f(x = k \mid \theta)\pi(\theta)}{\int_\theta f(x = k \mid \theta)\pi(\theta)} = \frac{\binom{n}{k}\theta^k (1-\theta)^{n-k} 21_{0 \le \theta \le \frac{1}{2}}}{2\int_{\frac{1}{2}}^{1} \binom{n}{k}\theta^k (1-\theta)^{n-k}} \tag{6.5}$$

From Appendix II, we can write

$$\frac{\theta^k (1-\theta)^{n-k} 1_{0 \le \theta \le \frac{1}{2}}}{\int_0^{\frac{1}{2}} \theta^k (1-\theta)^{n-k}} = \frac{\theta^k (1-\theta)^{n-k} 1_{0 \le \theta \le \frac{1}{2}}}{\sum_{i=0}^{n-x} \binom{n-x}{i}(-1)^i \left(\frac{1}{2}\right)^{x+i+1}}.$$

Now assume that in 100 patients, there was 1 patient with an abscess. The posterior distribution for $n = 100$ and $k = 99$ is now

$$\pi(\theta \mid x = 99) = \frac{\theta^{99}(1-\theta)^1 \, \mathbf{1}_{0 \le \theta \le \frac{1}{2}}}{\sum_{i=0}^{1}\binom{1}{i}\frac{(-1)^i}{99+i+1}\left(\frac{1}{2}\right)^{100+i}} = \frac{\theta^{99}(1-\theta)^1 \, \mathbf{1}_{0 \le \theta \le \frac{1}{2}}}{\binom{1}{0}\frac{(-1)^0}{100+0}\left(\frac{1}{2}\right)^{100}+\binom{1}{1}\frac{(-1)^1}{100+1}\left(\frac{1}{2}\right)^{101}}$$

$$= \frac{\theta^{99}(1-\theta)^1 \, \mathbf{1}_{0 \le \theta \le \frac{1}{2}}}{\dfrac{1}{100\left(2^{100}\right)} - \dfrac{1}{101\left(2^{101}\right)}} = \frac{\theta^{99}(1-\theta)^1 \, \mathbf{1}_{0 \le \theta \le \frac{1}{2}}}{\dfrac{102}{(101)(100)\left(2^{101}\right)}}.$$

$$(6.6)$$

Now note that we observed 99 infections in 100 patients, an empirical probability of infection of 0.99, substantially greater than the prior belief that the event rate was no higher than 0.50. However, the following computation demonstrates that the posterior probability of the event rate being greater than 0.50, a result that is clearly supported by the data, is zero!

$$P[\theta \ge 0.50] = \int_{0.50}^{1} \pi(\theta \mid x = k) = \frac{1}{\dfrac{102}{(101)(100)\left(2^{101}\right)}} \int_{0}^{0.50} \theta^{99}(1-\theta)^1 \, \mathbf{1}_{\frac{1}{2} \le \theta \le 1} = 0.$$

The only region of θ for which the integrand is nonzero is the region in which the data did not occur. Thus, the computation rejects any information from the experiment when it has no support from the prior distribution. Basically, the actual proportion of patients with endpoints occurred in a region that had no support from the prior distribution. Since the prior distribution said the result was "impossible," this impossible result was not folded into the posterior distribution, and no update took place.

However, the incorporation of a counterintuitive component to the prior distribution remedies this. If the investigator had chosen

$$\pi(\theta) = 2p\mathbf{1}_{0 \le \theta \le 0.50} + 2(1-p)\mathbf{1}_{0.50 \le \theta \le 1}, \tag{6.7}$$

he would have balanced his strong belief that the probability of an abscess was less than 50% by the probability that his assessment was incorrect. In this case, the posterior probability distribution would be

$$\pi(\theta \mid x = k) = \frac{f(x = k \mid \theta)\pi(\theta)}{\int_\theta f(x = k \mid \theta)\pi(\theta)} = \frac{\binom{n}{k}\theta^k(1-\theta)^{n-k} 2\left(p1_{0\le\theta\le 0.50} + (1-p)1_{0.50\le\theta\le 1}\right)}{2p\int_0^{\frac{1}{2}}\binom{n}{k}\theta^k(1-\theta)^{n-k} + 2(1-p)\int_{\frac{1}{2}}^1 \binom{n}{k}\theta^k(1-\theta)^{n-k}}$$

$$= \frac{\theta^k(1-\theta)^{n-k}\left(p1_{0\le\theta\le 0.50} + (1-p)1_{0.50\le\theta\le 1}\right)}{p\int_0^{\frac{1}{2}}\theta^k(1-\theta)^{n-k} + (1-p)\int_{\frac{1}{2}}^1 \theta^k(1-\theta)^{n-k}}.$$

Using the results of Appendix B, this becomes

$$\pi(\theta \mid x = k) = \frac{\theta^k(1-\theta)^{n-k}\left(p1_{0\le\theta\le\frac{1}{2}} + (1-p)1_{\frac{1}{2}\le\theta\le 1}\right)}{p\sum_{i=0}^{n-x}\binom{n-x}{i}(-1)^i\left(\frac{1}{2}\right)^{x+i+1} + (1-p)\sum_{i=0}^{n-x}\binom{n-x}{i}(-1)^i\left(1-\frac{1}{2}\right)^{x+i+1}}$$

which, for $n=100$ and $x = 99$ becomes

$$\pi(\theta \mid x = 99)$$

$$= \frac{\theta(1-\theta)^{99}\left(p1_{0\le\theta\le\frac{1}{2}} + (1-p)1_{\frac{1}{2}\le\theta\le 1}\right)}{p\left[\binom{1}{0}\frac{(-1)^0}{100+0}\left(\frac{1}{2}\right)^{100} + \binom{1}{1}\frac{(-1)^1}{100+1}\left(\frac{1}{2}\right)^{101}\right] + (1-p)\left[\binom{1}{0}\frac{(-1)^0}{100+0}\left(1-\frac{1}{2}\right)^{100} + \binom{1}{1}\frac{(-1)^1}{100+1}\left(1-\frac{1}{2}\right)^{101}\right]}$$

$$= \frac{\theta(1-\theta)^{99}\left(p1_{0\le\theta\le\frac{1}{2}} + (1-p)1_{\frac{1}{2}\le\theta\le 1}\right)}{p\left[\frac{1}{100(2^{100})} - \frac{1}{(101)(2^{100})}\right] + (1-p)\left[\frac{1}{100} - \frac{1}{101}\right]}$$

with the approximation that $1 - \left(\frac{1}{2}\right)^n \approx 1$ for large n. The posterior probability that θ is less than 50% is now

$$P[\theta \ge 0.50 \mid x = 99] = \frac{(1-p)\left[\frac{1}{100} - \frac{1}{101}\right]}{p\left[\frac{1}{100(2^{100})} - \frac{1}{(101)(2^{100})}\right] + (1-p)\left[\frac{1}{100} - \frac{1}{101}\right]}$$

which we can evaluate for different values of p (Figure 6.11).

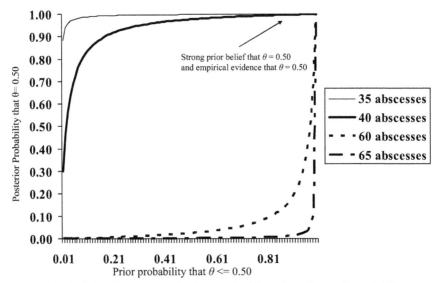

Figure 6.11. Relationship between role of counterintuitive prior and posterior probability as a function of the number of abscesses.

Figure 6.11 demonstrates the relationship between the posterior probability, and the prior probability that the number of abscesses identified in 100 patients is less than 0.50. There are four curves each depicting the relationship between the prior and posterior distribution of $P[\theta \leq 0.50]$ for different findings.

The further to the right one proceeds on the x-axis, the more extreme is the prior belief that $\theta \leq 0.50$. Note that when there are a relatively small number of patients with abscesses (i.e., 35 patients in 100 or 40 patients in 100), then the posterior probability is very high when the prior probability that $\theta \leq 0.50$ is large. This is a perfectly reasonable conclusion because both the prior probability and the data strongly suggest that $\theta \leq 0.50$. However, note that, when the prior belief that $\theta \leq 0.50$ is extremely high ($p > 0.90$ on the x-axis), the posterior probability that $\theta \geq 0.50$ is also high even when the current evidence suggests otherwise (i.e., there are 60 or 65 patients with absences out of 100 patients. By diminishing the extreme prior belief that $\theta \leq 0.50$ to a more moderate level, e.g., 0.66, the posterior probability can more realistically reflect the counterintuitive findings of the data. Decreasing the prior $P[\theta \leq 0.50]$ from 1 to 0.66 introduces a counterintuitive component.

This plays an important role in allowing a important update in the prior probability in the face of unexpected experimental information.

6.7 Conclusions

These examples are not to denigrate the use of prior information in clinical trials. To the contrary, clinical trials are perhaps the best findings and results on which clinical trials resides. However, clinical trials, while the best source of information, must be carefully designed, with appropriate circumscription of its conclusions. The example of ELITE I and II, as with the examples of the Vesnarinone studies and PRAISE I and II demonstrate the ephemeral nature of clinical trial results when they are perturbed by data-based protocol changes [14]. However, in these circumstances, the appropriate prior distributions should include a healthy dose of skepticism about the insight of the medical community. if the basis of prior information is unhelpful, then the Bayesian analysis is undermined. If we are to rely on clinical trials for prior information, those trials must be expertly conducted. In addition, prior information must be counterbalanced by an important and influential counterintuitive component to reflect the inherent uncertainty in clinical observations and research findings.

As long as it is true that what we believe in health care can be markedly different than what we ought to believe, there must be room for the use of the counterintuitive prior distribution.

Problems

1. Articulate the difference between a noninformative prior distribution, and a counterintuitive prior distribution in the Bayes paradigm.

2. What is the justification for the implementation of a counterintuitive prior distribution in health care research?

3. The beta distribution is very popular distribution among Bayesian workers. Its form is

$$\pi(\theta) = \frac{\Gamma(\alpha+\beta)}{\Gamma(\alpha)\Gamma(\beta)} \theta^{\alpha-1} (1-\theta)^{\beta-1} \mathbf{1}_{0 \le \theta \le 1}$$

where α and β are constants. Can you show using Appendix K, that the binomial distribution with parameters n and θ is a form of the beta distribution?

4. Demonstrate using Appendix K, that if the prior distribution is beta, and the conditional distribution is beta, than the posterior distribution is beta. A distribution that has this property is known as a conjugate family of distributions.

5. Demonstrate that the normal distribution is a member of the conjugate family of distributions.

References

1. Ramsey F. (1926). Truth and Probability in Ramsey 1931 The Foundations of Mathematics and other Logical Essays, Ch VII, p.156–198, edited by R.B. Braithwaite, London. Degan, Paul, Trench, Trubner & Co., New York: Harcourt, Brace, and Company. (1999 electronic edition).
2. Feldman A.M., Bristow M.R., Parmley, W.W. et al. (1993). Effects of vesnarinone on morbidity and mortality in patients with heart failure. *New Engand Journal of Medicine* **329**:149–55.
3. Cohn J., Goldstein S.C., Feenheed S. et al. (1998). A dose dependent increase in mortality seen with vesnarinone among patients with severe heart failure. *New England Journal of Medicine* **339**:1810–16.
4. Egger M., Smith G.D., Phillips A.N. (1997). Meta-analyses: principles and procedures. *British Medical Journal* **315**:1533–1537.
5. Alderson P., Roberts I. (1997). Corticosteroids in acute traumatic brain injury: systematic review of randomised controlled trials. *British Medical Journal* **314**: 1855–1859.
6. Gregson B., Todd N.V., Crawford D., Gerber C.J., Fulton B., Tacconi L., et al. (1999). CRASH trial is based on problematic meta-analysis. *British Medical Journal* **319**: 578.
7. Shepherd J., Cobbe, S.M., Ford, I., et al. (1995). Prevention of CAD with pravastatin in men with hypercholesterolemia. *New England Journal of Medicine* **333**:1301–7.
8. Sacks, F.M., Pfeffer, M.A., Moyé, L.A., Rouleau, J.L., Rutherford, J.D., Cole, T.G., Brown, L., Warnica, J.W., Arnold, J.M.O., Wun, C.C., Davist, B.R., Braunwald. E. (1996). The effect of pravastatin on coronary events after myocardial infarction in patients with average cholesterol levels. *New England Journal of Medicine* **335**:1001–9.
9. Long-Term Intervention with Pravastatin in Ischaemic Disease (LIPID) Study Group. (1998). Prevention of cardiovascular events and death with pravastatin in patients with CAD and a broad range of initial cholesterol levels. *New England Journal of Medicine* **339**:1349–1357.
10. The PPP Project Investigators (1995). Design, rationale, and baseline characteristics of the prospective pravastatin pooling (PPP) project; a combined analysis of three large-sclae randomized trials: Long-Term Intervention with Pravastatin in Ischaemic Disease (LIPID), Cholesterol and Recurrent Events (CARE), and West of Scotland Coronary Prevention Study (WOSCOPS). *American Journal of Cardiology* **76**:899–905.

11. Simes J., Furberg C.D., Brawnwald E., Davis B.R., Ford I., Tonkin A., Shepherd J., for the Prospective Pravastatin Pooling project investigators (2001). Effects of pravastatin on mortality in patients with and without coronary heart disease across a broad range of cholesterol levels. *European Heart Journal* **23**:207–215.

12. Moyé L.A. for the SAVE Cooperative Group. (1991). Rationale and Design of a Trial to Assess Patient Survival and Ventricular Enlargement after Myocardial Infarction. *American Journal of Cardiology* **68**:70D–79D.

13. UK Prospective Diabetes Study Group. (1991). UK Prospective Diabetes Study (UKPDS) VIII. Study, design, progress and performance. *Diabetologia* **34**:877–890.

14. Moyé L.A. (2003). *Multiple Analyses in Clinical Trials: Fundamentals for Investigators*. New York. Springer. Chapter 8.

15 UKPDS Study Group. (1998). Intensive blood glucose control with sulphonylureas or insulin compared with conventional treatment and risk of complications in patients with type 2 diabetes. *Lancet* **352**:837–853.

16. Turner, R.C., Holman, R.R. on behalf of the UK Prospective Diabetes Study Group. (1998). The UK Prospective Diabetes Study. Finnish Medical Society DUOCECIM, *Annals of Medicine* **28**:439–444.

17 UKPDS Study Group. (1998). Intensive blood glucose control with sulphonylureas or insulin compared with conventional treatment and risk of complications in patients with type 2 diabetes. *Lancet* **352**:837–853.

18. Moore T. (1995) *Deadly Medicine*. New York: Simon and Schuster.

19. The CAST Investigators. (1989). Preliminary Report: effect of encainide and flecainide on mortalithy in a randomized trial of arrhythmia suppression after myocardial infarction. *New England Journal of Medicine*. **321**:406–412.

20. Pitt, B, Segal, R., Martinez, F.A. et al. on behalf of the ELITE Study Investigators (1997). Randomized trial of losartan versus captopril in patients over 65 with heart failure. *Lancet* **349**:747–52.

21. Jensen, B.V., Nielsen, S.L. (1997). Correspondence: Losartan versus captopril in elderly patients with heart failure. *Lancet* **349**:1473.

22. Fournier A., Achard J.M., Fernandez L.A. (1997). Correspondence: Losartan versus captopril in elderly patients with heart failure. *Lancet* **349**:1473.

23. Pitt, B., Poole-Wilson P.A., Segal, R., et. al (2000). Effect of losartan compared with captopril on mortality in patients with symptomatic heart failure randomized trial–The losartan heart failure survival study. ELITE II. *Lancet* **355**:1582–87.

Chapter 7
Using Posterior Distrib tions:
Loss and Risk

7.1 Introduction

Our discussion of Bayes procedures have focused on the technique (and pitfalls) of updating prior information to posterior knowledge. The investigator begins with a prior information encompassing knowledge, belief, and the possibility that his belief may be wrong. We have concentrated on this prior belief's motivation, its development, and its mathematical incorporation into the decision-making process. Bayes theorem brings this prior information together with the current data, generating a posterior distribution.

The posterior distribution has been our goal thus far, but that is just a temporary way station. Our actual goal is to wield this posterior distribution in order to make the correct decision. To guide this mobilization, we must understand the concept of loss and risk.

7.2 The Role of Loss and Risk

Both frequentists and Bayesians have the same goal — to estimate and infer accurately. We wish to know the incidence rate of an adverse event believed to be due to a drug, or to make a decision about whether an effect of an intervention produces a large enough benefit to proceed with its development. Each of these processes involves making a decision — we decide to select an event rate estimate, or we decide to move ahead with the product's development.

However, with each possible choice, the decision maker must acknowledge the possibility that the selected decision was wrong; for a wrong decision, a penalty or price must be paid. For example, underestimating a diabetic patient's blood sugar when the patient has missed their daily insulin injections can lead to new symptoms of their disease, requiring hospitalization. Alternatively, overestimating a patient's blood sugar when they have taken too much insulin and missed a meal can generate inaction that produces convulsions, coma, and death.

These consequences of inappropriate decisions must be embedded into the decision process. In Bayesian statistics, this incorporation takes place through the loss function. Loss functions are mathematical representations of the loss debited or the gain credited by a decision. Bayesian statisticians overtly incorporate these prices and penalties into the decision process itself. We will define $L(\theta, a)$ as the loss associated by taking action a in the presence of the true value of θ.

A Bayesian uses the loss function to guide her interpretation of the posterior distribution. A natural action is to measure the average value of the loss over the posterior distribution; this average is known as the posterior risk $R(\theta, a)$. Every possible decision a has a posterior risk linked to it.

The Bayes procedure is that action or estimate δ_B which produces the lowest risk, i.e., the smallest average loss. The risk of the Bayes procedure is termed the *Bayes risk*, $R(\theta, \delta_B)$.

Thus the new adaptation of our work is to construct a reasonable loss function, $L(\theta, a)$, then to find the procedure or action, δ_B (i.e., the estimate or decision) that minimizes this loss over the posterior distribution (Figure 7.1).

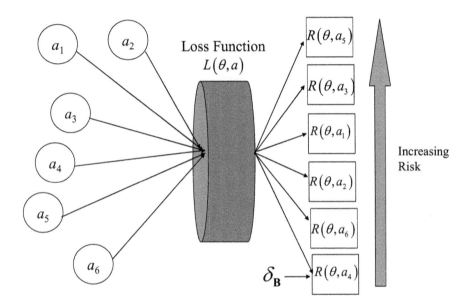

Figure 7.1. Several possible actions are ranked by the risk that each produces. The action with the lowest risk is the Bayes action, in this case, action a_4.

Since there are two classes of Bayes procedures, decision making and estimation, there is a class of loss function attached to each of them. We will explore the use of each of them separately, beginning with the simplest examples, and advancing to more realistic scenarios.

7.3 Decision Theory Dichotomous Loss
The use of loss functions can greatly inform the decision process. In many circumstances, loss functions can make all of the difference. We see the use of loss functions in our daily lives that reflect the value of trade offs, loss functions that evolve over time. Thus, the loss incurred by passengers who are inconvenienced by additional security requiring them to be electromagnetically screened, physically searched made such procedures impossible twenty-five years ago. However, the

loss of allowing passengers onto planes who have the means to destroy the plane have eclipsed the "convenience loss," and passengers accept the loss of their convenience to ensure the greater loss (i.e., loss of life) is not incurred.

Bayesian loss functions quantify this information. We use the notation $L(a_i \mid a_j)$ to denote the loss sustained if action a_i is taken when action a_j is correct. Consider the circumstance where a decision maker must choose between two options a_1 and a_2. Action a_1 will incur some gain if it appropriate, and a loss if it is not. Similar consequences accrue for action a_2 (Table 7.1).

Table 7.1. Loss function for a two action problem. Each of actions a_1 and a_2 are associated with a loss when they are selected.

| | | Decision | |
		Take action a_1	Take action a_2
	Action a_1 correct	$L(a_1 \mid a_1)$	$L(a_2 \mid a_1)$
Reality			
	Action a_2 correct	$L(a_1 \mid a_2)$	$L(a_2 \mid a_2)$

$L(a_i \mid a_j)$ signifies the loss sustained by taking action a_i when action a_j was appropriate.

The loss associated with action a_1 has two components. The first is the loss associated when a_1 is appropriate (this actually may be considered gain); the second is the loss with action a_1 is inappropriate. However, what must also be considered is the probability that the actions are correct. This probability is factored in by considering the likelihood that their actions are correct. Thus, the risk associated with action a_1, $R(a_1)$ is

$$R(a_1) = P[\text{action } a_1 \text{ correct}] L(a_1 \mid a_1) + P[\text{action } a_2 \text{ correct}] L(a_1 \mid a_2).$$

Analogously, the risk associated with action a_2 is

$$R(a_2) = P[\text{action } a_1 \text{ correct}] L(a_2 \mid a_1) + P[\text{action } a_2 \text{ correct}] L(a_2 \mid a_2).$$

The decision rule decides in favor of action a_1 if $R(a_1) \le R(a_2)$. Denote $P[a_1]$ as the probability that action a_1 is correct, and $1 - P[a_1]$ as the probability that action a_2 is correct. Then $R(a_1) \le R(a_2)$ implies

$$P[a_1]L(a_1 \sim a_1)+(1-P[a_1])L(a_1 \sim a_2) \leq P[a_1]L(a_2 \sim a_1)+(1-P[a_1])L(a_2 \sim a_2).$$

We can solve this inequality for $P[a_1]$ to find

$$P[a_1] \geq \frac{L(a_1 \sim a_2)-L(a_2 \sim a_2)}{L(a_1 \sim a_2)+L(a_2 \sim a_1)-L(a_1 \sim a_1)-L(a_2 \sim a_2)} \quad (7.1)$$

Thus we would choose action a_1 if inequality (7.1) is satisfied. Before we apply this result, note that this expression makes no assumption about the form of the posterior distribution. In fact, as we will see this risk expression can be evaluated with respect to the prior distribution as well. The selection of the loss function, and the computation of the region over which the probability will be assessed is a calculation that is separate and apart from the form of the probability distribution itself.

Example 7.1: Loss Functions and Hypothesis Testing

Assume that a frequentist investigator is carrying out a classical hypothesis test for the mean θ of a normal distribution. Following the established rules, she formulates a null hypothesis H_0: $\theta = \theta_0$ and an alternative hypothesis H_a: $\theta \neq \theta_0$. She intends to collect data, and reject the null hypothesis if the test statistic falls in the critical region.

In the traditional hypothesis testing paradigm there are two possible correct decisions (rejecting H_0 appropriately; rejecting H_1 appropriately; and two incorrect decisions (rejecting H_0 inappropriately; rejecting H_1 inappropriately) (Table 7.2).

The incorrect decisions are well known to frequentists who have identified these errors as Type I and Type II errors. In our current decision-theoretic paradigm, the investigator pays a penalty for committing each of these two mistakes. No loss is incurred when H_1 is appropriately rejected, and H_2 is appropriately rejected.

In Table 7.2, we hypothesis that no loss (or gain) is incurred with a correct decision. However, losses are sustained for an incorrect decisions. Action a_1 is the decision not to reject the null hypothesis. How does the scientist know when to reject H_0? The investigator can use equation (7.1) to conclude that nonrejection of the null hypothesis is appropriate when

Table 7.2. Loss function construction for the traditional hypothesis testing paradigm.

		Decision	
		a_1 Do not reject H_0	a_2 Reject H_0
Reality	H_0 correct	0	19
	H_0 incorrect	1	0

$$P[H_0 \text{ is correct}] \geq \frac{L(a_1 \mid a_2) - L(a_2 \mid a_2)}{L(a_1 \mid a_2) + L(a_2 \mid a_1) - L(a_1 \mid a_1) - L(a_2 \mid a_2)} = \frac{1}{20}$$

Thus the action of not rejecting the null hypothesis is optimal if the probability that the null hypothesis is correct is greater than 0.05, the traditional threshold for a type I error.[*]

∎

From this example, we see that the decision theoretic model subsumes the frequentist approach to the standard hypothesis test. However, it also reveals an obscure underpinning of the commonly used 0.05 threshold. Clearly the 0.05 level is motivated by the (tacit) belief that it is nineteen times more costly to commit a Type I error than a Type II error. While it is natural to argue for a level other than 0.05, the decision-theoretic approach provides a rationale and a defense for other type I error levels. For example, if the Type I error loss was not 19 times as costly, but only 10 times as costly as the Type II error level, then the threshold value for $P[H_0 \text{ is correct}]$ is $1/11 = 0.091$, almost twice as large as the Fisherian 0.05 standard. The relationship between the ratio of the loss for a Type I and Type II error and the "p-value" is easily generated (Figure 7.2).

---

[*] The 0.05 level is principally motivated by tradition. Its original source was an experiment Ronald Fisher was asked to conduct to assess the effect of manure on crop yield. See Chapter Five.

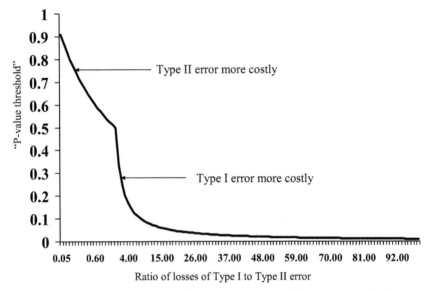

Figure 7.2. Threshold for rejecting the null hypothesis as a ratio of the loss associated with a Type I error to a Type II error.

Figure 7.2 depicts the ratio in the threshold for taking action a_1 (i.e., accepting the null hypothesis) as a function of the ratio of the losses sustained by a Type I error to that paid for a Type II error. We see that if the ratio of losses is less than one (i.e., the left-most region on the abscissa), then the Type II errors are more costly, then the p-values are very high; in fact, defensible values larger than the 0.50 level are permissible. This probability falls to the value of 0.50 level when the ratio of the losses is 1.

However, as the relative penalty paid for a type I error increases, the "p-value" threshold decreases. For a ratio of 19, the ratio is 0.05 as demonstrated earlier in this section. Thus, the Bayesian perspective on the traditional frequentist hypothesis-testing scenario raises the possibility of setting loss functions not just based on the traditional 0.05 level, but on the relative loss associated with either of the two type I and type II sampling errors.

The second point in this development is the identification of $P[H_0 \text{ is correct}]$. This is not the p-value on which frequentists have come to place such reliance. The p-value is the probability that sampling error generated the data result, i.e., it is the probability that the sample would generate its evidence that the population mean θ was not equal to θ_0 given that the population mean is in fact θ_0. These are complicated events for the investigator to understand.

Alternatively, the Bayesian perspective focuses on the simple probability that the population mean is θ_0. Since this information is available from both the prior distribution and the posterior distribution, either of these distributions can be used to assess this probability, using the same formulation of the loss function.

For example, recall from Chapter Four that if a selection of n observations $x_1, x_2, x_3,\ldots x_n$ follow a normal distribution with mean θ and variance σ^2, and the prior distribution of θ is normal with mean μ and variance υ^2, then the posterior distribution is normally distributed with mean μ_p and variance v_p^2, where

$$u_p = \frac{\upsilon^2}{\upsilon^2 + \sigma^2}\bar{x}_n + \frac{\sigma^2}{\upsilon^2 + \sigma^2}\mu;$$

$$(7.2)$$

$$v_p^2 = \frac{\upsilon^2\sigma^2}{\upsilon^2 + \sigma^2}.$$

Thus, one can compute the prior probability that θ falls in a particular region of interest, and compare the solution to that obtained from the posterior probability.

Example 7.2: Discrete Loss Functions and HDL Levels

Assume the investigator is interested in assessing the probability that the high density lipoprotein (i.e., the "good" cholesterol) level θ is less than 35 mg/dl. Her prior distribution suggests that θ follows a normal distribution with mean 35 and variance 30. Her loss function places the loss of incorrectly concluding that the HDL level is less than 35 mg/dl at eight times the loss of inappropriately deciding that θ > 35 mg/dl. Using equation (7.1) she concludes that she should only conclude $\theta \le$ 35 mg/dl when

$$P[\theta \le 35\,\text{mg/dl}] \ge \frac{1}{1+8} = 0.111.$$

Using the prior distribution, she finds the value of this probability is 0.50, suggesting that, in the absence of the data, it would be appropriate for her to conclude that $\theta \le 35$ mg/dl.

She now collects a sample of 10 subjects, and discovers that the mean is 39 mg/dl and the variance is 50. Using the expressions from (7.2), she computes μ_p = 38.43 mg/dl and υ_p = 4.29. Thus, using this posterior information, she calculates

$$P[\theta \le 35 \text{ mg/dl}] = P[\,N(38.43, 4.29) \le 35\,\text{mg/dl}] = 0.048.$$

Since this is less than the 0.111 threshold set by consideration of the loss function, she now concludes based on her data that θ is less than 35 mg/dl. If she is criticized for drawing this conclusion, her best defense resides in the selection of the loss function, and selection of the prior distribution for the HDL level.

7.4 Generalized Discrete Loss Functions

We can easily extend our results from section 7.3 to consider more complex loss functions that involve more than two actions. Here, the decision maker must select one action from a large collection of them, each associated with a loss. As in the previous section, we can quickly lay out a loss function table that demonstrates the losses sustained for a given action a_i, $i = 1$ to a. (Table 7.3)

Table 7.3. Loss function construction for categorical decision analysis

		Decision				
		a_1	a_2	a_3	...	aa
	a_1 correct	$L(a_1 \sim a_{1)}$	$L(a_2 \sim a_{1)}$	$L(a_3 \sim a_{1)}$	...	$L(a_a \sim a_{1)}$
Reality	a_2 correct	$L(a_1 \sim a_{2)}$	$L(a_2 \sim a_{2)}$	$L(a_3 \sim a_{2)}$	...	$L(a_a \sim a_{2)}$
	a_3 correct	$L(a_1 \sim a_{3)}$	$L(a_2 \sim a_{3)}$	$L(a_3 \sim a_{3)}$	...	$L(a_a \sim a_{3)}$
	$\vdots$	$\vdots$	$\vdots$	$\vdots$		$\vdots$
	a_a correct	$L(a_1 \sim a_{a)}$	$L(a_2 \sim a_{a)}$	$L(a_3 \sim a_{a)}$	...	$L(a_a \sim a_{a)}$

Selecting one action from a collection of possible choices, each associated with a loss leads to a matrix of loss functions which much all be considered.

Following the development from the previous section, we can compute the risk of action $R(a_i)$, as

$$R(a_i) = \sum_{j=1}^{a} P[a_j] L(a_i \mid a_j). \qquad (7.3)$$

Thus, we can compute the risk of each of the a possible actions. The Bayes action, δ_B, is the action that minimizes the risk.

While this procedure is easily stated, the actual procedure can lead to mathematical complications as demonstrated in the following example.

Example 7.3: Multiple Discrete Loss Functions: Alzheimer's Disease

Alzheimer's disease is the progressive loss of mental abilities with advancing age. It can manifest itself as loss of cognitive function, memory loss, disorientation, and the new incapacity to make rationale decisions. As the average age of the U.S. population increases, the prevalence of this pervasive disorder is also on the rise.

Preventing the occurrence or delaying the progression of Alzheimer's disease is a public health imperative. These abilities require the presence of accurate tools that can quickly and precisely diagnosis the presence of this disease at an early age. Currently, investigators have developed an assay that they believe will accurately predict the presence of Alzheimer's disease. Its most useful deployment will aid the physicians as they take one of there actions

Action 1 (a_1): Decide that the patient does not have Alzheimer's disease
Action 2 (a_2): Decide that additional testing is necessary
Action 3 (a_3): Decide that the patient has Alzheimer's disease

Based on this universe of possible responses, investigators have constructed the following loss function (Table 7.4).

Table 7.4. Loss function for Alzheimer's disease based on a new test

		Decision		
		No Alzheimer's Disease	More testing required	Alzheimer's Disease
	No Alzheimer's disease	-20	1	75
Reality	More testing required	1	0	25
	Alzheimer's disease present	: 26	: 5	: -10

In this scenario there are gains and losses associated with any decision.[*] In each scenario where the physician makes a correct diagnosis, the negative value of the loss function appropriately reflects a gain; the loss function is neutral if the physician appropriately chooses to select the need for additional testing. Alternatively, there is a substantial penalty for an incorrect diagnosis. The risk functions are complicated (Figure 7.3).

---

[*] The fact that a loss function can reflect gain is why some workers refer to these relationships as *utility* functions.

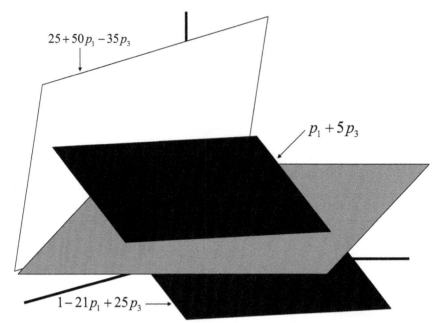

Figure 7.3. The three regions of risk that must be evaluated to find the Bayes procedure.

We can write the risks of each of the three actions as

$$R(a_1) = \sum_{j=1}^{a} P[a_j] L(a_1 \mid a_j) = -20p_1 + p_2 + 26p_3.$$

$$R(a_2) = \sum_{j=1}^{a} P[a_j] L(a_2 \mid a_j) = p_1 + 5p_3.$$

$$R(a_3) = \sum_{j=1}^{a} P[a_j] L(a_3 \mid a_j) = 75p_1 + 25p_2 - 10p_3.$$

We can simplify by requiring $p_1 + p_2 + p_3 = 1$, permitting

$$R(a_1) = 1 - 21p_1 + 25p_3.$$
$$R(a_2) = p_1 + 5p_3. \qquad (7.4)$$
$$R(a_3) = 25 + 50p_1 - 35p_3.$$

We might expect that the Bayes procedure will depend on the values of p_1 and p_3, the probabilities that the patient does and does not have Alzheimer's disease, respectively.

We can use the expressions in (7.4) to find the regions of p_1 and p_3 for which action a_1 is the Bayes procedures (Figures 7.4 and 7.5).

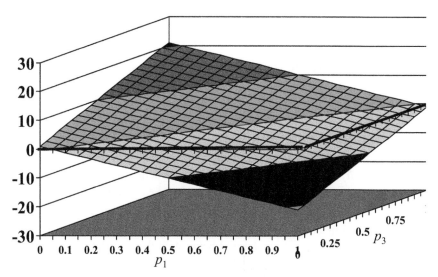

Figure 7.4 Deciding the patient is Alzheimer's disease free is preferred to additional testing.

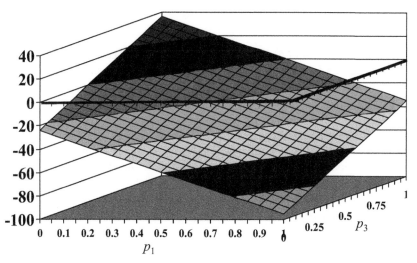

Figure 7.5 Deciding the patient is Alzheimer's disease free has lower risk than deciding the patient has the disease.

Thus the Bayes action is a_1,(i.e. $\delta_B = a_1$) if $R(a_1) \leq R(a_2)$ and, simultaneously $R(a_1) \leq R(a_3)$, which implies

$$1 - 21p_1 + 25p_3 < p_1 + 5p_3$$
$$1 - 21p_1 + 25p_3 < 25 + 50p_1 - 35p_3.$$

Similar inequalities must be solved to find the regions for which $\delta_B = a_2$ and $\delta_B = a_3$.

∎

7.5 Continuous Loss Functions

Continuous values loss functions, commonly expressed as $L(\theta, \delta_B)$, play an important role in identifying Bayes procedures. The Bayes actions generated by continuous loss functions are typically actions of estimation, i.e., "estimate θ by δ_B". Here, δ_B is a function of the posterior distribution of θ. For continuous valued loss functions, tables of loss function values are usually not informative.

As has been our custom, we will begin with the simplest formulations of these continuous loss functions, building our intuition as we add increasing layers of sophistication and realism to the loss function.

7.5.1 Linear Loss

We begin with simplest loss function, linear loss

$$L(\theta, \delta_B) = \theta - \delta_B. \tag{7.5}$$

While the simple form of (7.5) is attractive, its utility is reduced by the observation that minimizing this loss function (and the associated risk) is simply achieved by choosing the largest value of δ_B possible. In reality, this is commonly an unacceptable option.

Example 7.4: West Nile Virus Infection Rates

The prevalence of West Nile viral infections in West Texas is low, primarily because of this region's exceedingly dry climate. Let θ be the prevalence of this condition. The investigators believe that the true prevalence is less than 5 per million subjects, but have no real idea how small it is within this interval. They assume that the prior distribution $\pi(\theta) = 200,0001_{\theta \in [0,.000005]}$, i.e., the uniform distribution on the interval $[0, 5/1,000,000]$. Minimizing the risk with respect to (7.5) simply requires us to choose the largest value of δ_B possible, or $\delta_B = 0.000005$.

If the number of subjects in this region infected with West Nile virus were believed to follow a Poisson distribution with parameter θ, then the posterior distribution loss function with respect to this distribution is

$$\pi(\theta \mid x) = \frac{\left(\dfrac{\theta^x}{x!}e^{-\theta}\right)(200,000)\mathbf{1}_{\theta \in [0,.0.000005]}}{\displaystyle\int_0^{0.000005}\left(\dfrac{\theta^x}{x!}e^{-\theta}\right)(200,000)\mathbf{1}_{\theta \in [0,.0.000005]}\,d\theta}.$$

Now, assume that, during the observation period, no patient has arrived with West Nile virus infection. In this case, the posterior distribution simplifies to

$$\pi(\theta \mid x = 0) = \frac{(200,000)e^{-\theta}\mathbf{1}_{\theta \in [0,.0.000005]}}{\displaystyle\int_0^{0.000005}(200,000)e^{-\theta}\,d\theta} = \frac{e^{-\theta}\mathbf{1}_{\theta \in [0,.0.000005]}}{1 - e^{-0.000005}} \qquad (7.6)$$

$$= (200,000)e^{-\theta}\mathbf{1}_{\theta \in [0,.0.000005]}$$

which is just a simple exponential distribution scaled to the [0, 0.000005] interval. However, using linear loss, the best estimator of the infection rate θ remains the maximum possible value, $\delta_B = 0.000005$. In this case, assuming a linear loss function leads to the conclusion that we should choose the highest possible infection rate regardless of the new evidence presented by the data. This is a rarely useful assumption in biostatistics.[*]

7.5.2 Weighted Linear Loss
A much more useful relationship that preserves the simple linearity of loss function is weighted linear loss, expressed as

$$L(\theta, \delta_B) = K_1(\theta - \delta_B)\mathbf{1}_{\theta > \delta_B} + K_2(\delta_B - \theta)\mathbf{1}_{\theta \le \delta_B}. \qquad (7.7)$$

Here, K_1 and K_2 are known weights, assigned much like weights were assigned in the dichotomous loss function tables of section 7.3. In this formulation, loss $K_1(\theta - \delta_B)$ is assigned when δ_B underestimates θ, and loss K_2 multiplies the linear loss assigned for overestimates (Figure 7.6).

---

[*] However, there are procedures, called minimax rules which choose as the action the procedure that minimizes the probability of the worst possible outcome (i.e., the outcome with the worst loss).

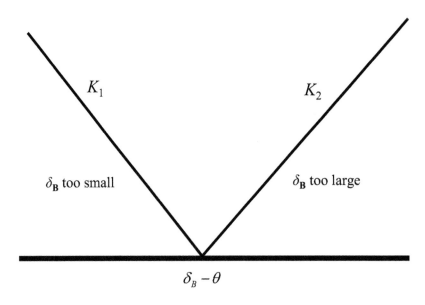

$$\delta_B - \theta$$

Figure 7.6. Characteristics of weighted linear loss

Before we do any formal calculations, consideration of (7.7) can generate some useful insight into the identity of the Bayes procedure.

When $K_1 > K_2$, the investigator plays a greater price for underestimating θ, suggesting that larger values of δ_B should be selected. Assume from Figure 7.6 that $K_1 = 40$ and $K_2 = 10$, and $\theta = 70$. If the investigator chooses to estimate θ by a value less than 70, e.g., $\delta_B = 60$, then the loss that she sustains is $L(\theta, \delta_B) = 40(70 - 60) = 400$. However, should she choose to estimate θ by a value greater than 70 e.g., $\delta_B = 80$, the value of the sustained loss is less, i.e., $L(\theta, \delta_B) = 10(80 - 70) = 100$. The immediate conclusion from this example is that when underestimation of θ produces a larger loss, the investigator is driven to select larger values of δ_B (Figure 7.7). Thus, from Figure 7.7, the price the investigator pays for underestimating the parameter θ increases drives the investigator to choose a larger value for δ_B.[*]

In the reverse situation, when the loss function requires a heavy penalty for overestimating θ by δ_B, the investigator is motivated to reduce the loss function by choosing a smaller value of δ_B (Figure 7.8). When underestimation and overes-

---

[*]If K_1 was 10,000, and K_2 is 0.001, the price the investigator pays for underestimating θ is so large, that they may want to choose the maximum possible value for δ_B.

timation of θ by the same amount produce equal loss, then a value of δ_B that is close to the center of the distribution appears more appropriate.

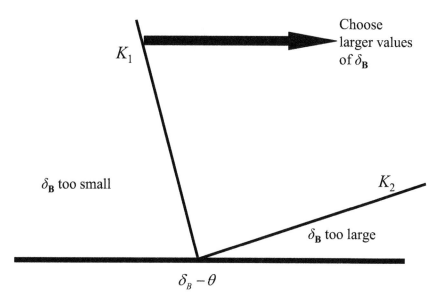

Figure 7.7. As the loss for choosing a value of δ_B less than θ grows, the drive to select a larger value δ_B increases.

that when $K_1 = K_2$, δ_B is the median of the distribution of θ.

Example 7.5: Reactive Airway Disease

Asthma is a reactive airway disease. When exposed to an irritant, the immune cells in the bronchial linings release a substance that causes the muscles in these airways to constrict, restricting the airflow to the alveoli where gas exchange takes place. In one context, these actions can be viewed as protective since they keep the allergen from getting deeper into the lung tissue, while sending a clear signal to the person that they should immediately go to an area where they can breathe. However, the chronic effects of asthma include discomfort, reduced activity level, low blood oxygen level, and in *status asthmaticus*, can produce death.

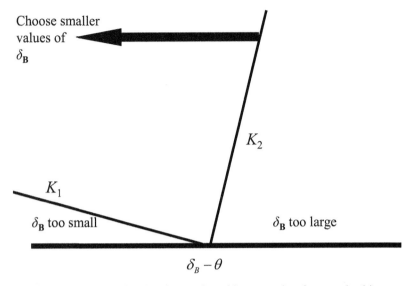

Choose smaller values of δ_B

K_2

K_1

δ_B too small

δ_B too large

$\delta_B - \theta$

Figure 7.8. As the loss for choosing a value of δ_B greater than θ grows, the drive to select a smaller value δ_B increases.

This line of reasoning is the motivation for the selection of the Bayes procedure for weighted linear loss.

For a loss function of

$$L(\theta, \delta_B) = K_1(\theta - \delta_B)1_{\theta > \delta_B} + K_2(\delta_B - \theta)1_{\theta \leq \delta_B},$$

then δ_B **is the** $\dfrac{K_1}{K_1 + K_2}$ **percentile value of the distribution of** θ.

The formal proof of this is readily available [1]. We can use this result to conclude

One of the measures of lung function in patients with asthma is the forced expiratory volume at one second (FEV$_1$). The patient is strongly encouraged to exhale as much air as possible from their lungs in one second. The smaller the FEV$_1$, the smaller the force of the air generated by the patient, the greater the impediment offered to normal lung function by their asthma.

A physician is caring for a 23 year old Hispanic female with asthma. The patient is 56 inches (1.4 meters) tall. Her predicted FEV$_1$ in liters [2] (f_p) is

$$f_p = (3.2138 * (\text{height in meters})) - (0.0243 * (\text{age in years})) - 1.4184$$
$$= 3.2138(1.4) - 0.0243(23) - 1.4184$$
$$= 2.52.$$

An FEV_1 is considered normal if it exceeds 80% of its predicted value. The investigator is interested in estimating his patient's FEV_1 and determining if it is in the normal range.

In his careful deliberation, this physician must balance the import of underestimations and overestimations of the FEV_1, θ. If he underestimates the FEV_1 he runs the risk of over-medicating his patient. Since all medications have risks associated with them, the unnecessary use of a medication (and the financial cost that his patient must bear for the medication) must be considered.

However, overestimating the FEV_1 poses its own share of difficulties. In this circumstance the physician would conclude that the patient's lung function was better than it actually was. This would lead to under treatment of the asthma, permitting the patient's condition to "break through" the prescribed therapy. The consequences of this would be an urgent trip to the emergency room, and the new prescription of emergency medications to get the patient's asthma under control. He has decided that this risk of missing an abnormally low FEV_1 is 5 to 10 times greater than underestimating its value. He chooses the ratio of the risks as 8. Therefore, his Bayes estimator will be the $1/(1+8) = 0.11$ of the 11th percentile of the posterior distribution.

Assume that the prior distribution, $\pi(\theta)$ is normal with known mean μ and variance v^2. The physician has one measurement of FEV_1 (x) which he assumes is normally distribution with mean θ and variance σ^2. Then we know the posterior distribution of θ is normal with mean u_p and variance v_p^2 where

$$u_p = \frac{v^2}{v^2 + \sigma^2} x + \frac{\sigma^2}{v^2 + \sigma^2} \mu;$$

$$(7.8)$$

$$v_p^2 = \frac{v^2 \sigma^2}{v^2 + \sigma^2}.$$

Previous measurements of this asthmatic patient suggest that the mean of the prior distribution is 2.10 with standard deviation of 0.40, reflecting the patient's difficulty with sustaining a normal FEV_1 and her continued need for medication. A new assessment reveals a substantial improvement in her FEV_1 with $x = 2.70$. The standard deviation of this reading, σ, is 0.40. Using equation (7.8) the posterior distribution of the patient's FEV_1 has a mean FEV_1 of 2.32 with standard deviation 0.24 (Figure 7.9).

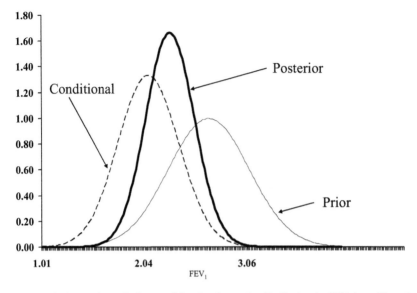

Figure 7.9. Comparison of prior, conditional and posterior distribution for FEV_1 in an Hispanic female with asthma.

The 11th percentile of this posterior distribution is 2.02, which is just at the lower bound of normal (80% of the predicted FEV_1). Thus, the physician decides to leave the patient's medications, initiated when her FEV_1 was clearly below normal, at their current level despite her apparent improvement because of the loss function's emphasis on avoiding an overestimation of her breathing capacity.   ∎

7.5.3 Square Error Loss

The loss function $L(\theta, \delta_B) = (\theta - \delta_B)^2$, known as squared error loss is the most popular loss function for Bayes procedures. Its symmetry is attractive in many estimation problems, and the identity of the Bayes procedures for this loss function is tractable for many recognizable probability distributions. The simple application of calculus reveals that for squared error loss, the Bayes procedure is simply the mean of the posterior distribution.

For a loss function of

$$L(\theta, \delta_B) = (\theta - \delta_B)^2,$$

then δ_B is the mean of the posterior distribution of θ

This result follows from the elementary application of calculus. We wish to find the value of δ_B that minimizes the risk $R(\theta,\delta_B) = \sum_\theta (\theta - \delta_B)^2 \pi(\theta \mid x_1,x_2,x_3,...x_n)$.

Expanding the quadratic term, we write

$$R(\theta,\delta_B) = \sum_\theta (\theta - \delta_B)^2 \pi(\theta \mid x_1,x_2,x_3,...x_n)$$
$$= \sum_\theta (\theta^2 - 2\theta\delta_B + \delta_B^2) \pi(\theta \mid x_1,x_2,x_3,...x_n)$$

In order to minimize $R(\theta,\delta_B)$, we need to take a derivative of the risk. However, since we will be taking a derivative with respect to δ_B, the derivative will pass through the summation with respect to θ. We can therefore write

$$\frac{dR(\theta,\delta_B)}{d\delta_B} = \sum_\theta \frac{d(\theta^2 - 2\theta\delta_B + \delta_B^2)}{d\delta_B} \pi(\theta \mid x_1,x_2,x_3,...x_n)$$
$$= \sum_\theta (-2\theta + 2\delta_B) \pi(\theta \mid x_1,x_2,x_3,...x_n).$$

We set this equal to zero to find where the slope changes and solve

$$\sum_\theta (-2\theta + 2\delta_B) \pi(\theta \mid x_1,x_2,x_3,...x_n) = 0$$
$$2\delta_B \sum_\theta \pi(\theta \mid x_1,x_2,x_3,...x_n) = 2\sum_\theta \theta\pi(\theta \mid x_1,x_2,x_3,...x_n)$$
$$\delta_B = \sum_\theta \theta\pi(\theta \mid x_1,x_2,x_3,...x_n).$$

Taking the second derivative and observing that it is positive for this value of δ_B allows us to conclude that the mean of the posterior distribution minimizes the risk.

Example 7.6: Modeling Drug Approval Activity

An executive at a major pharmaceutical company is interested in modeling the drug approval activity of the Federal Food and Drug Administration (FDA) advisory committees. The FDA is charged by federal law to determine whether drugs and devices are safe and effective for maintaining the good health and well being of the US population. Drug companies submit a new drug application (NDA) to the FDA for its review, and ultimately, the FDA decides to either approve the drug for use or not. Frequently, the agency will ask for the advice of a standing committee of outside specialists on whether a product should receive approval for a specific new use (known as an indication). Let the probability that an advisory committee will vote for approval of a drug or device be θ.

The drug approval process can be complex and the probability of approval is based on many factors including, but not limited to 1) the evidence for the effectiveness of the compound, 2) the constellation of adverse events[*] associated with the intervention, 3) the state of knowledge about the disease, 4) the natural history of the disease, 5) the availability of other treatments and their safety record.

The worker chooses a beta distribution for $\pi(\theta)$, whose form is

$$\frac{\Gamma(\alpha+\beta)}{\Gamma(\alpha)\Gamma(\beta)}\theta^{\alpha-1}(1-\theta)^{\beta-1}\mathbf{1}_{0\leq\theta\leq1}.$$

The beta distribution is a rich family of distributions, with a wide variety of shapes on the [0,1] interval (Figure 7.10).

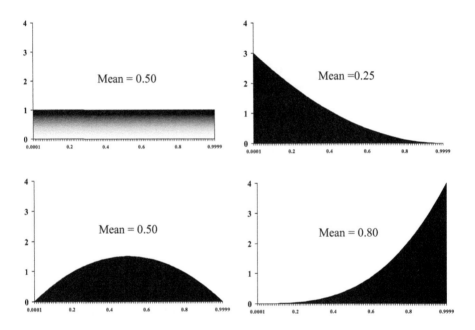

Figure 7.10. Members of the beta family of distributions.

Its mean is $\alpha/(\alpha+\beta)$.

It is important to understand the context in which this distribution is used. The scientist does not necessarily believe that the probability distribution of θ actually follows this complicated, functional form. He does believe that the character of the prior information is captured by this family of distributions. As the prior infor-

---

[*] Adverse events are side effects reasonably believed to be associated with the drug or device under consideration.

mation for θ changes over time with the accumulation of additional data and accompanying new insight, it might become useful to change from the beta family of distributions to another functional form, or to combine the beta distribution with other probability distributions. The purpose therefore is to accurately capture the relevant information about the prior information, not just cleave to a convenient functional form of the distribution. In this circumstance, the worker believes that the mean of the distribution is 0.667, and selects $\alpha = 10$, and $\beta = 10$.

The observer uses the binomial distribution to capture the conditional distribution of the number of approved projects. In this case

$$P[X = x] = \binom{n}{x} \theta^x (1-\theta)^{n-x}. \tag{7.9}$$

Appendix K reveals that when the prior distribution is beta with parameters α and β, and the conditional distribution is binomial, represented by (7.9), then the posterior distribution may be written as

$$\pi(\theta \mid x) = \frac{\Gamma(n+\alpha+\beta)}{\Gamma(\alpha+x)\Gamma(n-x+\beta)} \theta^{\alpha+x-1} (1-\theta)^{n-x+\beta-1} 1_{0 \leq \theta \leq 1}$$

which is a beta distribution with parameters $\alpha + x$ and $n - x + \beta$. The mean of the beta distribution is $\dfrac{\alpha + x}{n + \alpha + \beta}$. The squared error loss function tells us that the Bayes procedure, δ_B, is the mean of the posterior distribution. Note the mean has been updated from that of the prior, $\dfrac{\alpha}{\alpha + \beta}$, to now include the conditional data in the form of x and n.

The worker learns that from a random selection of advisory committees, 89 products were considered for approval of which 70 received a vote for approval. This permits the construction of the posterior distribution, and the Bayes procedure under this squared error loss is 0.769 (Figure 7.11).

Figure 7.11 reveals the upward translation of the distribution of FDA advisory committee approval vote proportion. However although squared error loss produced a convenient Bayes estimator, its foundation assumption that overestimation and underestimation of equal magnitudes share equal loss, would draw serious criticism from industry workers who understand just how expensive the drug development and approval process is. A more realistic loss function might more heavily weight the loss generated by overestimation of the advisory committee's propensity to provide an affirmative approval vote.

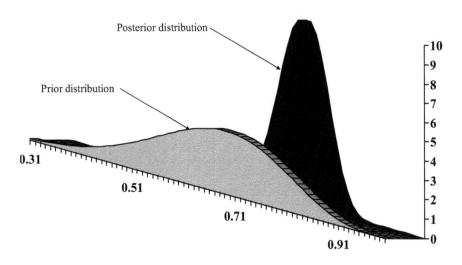

Figure 7.11. The prior and posterior distribution for the percent of products approved by a random selection of FDA advisory committees from 1998 to 2005. Each distribution is from the beta family.

7.6 The Need for Realistic Loss Functions

Loss functions used in didactic treatment of Bayes procedures are commonly simple formulations that demonstrate their utility without the introduction of complex formulations. However, these demonstrations must not be considered adequate substitutions for reality.

Typically, loss functions are quite complex, requiring flexibility and an understanding of the complications of the underlying circumstances. This real life complexity can require mathematical complications as the following example illustrates.

Example 7.7: Loss Function for Blood Sugar Measurement

A diabetology clinic is a clinic that focuses on the screening of patients for diabetes mellitus and their treatment. Modern medicine currently accepts blood sugar measurement as a critical measure to follow in patients with diabetes mellitus, a disease of abnormal glucose metabolism. The clinic is interested in incorporating Bayes procedures into its measurements of patient blood sugar.

Normally, blood sugar levels tend to remain between 60–100 milligrams per deciliter (mg/dl), increasing after a meal containing large quantities of sugar, and steadily declining until the next glucose ingestion. The blood sugar level decline is the result of the body cells absorbing and utilizing glucose (the body's principle source of chemical energy). In diabetes mellitus, the cells are unable to absorb blood glucose that is provided by food ingestion. The blood glucose levels slowly rise over months and years, as the body's ability to successfully absorb sugar into the cells declines. When the blood sugar rises to over 200 mg/dl, there is so much unutilized glucose in the blood that it actually filtered out by the kidneys into the urine.[*] It if rises to levels substantially higher than that, coma and death can follow. Thus accurate assessments of patients with high blood sugar levels are critical, and underestimates are to be avoided.

However, diabetic patients who are treated with insulin to reduce their blood sugar commonly have the reverse problem — abnormally low blood sugar. While insulin is an effective treatment tool for diabetes management, it can be a difficulty medicine to manage successfully, producing large swings in the blood sugar level if too much is given, or the dose is self-administered by the patient too early. In addition, any changes in the patient's eating or exercise pattern can amplify the effect of the patient's standard insulin dose. Decreases in blood glucose levels to 20 mg/dl or less produce convulsions, coma and death from hypoglycemia.[†]

Thus, both underestimation of abnormally high blood sugars, and overestimation of abnormally low blood sugar can each produce important delays in response to the diabetic patient. However, if one were to construct a loss function for the estimation of blood sugar θ, the loss function's shape actually depends on the location of θ, the patient's blood sugar level. In a patient who is recognized to be hypoglycemic, with frequent excursions of blood sugar into the abnormally low range, than the worst error in blood sugar assessment is overestimation. The loss function in this case should be more heavily weighted to Bayes procedures that are in the lower tail of the distribution.

Alternatively, patients whose blood glucose levels frequently are much greater than normal pay no profound price if their blood sugar level is overestimated. However, should their blood sugar be assessed at a lower level than it actually is, a critical opportunity to reduce blood glucose level from a dangerously high level may be lost. For these patients, a greater loss is paid for underestimation of blood glucose levels.

Patients who are screened for diabetes will have yet a different loss function. This may be more equally balanced between underestimation and overestimation of blood glucose levels.

For each of these loss functions, there will be a different Bayes procedure.

This more realistic loss function would be written as

$$L(\theta, \delta_{\mathbf{B}}) = K_1(\theta - \delta_{\mathbf{B}})\mathbf{1}_{\delta_{\mathbf{B}} \leq \theta \leq \theta_1} + K_2(\delta_{\mathbf{B}} - \theta)\mathbf{1}_{\theta \leq \delta_{\mathbf{B}} \leq \theta_1} + (\theta - \delta_{\mathbf{B}})^2\mathbf{1}_{\theta_1 \leq \theta \leq \theta_2}$$
$$= + K_3(\theta - \delta_{\mathbf{B}})\mathbf{1}_{\theta_1 \leq \delta_{\mathbf{B}} \leq \theta \leq \theta_2} + K_2(\delta_{\mathbf{B}} - \theta)\mathbf{1}_{\theta_1 \leq \theta \leq \delta_{\mathbf{B}} \leq \theta_2}.$$

---

[*] In fact, the diabetes mellitus means "sweet urine."
[†] Deliberate induction of hypoglycemia-induced convulsions used to be an accepted treatment for schizophrenia.

where θ_1 and θ_2 are the values of the blood glucose the values at which the loss function changes shape (Figure 7.12).

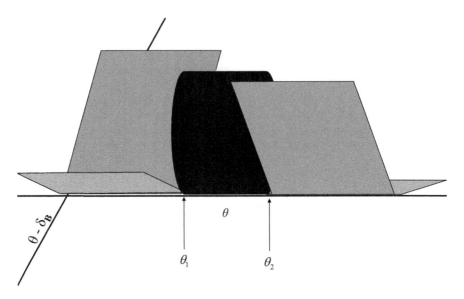

Figure 7.12. Proposed combined loss function for measuring blood glucose in a population of patients with diabetes mellitus.

We will see other examples of realistic loss functions in Chapter Eight.

Problems

1. A project manager for a clinical trial designed to assess the impact of therapy on elevations in diastolic blood pressure (DBP) is interested in devising a decision tool for screening incoming patients. The protocol of the study says that patients with a true DBP of greater than or equal to 85 mm Hg should be included. She pays a loss of 10 if she inappropriately admits a patient to the study when that patient does not have elevated DBP, and a loss of 8 if she inappropriately denies entry of a patient to the screening program. There is no loss sustained (i.e., $L(\theta, \delta_B) = 0$) for a correct decision. Assume that the posterior distribution of the true DBP (θ) is normal with a mean 82 mm Hg and standard deviation 7. Compute the minimum probability that a patient's DBP should be greater than 85 mm Hg before the patient is entered into the study.

2. A clinical trial is being monitored by an external monitoring group with the power to prematurely end the study. If they appropriately decide to end the study prematurely, the loss incurred by the study is -50. However, if they decide to prematurely end the study, proclaiming a therapy benefit when one does not exist, the loss to the study is 500. By inappropriately deciding that the study should be permitted to its schedule conclusion, the investigators would pay a loss of 100. Appropriately deciding the study should run its course produces a loss of zero. The investigators generate a test statistic that follows a standard normal distribution, large values supporting that the study should be discontinued, small values suggesting that the study should be continued. Find the smallest value of this normally distributed random variable that would suggest the study should be discontinued early.

3. A worker is interested in identifying the rate at which young men and women at a small college were not vaccinated for measles as children. The posterior distribution of the vaccination rate follows a beta distribution with parameters $\alpha = 0.5$ and $\beta = 6$. Assume the loss function is weighted linear loss where the risk of underestimating θ if five times greater than the loss of overestimating θ. Find the Bayes procedure, δ_B .

4. The "funding line" at national organizations that sponsor research is the score below which funds are granted to research application. Researchers submit applications whose contents are reviewed by these agencies. Upon completion of the review, the application is given a score, ranging from 0 to 1. The lowest score (0) reflects the highest caliber of research, and the highest score (1) reflects the worst research. Assume that no loss is paid for research that is high quality and funded, nor is a loss paid for lower quality research that isn't funded. Assume, however, that the loss of funding low quality research is 15 times greater than the loss of not funding high quality research. Assume the research score follows a beta distribution with $\alpha = 1$ and $\beta = 5$. Compute the funding line, that is the maximum research score for funding.

5. A neurologist examines a patient with symptoms suggesting that the patient is having either a transient ischemic attack (TIA) or a stroke. A TIA produces symptoms that will resolve within 24 hours, while a stroke generates permanent brain damage. Assume the posterior distribution of the duration of time this patient's symptoms persist follows a gamma distribution with $\alpha = 2$ and $r = 0.1$.
    a. Using squared error loss, compute the duration of symptoms for this patient.
    b. Using weighted linear loss where underestimation and overestimation of the patient's symptoms are believed to be equally costly, compute the duration of this patient's symptoms.

c. Using weighted linear loss where overestimation of the patient's symptoms are believed to be twice as costly as underestimation, compute the duration of this patient's symptoms.

References

1. Berger J.O. (1980). *Statistical Decision Theory: Foundations, Concepts, and Methods*. New York. Springer. P. 111–112.
2. Coultas D.B., Howard C.A., et al. (1988). Spirometric prediction equations for Hispanic children and adults in New Mexico. *American Review of Respiratory Disease* **138**: 1386–1392. (Table 4, page 1390).

Chapter 8
P tting It All Together

8.1 Introduction

We can now assemble a complete Bayes procedure. Our coverage of the law of total probability and Bayes theorem (Chapters Two and Three), discussions about prior distribution assembly, and the conversations concerning the loss function and Bayes risk (Chapter Seven) place us in the perfect position to construct a Bayes procedure from beginning to end in biostatistical settings.

In this chapter, we will consider two Bayes procedures, one from stoke neurology, and the second from the epidemiology of viral disease. Each case will begin with a discussion of background material to build up some intuition concerning the medical issue at hand. This will be followed by development of the prior distribution, the conditional distribution, and the loss function. From this step we will construct the Bayes procedure, examine some of its properties, and see how it changes based on small alterations in the prior distribution.

8.2 Illustration 1: Stroke Treatment

This example illustrates the construction of a Bayes estimate for the treatment of acute stroke with tissue-plasminogen activator (tPA).

8.2.1 Background

Cerebrovascular accidents (CVAs or strokes) are abrupt interruptions of blood flow to the brain. These interruptions lead to massive brain cell death, producing paralysis, loss of cognitive function, and, in extreme cases, coma and death.

Stroke is the number one cause of adult disability in the United States and the third leading cause of death. Approximately 600,000 people have a new or recurrent stroke each year in the U.S. Of these 500,000 are first attacks, and 100,000 are recurrent attacks. More men than women have strokes [1]. In the United States, stroke mortality fell by 15.1% from 1988 to 1998, but the actual number of stroke deaths rose 5.3% [1,2].

In many respects, strokes are similar to heart attacks. Both strokes and heart attacks commonly have the same mechanism of production, i.e., the initiation and development of atherosclerotic plaques in major arteries that supply these two end organs (the brain and the heart) with nutrients and oxygen rich blood. The atheromatous gruel grows over time, fed by lipid rich macrophages, aggravated by high vascular pressures, and the vasoactive effects of smoking. The creation of a fissure in the plaque can activate the intricate collection of clotting mechanisms that leads to the rapid development of a thrombus, further narrowing the lumen of the blood vessels, leading to death of the supplied tissue.

The risk factors for stroke (older age, hypertension, unfavorable lipid panels, smoking) are closely related to those of heart attacks. In addition, treatment is the same. The first treatment, prevention, requires the modulation of risk factor levels. A second is the identification of major blood vessels that are at risk (carotid vessels for the brain, coronary arteries for the heart) including bypassing the lesions or end-arterectomy.

Finally, acute treatment for each includes the use of clot lysis therapy including tissue plasminogen activator or tPA. Tissue plasminogen activator is an anti-clotting medication. When administered during the first few hours of a stroke's symptoms, it can stop the formation of (and even break up) a stroke-producing blood clot that develops in the brain. However, tPA has its own risks.

The tendency of blood to clot must be carefully balanced. Blood that does not clot loses the ability to repair damaged blood vessels that are commonly injured or worn down in the process of daily living. Blood that does not clot quickly enough leads to a painfully debilitating and short life, as revealed by the natural history of patients with untreated hemophilia.

Alternatively, blood that is too likely to clot (i.e., it exists in a hypercoagulable state) leads to blood clot formation where they are neither required nor helpful. Such clots can break off, be carried though the blood stream, and lodge in small (and sometimes large) vessels. The blockage of blood flow leads to death of the tissue that relies on the blood flow, now impeded by the clot. The results of these clots are pulmonary embolisms (if the arteries to the lungs are blocked), and heart attacks (if a coronary artery, a vessel supplying the cardiac muscles own blood supply is blocked) or strokes (if the blood supply to the brain is blocked).

The mechanism by which blood clots form is one of most studied and complex biochemical mechanisms known, involving literally hundreds of reagents, enzymes, and coenzymes. However, tPA can potentially tip the balance of coagulation too far, producing dangerous bleeding in joints and internal organs, including the brain. Thus, great care must be used in its use.

Current recommendations are that tPA be given within three hours of the stroke's onset of symptoms. The risk of bleeding is always present. However, the clot-busting effects of tPA have been shown to be effective in reducing the size of strokes, thereby improving patient outcome if it is administered within three hours of a stroke. The feeling is that the earlier tPA is provided the less severe the patient's stroke is likely to be. Thus an important monitoring tool for how well a hospital is performing in stroke treat is the percent of patients who receive tPA treatment for their stroke therapy. The duration of time between the patient's first symptoms and the time the tPA is injected is known as the "symptom-to-needle" time.

While it is relatively easy for units to monitor the use of tPA in their own emergency rooms, it is almost impossible to learn the precise sequence of events for patients who have been transferred to the ER from another facility (transfer hospital). Typically, the patient is stabilized at the initial hospital, a stabilization procedure that commonly involves the treatment with tPA. However, rarely is the time that has elapsed between the patient's symptoms and the dose of tPA reported. Thus, when the patient arrives at the second hospital for definitive treatment, the doctor at the receiving institution knows that tPA has been given, but does not know the symptom to treatment time. In this example, health care workers will compute based on the severity of the stroke, the distribution of symptom-to-needle times.

8.2.2 Parameterization of the Problem
We will let θ be the symptom-to-needle time of a particular patient who had their stroke symptoms treated with tPA at an outlying hospital and were transferred to our institution where they were hospitalized. Let x be the number of days for which the patient is hospitalized. In this circumstance, $\pi(\theta)$ is the prior belief about the distribution of symptom to needle time at the outlying hospital. The conditional distribution $f(x|\theta)$ is the probability distribution of the duration of days hospitalized at our hospital. We must compute $\pi(\theta|x)$, the probability distribution of the symptom-to-needle time at the transferring institution given the duration of the patient's hospitalization in days at our hospital.

8.2.3 The Prior Distribution
There is substantial discussion about the distribution of the symptom-to-needle time θ at a transferring hospital. Several stroke neurologists believe that the exponential distribution, introduced in Chapter Three, characterizes their beliefs about the distribution of symptom-to-needle time (Figure 8.1). However, this distribution has a variety of shapes governed by the parameter λ. Fortunately, since the mean of the distribution is λ^{-1}, they can use the average value of the mean tPA time to guide the selection of λ. Although these scientists believe the mean tPA time is relative late (2.5 hours, corresponding to $\lambda = 0.40$), they think that, everything being equal, the probability of earlier tPA administration is greater than that of a later injection. In addition, since the symptom-to-needle time can only be between zero and three hours, the probability distribution must be normed so that it integrates to one over this finite range. This is easily accomplished by dividing the probability function by the $P[X \leq 3] = 1 - e^{-0.40(3)} = 1 - e^{-1.2}$. Thus, their prior distribution of

choice is $\dfrac{0.40e^{-0.40\theta}}{1 - e^{-1.2}}$ for $0 \leq X \leq 3$.

However, other experts reject this distribution's shape, arguing that it is difficult to deliver tPA early. The time it takes for patients to 1) recognize that their symptom complex requires emergency care, and 2) transit to the emergency room for care precludes early hospital arrival, making early tPA distribution impossible. Thus this group of neurologists believes that the distribution of symptom to treatment time follows a exponential distribution scaled to have all times be between 0 and 3, but with the maximum probability occurring at time $t = 3$ not $t = 0$.

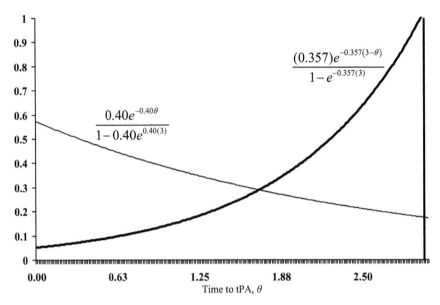

Figure 8.1. Competing beliefs about the symptom-to-needle time for tPA use. Some stroke neurologists believe that outlying hospitals are more likely to provide tPA therapy early, while others believe these institutions tend to give it later. The maximum permissible time is three hours.

They also believe that the mean symptom-to-onset time is somewhat later, 2.8 hours, corresponding to $\lambda = 0.357$. Thus, their form for the prior distribution is $\dfrac{(0.357)e^{-0.357(3-\theta)}}{1-e^{-0.357(3)}}$, also normalized so that the probability that the symptom to nee-dle time θ is within three hours (Figure 8.1).

.   Other experts react, claiming that the patients who arrive late fall outside the three hour window and never receive tPA. These discussions continue, leading to the compromise position of mixing the two distributions. They eventually decide on the following prior distribution mixture for θ,

$$\pi(\theta) = 0.30\frac{0.40e^{-0.40\theta}}{1-e^{-0.40(3)}} + 0.70\frac{(0.357)e^{-0.357(3-\theta)}}{1-e^{-0.357(3)}} \tag{8.1}$$

the weights 0.30 and 0.70 reflecting the final consensus beliefs in the likelihood of the two philosophies about the symptom-to-needle time (Figure 8.2).

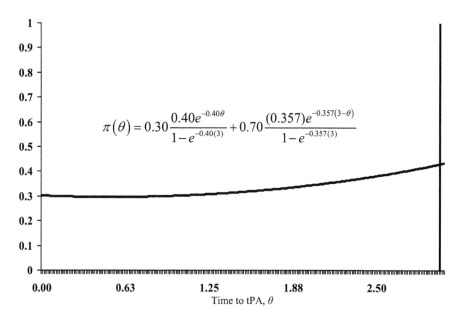

Figure 8.2. Consensus *a priori* belief about the symptom-to-needle time, with weights 0.30 and 0.70.

8.2.4 Conditional Distribution

It is generally accepted that early tPA use produces reduced stroke size, with consequent lower stroke death rates, and reduced hospitalizations. In patients who do not die during the hospitalization, the distribution of hospitalization stay follows a Poisson distribution with parameter $g(\theta)$, where θ is the symptom-to-needle time.

In this circumstance $g(\theta) = \dfrac{72\theta}{24\,\text{hours day}^{-1}} = 3\theta$. For example, if $\theta = 3$ hours, then

the mean duration of stay is (72)(3)=216 hours, or $216\!\!\big/\!\!24 = 9\,\text{days}$. Thus the conditional distribution of the duration of hospital stay in days is

$$f(x\mid\theta) = P[x = k \mid \theta] = \frac{(3\theta)^k}{k!}e^{-3\theta} \tag{8.2}$$

(Figure 8.3).

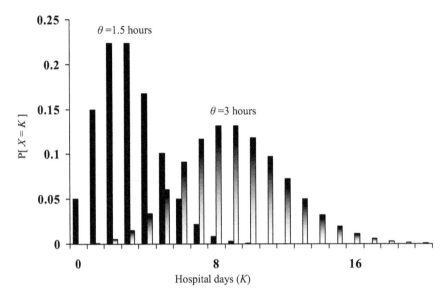

Figure 8.3. Distribution of hospital stay as a function of symptom-to-needle time, θ

8.2.5 Loss Functions

The investigators are interested in two interrogations. The first is to compute the Bayes estimate, δ_B, of the symptom-to-needle time from the transfer hospital, given the duration of hospital stay, k. In this circumstance, squared error loss is inappropriate, given that the penalty for underestimation are different than that of an equivalent overestimation.

If θ is large, the investigators intend to work with the transferring hospital in an attempt to reduce it. This includes contacting the transferring hospital to collect additional data concerning their symptom-to-needle time and also to educate the hospital's emergency room staff about this procedure. This effort would be wasted when the investigators believe the symptom-to-needle time is longer than it is. However, if θ if underestimated, then the transferring hospital may be treating stroke patients sub-optimally, a state of affairs that would produce avoidable morbidity and mortality. The loss in this case is substantially greater than that of underestimation. The investigators decide that the loss of an underestimation is twenty times greater than that of overestimation. Using the results from Chapter Seven, the Bayes procedure will be the $20\big/(20+1) = $ 95th percentile of the posterior distribution of θ.

8.2.6 Identifying the Posterior Distribution

With the prior distribution identified, and the loss function in place, we are in a position to find and evaluate the posterior distribution.

Recall that

$$\pi(\theta \mid x) = \frac{f(x \mid \theta)\pi(\theta)}{\sum_\theta f(x \mid \theta)\pi(\theta)} \tag{8.3}$$

which here becomes

$$\pi(\theta \mid x) = \frac{\dfrac{(3\theta)^k}{k!}e^{-3\theta}\left[0.30\dfrac{0.40e^{-0.40\theta}}{1-e^{-0.40(3)}} + 0.70\dfrac{(0.357)e^{-0.357(3-\theta)}}{1-e^{-0.357(3)}}\right]1_{\theta\in[0,3]}}{\displaystyle\sum_\theta \dfrac{(3\theta)^k}{k!}e^{-3\theta}\left[0.30\dfrac{0.40e^{-0.40\theta}}{1-e^{-0.40(3)}} + 0.70\dfrac{(0.357)e^{-0.357(3-\theta)}}{1-e^{-0.357(3)}}\right]1_{\theta\in[0,3]}} . \tag{8.4}$$

The only real challenge in expression (8.4)'s evaluation is the denominator. We use Appendix L to see that the denominator can be simplified to

$$0.429\frac{3^k}{k!}\int_0^3 \theta^k e^{-3.4\theta}d\theta \; + \; 0.365\frac{3^k}{k!}\int_0^3 \theta^k e^{-2.64\theta}d\theta,$$

which can be computed for values of k, allowing us to write the posterior distribution as

$$\pi(\theta \mid x) = \frac{\dfrac{3^k}{k!}\left[(0.172)\theta^k e^{-3.4\theta} + (0.130)\theta^k e^{-2.64\theta}\right]}{0.172\dfrac{3^k}{k!}\int_0^3 \theta^k e^{-3.4\theta}d\theta \; + \; 0.130\dfrac{3^k}{k!}\int_0^3 \theta^k e^{-2.64\theta}d\theta}$$

$$= \frac{\left[(0.172)\theta^k e^{-3.4\theta} + (0.130)\theta^k e^{-2.64\theta}\right]1_{\theta\in[0,3]}}{0.172\int_0^3 \theta^k e^{-3.4\theta}d\theta \; + \; 0.130\int_0^3 \theta^k e^{-2.64\theta}d\theta} \tag{8.5}$$

The distribution of the symptom-to-treatment time as a function of k, the duration of the hospital stay is easily produced from the last line of expression (8.5) (Figure 8.4). Each curve represents the distribution of symptom to treatment time for a different duration of hospital stay in days, k. For $k = 4$, indicating that a patient had a short hospital stay, the probability distribution of the symptom to needle time is clustered to the left, suggesting that tPA was most likely given early after symptom onset. As k increases from 4 days, to 7 days, to 12 days, the probability of the symptom to needle time shifts to the right, indicating that it took longer for patients to receive their tPA at the outlying hospital.

We can compute the probability that patients received tPA within one hour of symptom onset $P[\theta < 1]$, and the δ_B which the investigators stated was the 95th percentile of the posterior distribution of θ (Table 8.1).

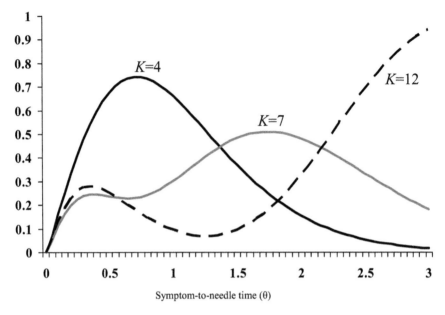

Symptom-to-needle time (θ)

Figure 8.4. Posterior distribution of symptom onset to tPA treatment time at a transferring hospital as a function of the duration of the hospital stay in days, K.

Table 8.1 Probability that symptom-to-needle time is less than one hour and the posterior estimate of symptom to onset time as a function of K the duration of hospital stay in days.

K	$P[\theta < 1]$	δ_B (days)
4	0.55	2.10
7	0.21	2.80
12	0.19	2.95

The posterior probability that the symptom-to-needle time is less than one hour decreases in an important and informative manner, demonstrating the large shift to longer symptom to onset times as the hospital duration increases.

Alternatively, the Bayes procedure does not produce a useful gradient as the hospital duration increases. Insisting on the 95th percentile for the Bayes estimate has essentially moved δ_B to the right extreme value of the symptom to treatment duration which can be no greater than three. This is a direct result of the loss function which placed a far greater loss on underestimating than overestimation of the symptom to treatment duration.

8.3 Illustration 2: Adverse Event Rates

A problem that bedevils the drug development industry is the identification of rare adverse events associated with a new, promising compound. We will develop a Bayes procedure that assists in the detection of an adverse event signal in the population at large after the drug has been approved and is in general use.

8.3.1 Background

Drug development programs of major pharmaceutical companies involve a substantial amount of energy as compounds are developed for human use. Beginning with chemical and biochemical assays, the compound must be rigorously tested in animals before it is permitted to enter human testing. Once in the human testing phase, the drug must first be demonstrated to be safe. This early evaluation takes place in what are Phase 1 studies, where normal volunteers are administered the compound under tightly controlled circumstances (typically in a special observation unit). Should the compound be deemed relatively safe in Phase I studies, it is then permitted to enter Phase II analyses, where it is tested in individuals who have the disease that the investigators believe will be ameliorated by the compound. Only after these Phase I and Phase II studies are successfully completed can the drug enter the pivotal Phase III studies, i.e., the clinical trials that reproduce on a larger scale the risk and benefits of the intervention that emerged from the Phase II studies. The demonstration of the intervention's safety and effectiveness at this level can lead to drug approval by the federal Food and Drug Administration (FDA).

The investigators, regulatory agency, and health practitioner community understand that all interventions have adverse effects[*] associated with them. These adverse effects range from minor symptoms (e.g., infrequent, mild nausea) to more serious problems (e.g., profound fatigue, blurred vision, palpitations, and diarrhea). Sometimes the side effects can be dangerous and life-threatening (e.g., heart attacks, toxic megacolon, primary pulmonary hypertension, cancer development, or birth defects).

Many times these adverse events occur so frequently that Phase II and Phase III clinical trials can identify them, producing estimates of their occurrence in the population. However, even though Phase III clinical trials typically recruit hundreds, if not thousands (and in some cases, tens of thousands of patients), it is

---

[*] According to the FDA, an adverse effect is defined as an undesirable side effect, reasonably believed to be associated with the drug. The agency does not require that the drug be shown to cause the adverse effect—only the association between the two needs to be demonstrated for a monitory to be required.

still possible that they will not reliably detect some adverse events. This detection inability occurs for two reasons.

First, the sample of patients selected for the Phase III studies may have different characteristics than those patients in the population in which the compound may ultimately be used. For example, a medication for the treatment of headaches may have produced only minor adverse effects in headache-prone, but otherwise healthy patients in a Phase III study, but produces an exacerbation of lung disease when used in patients who have asthma or bronchitis. Since only patients without these diseases were admitted to the Phase III study, the study was uninformative about all of the effects of the therapy in these patients. It is only after regulatory approval, when physicians are free to prescribe the medication widely to a population of patients with different medical histories and disease complexities that the full spectrum of the compound's effects become evident.

Secondly the Phase III studies may contain too few patients to discern the occurrence of rare but lethal adverse events. For example, severe, acute liver failure leading to either liver transplant or death occurs at the rate of 1 case per 1,000,000 patients per year in the United States. Assume that a new drug being evaluated in a pre-FDA approval clinical trial increases this incidence by tenfold, to 1 case per 100,000 patients exposed per year. The magnitude of this intervention's effect on the annual incidence of acute liver failure is a critical piece of information that both the private physician and the patient require as they jointly consider whether the risk of this drug is worth its benefits.

However, an important consequence of this tenfold increase in acute liver failure is that (on average) 100,000 patients would need to be exposed to this drug in order to be expected to see one case of acute liver failure per year. This sample size is much larger than the typical number of patients studied in Phase III clinical trials. Thus, the substantial increase in the rate of acute liver failure produced by the intervention would be invisible in smaller Phase III clinical trials which recruit and follow less than 1000 patients for 6 months. If this drug were approved and released for general dispersal through the population for which the drug is indicated, patients would unknowingly be exposed to a devastating, unpredicted adverse event. The fact that a clinical trial, not designed to detect an adverse effect, does not find the adverse effect is characterized by the saying "absence of evidence is not evidence of absence" [3]. This phrase summarizes the observation that the absence of evidence (within the clinical trial) that the drug is associated with a serious adverse event is not evidence that the compound will not generate this serious side effect in the population at large.

8.3.2 Statement of the Problem

A pharmaceutical company has developed a compound that it believes is effective in slowing the evolution of cardiovascular disease, and will reduce the occurrence of heart attacks. Since millions of patients are at risk of heart attack, the company understandably anticipates wide usage of its hypothetical drug, Clynym.

Phase II and Phase III testing demonstrate the effectiveness of the compound. However, the biochemistry of the drug suggest that it could have a harmful effect on the liver.

After the Phase II and III studies are complete, the company discusses the state of the relationship between Clynym and adverse effects affecting the liver. Not a single patient in either the Phase II study (consisting of 100 patients) or the Phase III study (consisting of 5,000 patients) developed liver disease after Clynym use. This, they argue, is the strongest sign that the drug is safe. However, others contend that the small sample sizes of the Phase II/III studies make it impossible to determine the effect on the liver. They note that the background rate of acute liver failure is one patient per million per year. A hundred fold, Clynym-generated increase in incidence of acute liver failure, would not be seen in a 5,000 patient study. However, the company does not have the resources to conduct a study involving the much larger number of patients needed to assure both itself and the FDA that the drug has no harmful liver effects.

The company has received approval to market Clynym; however, they have agreed to carry out a post approval evaluation of the effect of Clynym on the liver. The research design and biostatistics division of the company convinces the company to take a Bayesian approach to the estimate of the incidence of acute liver failure associated with their drug.

Let θ be the rate of occurrence of acute liver failure of patients taking Clynym. If the drug is not associated with this disease, then θ is 1 per million patients exposed per year. The goal is to estimate θ given the observed number of patients in the study *(K)* with acute liver failure.

8.3.3 Constructing the Prior Distribution

Assembly of the prior distribution for the incidence of Clynym-induced acute liver failure generates heated discussion within the company. In the absence of any patients identified in the Phase II/III evaluations, several scientists in the company argue that the prior distribution is simply that $\theta = 1$ per million per year. Others suggest that there should be variability around the belief that Clynym has no adverse effect on the liver, but that the distribution must focus attention on the strong conviction, supported by absence of data to the contrary, that the rate of acute liver failure is $\theta = 1$. The company scientists who believe Clynym is liver-safe put their support behind the distribution $\pi(\theta) = \dfrac{\alpha^r}{\Gamma(r)}\theta^{r-1}e^{-\alpha\theta}\mathbf{1}_{\theta\in[0,\infty]}$, selecting $\alpha = r = 0.0125$ (Figure 8.5). This prior has a mean value for θ of 1 patient per million per year. However it is tightly focused on the relatively smaller values of the incidence rate, consistent with the beliefs of many of the company's scientists. They vehemently lobby for this probability distribution, designated the conservative prior.

However, other scientists, alarmed by the plausibility of the suggested mechanism by which liver disease may be induced by Clynym, argue that this first proposed prior distribution puts too little emphasis on the distinct possibility that the drug may be hepatotoxic. They therefore suggest that the distribution should be shifted to the right, providing more support for the possibility of induced liver damage. They stay within the gamma family of distributions, but suggest different values of the distribution's parameters (Figure 8.6).

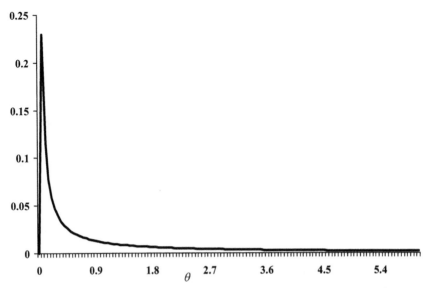

Figure 8.5. First suggested prior probability distributions for θ, the incidence of acute liver disease associated with Clynyn. The mean value θ under this distribution is one patient per million per year.

Figure 8.6 presents the alternative prior distributions for the rate of acute liver failure associated with Clynyn. Unlike the prior distribution displayed in the previous figure, these probability distributions place a greater probability on the possibility that the Clynyn may be hepatotoxic, as demonstrated by the larger mean values. However, even though the distribution places greater probability of the idea that the rate of Clynyn induced acute liver failure is larger than one patient per million exposed per year, the mean value of this rate, 1.34, is still small, a concession that they hope will win over the conservative prior's advocates.

However, the proponents of each figure's prior distribution become increasingly strident as the researchers painfully struggle to move toward a consensus. Those who argue for the conservative prior distribution that was tightly clustered around smaller values of the event rate θ claim that theirs is the only prior that is data-based, as opposed to "suspicion-based" perspective of the advocates of the priors of Figure 8.6. The proponents of the "vigilance priors" in Figure 8.6 state that the public must be protected from harm, and the company must be protected from lawsuits by patients claiming to sustain Clynyn-induced liver damage from their drug. The company, they argue, can be charged with negligence if its supports a prior distribution that ignores the warning provided by the Clynyn's mechanistic data suggesting an hepatotoxic effect of its drug.

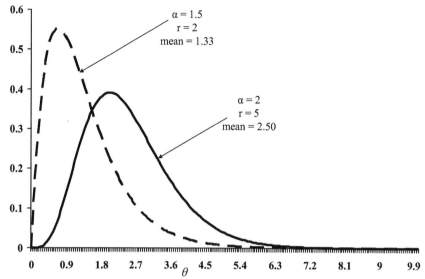

Figure 8.6. Alternative distributions for the prior probability of θ, the incidence of acute liver disease associated with Clynyn. These distributions assign greater probability to a hepatotoxic effect of the drug.

Each camp uses the argument that to give in the other is to allow the trial's results to be dictated by a self-fulfilling prophesy. Those who argue for the conservative prior of Figure 8.5 say that to support the vigilance priors in Figure 8.6 all but assures that the acute liver failure rate identified in the study will be larger than it actually is. To accept the vigilance priors is to feed the self-fulfilling prophesy that larger incidence rates for acute liver failure will be identified. Alternatively, advocates of Figure 8.6 argue that its conservative opponents wish to force the study results to conform with their false sense of security that derives from the results of Phase II/ III studies. All are conscious of the fact that hundreds of millions of dollars in the drug's development are at stake.

Finally, a consensus is reached. The official prior distribution of the study, $\pi(\theta)$, is

$$\pi(\theta) = (0.75)\frac{0.0125^{.00125}}{\Gamma(0.0125)}\theta^{0.0125-1}e^{-.0.01250} + (0.25)\frac{1.5^2}{\Gamma(2)}\theta^{2-1}e^{-1.50}. \qquad (8.6)$$

A mixture of two gamma distributions (Figure 8.9).

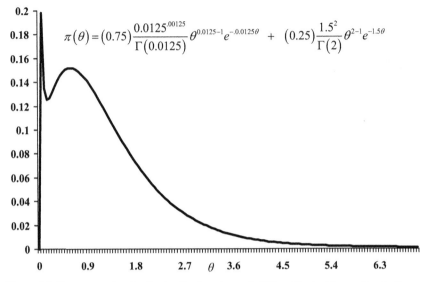

Figure 8.7. Consensus prior distribution for the prior probability of the incidence of acute liver disease associated with Clynyn. While most of the probability is concentrated at the smaller values of θ, there is a substantial tail probability supporting higher values.

The mixture is heavily weighted ($p = 0.75$) to the conservative prior distribution, but its heavy tail reflects the concerns of those who have argued for the vigilance prior.

8.3.4 Conditional Distribution
Settling on the form of the conditional distribution was uncontroversial. Since patients are assumed to develop acute liver failure independently of each other with an incidence rate of θ, the probability that there are k patients in 1,000,000 who develop acute liver failure is believed to follow a Poisson distribution with parameter θ,

$$P[X = k] = \frac{\theta^k}{k!} e^{-\theta}.$$

8.3.5 Loss Function
This is equally controversial, with the arguments for greater loss for overestimation balancing those for underestimation of the rate. The company settled on the median of the posterior distribution as their Bayes estimator.

8.3.6 Constructing the Posterior Distribution
The prior distribution is a mixture of two gamma distributions. To find the posterior distribution, we write

$$\pi(\theta \mid x = k) = \frac{f(k \mid \theta)\pi(\theta)}{\sum_{\theta} f(k \mid \theta)\pi(\theta)}$$

$$= \frac{\dfrac{\theta^k}{k!}e^{-\theta}\left[(0.75)\dfrac{0.0125^{.00125}}{\Gamma(0.0125)}\theta^{0.0125-1}e^{-0.0125\theta} + (0.25)\dfrac{1.5^2}{\Gamma(2)}\theta^{2-1}e^{-1.5\theta}\right]}{\sum_{\theta}\dfrac{\theta^k}{k!}e^{-\theta}\left[(0.75)\dfrac{0.0125^{.00125}}{\Gamma(0.0125)}\theta^{0.0125-1}e^{-.0125\theta} + (0.25)\dfrac{1.5^2}{\Gamma(2)}\theta^{2-1}e^{-1.5\theta}\right]}. \qquad (8.7)$$

The assessment of (8.7) begins with the recognition that the problem is simplified if we momentarily set aside its mixture component. Once we focus on a prior distribution with a single gamma density, namely,

$$\pi(\theta \mid k) = \frac{f(k \mid \theta)\pi(\theta)}{\sum_{\lambda} f(k \mid \theta)\pi(\theta)} = \frac{\dfrac{(\theta)^k}{k!}e^{-\theta}\dfrac{\alpha^r}{\Gamma(r)}\theta^{r-1}e^{-\alpha\theta}1_{0\le\theta\le\infty}}{\displaystyle\int_0^\infty \dfrac{\theta^k}{k!}e^{-\theta t}\dfrac{\alpha^r}{\Gamma(r)}\theta^{r-1}e^{-\alpha\theta}}.$$

We can write this posterior distribution using Appendix E

$$\pi(\theta \mid k) = \frac{(\alpha+1)^{k+r}}{\Gamma(k+r)}\theta^{\alpha+r-1}e^{-(\alpha+1)\theta}1_{0\le\theta\le\infty}$$

which is a gamma distribution with parameters $\alpha + 1$ and $k + r$. Thus, the posterior distribution for the Clynym's acute liver failure rate is a mixture of these posterior gamma distributions,

$$\pi(\theta \mid k) = (0.75)\frac{1.0125^{0.0125+k}}{\Gamma(0.0125+k)}\theta^{0.0125+k-1}e^{-1.0125\theta} + (0.25)\frac{2.5^{2+k}}{\Gamma(2+k)}\theta^{2+k-1}e^{-2.5\theta} \qquad (8.8)$$

and we can evaluate this as a function of k.

A post approval study is carried out on patients exposed to Clynyn. In a one-year period, there are 500,000 patients placed on this therapy, 2 of which have suffered fatal liver disease. This is a rate of 4 per million patients per year, or $k = 4$. Using this value in the posterior distribution (8.8) we can find the posterior distribution of θ.

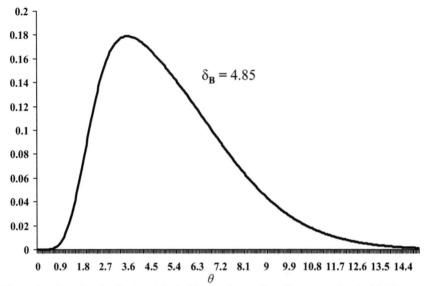

Figure 8.8. Posterior distribution of the incidence of acute liver disease associated with Clynyn when 2 events have occurred in 500,000 patients. The Bayes procedure, δ_B, is the median of the posterior distribution.

The median of this distribution is the Bayes procedure in accordance with the loss function selected for this example. For $k = 4$, $\delta_B = 4.85$.

From the posterior distribution, δ_B is clearly a function of the mix of the two gamma distributions as determined by p, and the number of cases of acute liver failure, denoted by k. While Figure 8.8 provides the posterior distribution for one value of p and k, it does not reveal how sensitive the Bayes procedure is to these values. Fortunately, the posterior distribution (8.8) allows us to examine the relationship between δ_B and these two parameters (Figure 8.9). Here we see that, as expected, the Bayes procedure gets larger as the number of patients with acute liver failure increase in the study. However the relationship between the mixture probability and δ_B is more complex. In fact, δ_B increases as function of p. This may seen counterintuitive, since the greater the value of p, the greater the influence of the conservative prior distribution in the mixture. However, the explanation for this unanticipated behavior becomes clear in an examination of the posterior distribution as a function of p (Figure 8.10).

This figure, shows the posterior distribution of θ, the incidence of acute liver failure as a function of p for $k = 2$. We see that as p increases, the tail probabilities increase. Since the Bayes procedure is the median, than we would expect the median to get larger as the tail probabilities increase.

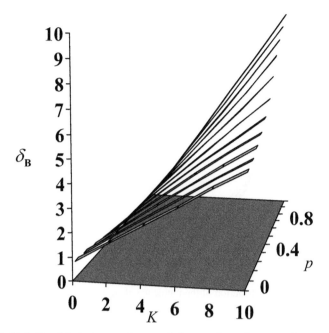

Figure 8.9. Relationship between δ_B, p and the number of cases of acute liver failure, K.

8.4 Conclusions

The two examples provided in this chapter illustrate some of the complexities in implementing Bayesian procedures in clinical trials. The selection of the prior distribution and loss function are commonly the focal point of intense discussion since the Bayes procedure depends on their choices. Once these selections have been made, a examination of the relationship between the Bayes procedure and these selections must be examined. One advantage of this sensitivity analysis is to expose the most critical assumptions needed to determine the location of δ_B. However, a second equally important dividend is that the initial conversations about these Bayes procedures incorporate many important diverse points of view, and in the process educate all investigators and interested parties in the assumptions underlying the final estimator.

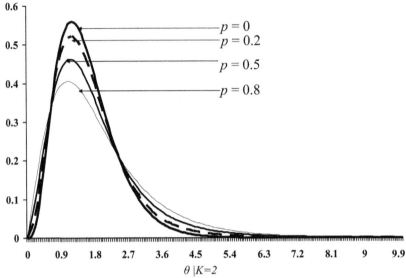

Figure 8.10. Posterior distribution of the incidence of acute liver disease associated with Clynyn for $K = 2$ as a function of the mixture probability p. Note that the tail probability increases with an increase in p, a trend that produces larger median values.

References

1. American Heart Association. (2000). Stroke Statistics. In: *2001 Heart and Stroke Statistical Update.* Dallas: American Heart Association.
2. American Heart Association.(2000). *2001 Heart and Stroke Facts*, Dallas: American Heart Association.
3. Senn, S. (1997). *Statistical Issues in Drug Development.* Chichester, Wiley, Section 15.2.1.

9
Bayesian Sample Size

9.1 Introduction

The sample size computation is required for small research studies and large clinical trials, for grant applications, new drug applications, and publications in peer-reviewed literature. It is ubiquitous in applied statistics.

The Bayesian sample size calculation is an active field of investigation, producing different perspectives for the best criteria to choose the number of subjects in a research effort. The incorporation of Bayes procedures in sample size calculations covers a broad spectrum. In some cases, they offer a simple adaptation of the frequentist approach to the sample size issue, requiring little new work and little new intuition to obtain a readily understood result. Alternatively, Bayes sample size procedures have been developed *de novo*, requiring a new perspective on the sample size issue [1]. In each of these calculations, the worker must balance accuracy with computational complexity to produce a useful and comprehensible result.

This chapter will focus on the development of Bayes sample size calculations. This introductory chapter begins at an elementary level, moving forward to complex Bayesian sample size calculation tools. Appendix M provides an introductory review of the basic sample size computation in the frequentist domain, and should be reviewed before beginning this chapter's discussion.

9.2 The Real Purpose of Sample Size Discussions

There are many different treatises on sample size calculations in clinical trials, e.g., [2–6]. Several of these discuss important and useful nuances of the sample size computation that are useful in complex clinical trial design. However, one of the most important lessons concerning sample size computation is that they are often not about sample size at all. The computations may have been initially motivated by stark concerns about type I and type II error in the frequentist domain, or about prior distributions for unknown parameters in the Bayesian thought process. However, these computations reflect other pressing considerations as well.

Sample size computations are the appropriate table over which important research agendas collide, ultimately deciding the purpose and direction of the effort. When the research agendas between investigators, statisticians, epidemiologists, and administrators are open for all to see, the investigational effort can be designed around a jointly supported consensus of the purpose of the study.

Concerns about funding, patient and investigator numbers, and in a clinical trial, the availability of the intervention must all be factored into the study design to provide a computation for an executable research effort that is worth carrying out [7].

9.3. Hybrid Bayesian-Frequentist Sample Sizes

The sample size formulas derived in Appendix M are the product of frequentist concerns. They provide, in the absence of any consideration for prior probabilities and loss functions, the minimum sample size for a research endeavor given the effect size and the magnitude of the type I and type II errors. Knowledge of other parameters such as event rates in the case of dichotomous endpoints, and standard deviations in the case of continuous endpoints are assumed to be both fixed and known.

Incorporating useful concepts from the Bayesian environment, e.g., the notion of a loss function for the sample size N is easily to imagine, since both underestimation and overestimation of N each have costs and therefore loss associated with them. However, the concept of a prior distribution for N at first blush seems artificial since there is no population of N's from which the investigator randomly selects. However, it is reasonable to assume that, although N is fixed, other parameters on which N depends may have important variability. Thus, an initial attempt to embed some of the Bayesian philosophy into sample size considerations begins with relaxing the assumption of total knowledge about the parameters on which the sample size depends.

9.3.1 One-Sample Test on a Proportion

Theoretically, this is straightforward computation. Assume that we collect a sample of observations that reflect dichotomous outcomes, e.g., mortality results. We are interested in carrying out a statistical hypothesis test for the value θ the mortality rate. The hypothesis test is

$$H_0: \theta = \theta_0 \qquad \text{versus} \quad H_a: \theta \neq \theta_0.$$

The investigators have chosen an *a priori* test-specific type I error level α, and the power of the statistical hypothesis test is $1 - \beta$. The hypothesis test will be two-sided, where Δ be the effect size (absolute rather than relative difference) in the proportion that the investigators wish to detect. From Appendix M, the minimum sample size N from the frequentist domain is

$$N = \frac{\theta(1-\theta)\left(Z_{1-\alpha/2} - Z_\beta\right)^2}{\Delta^2}. \tag{9.1}$$

Since the standard normal percentile values $Z_{1-\alpha/2}$ and Z_β are constants, we may write the sample size N as $N = g(\theta, \Delta)$.

Thus, far, this computation assumes that both the proportion θ and the effect size Δ are fixed. However, if we presume that they have a joint probability distribution $\pi(\theta, \Delta)$, then we compute not N, but instead its average or expected value N, denoted as $\mathbf{E}[N]$, where

$$\mathbf{E}[N] = \sum_{\theta, \Delta} g(\theta, \Delta) \pi(\theta, \Delta). \tag{9.2}$$

Essentially, we take an average of the sample size over the values of θ and Δ. This is identical to the notion of compounding that we discussed in Chapters Two and Three.

Averaging produces a hybrid computation. The sample size is based on Fisherian considerations of null and alternative hypotheses with their attendant type I and type II errors. Yet, building in the assumption of probability distribution for the proportion θ and the effect size Δ incorporates an unmistakable Bayesian flavor.

9.3.1.1 Providing a Probability Distribution for θ

We begin by assuming that Δ is fixed in the sample size formula for N in (9.1) but θ follows a probability distribution. Since $0 \le \theta \le 1$ and we would like a wide selection of individual distributions from which to choose, a natural selection is that this prior distribution be selected from the beta family of distributions. Thus,

$$\pi(\theta) = \frac{\Gamma(\alpha_1 + \beta_1)}{\Gamma(\alpha_1)\Gamma(\beta_1)} \theta^{\alpha_1 - 1} (1 - \theta)^{\beta_1 - 1} \tag{9.3}$$

This distribution offers important flexibility in the location of probability for θ for $0 \le \theta \le 1$. As demonstrated in Appendix K, we can identify the mean and variance of θ using only the prior distribution

$$\mathbf{E}[\theta] = \frac{\alpha_1}{\alpha_1 + \beta_1}$$

$$\mathbf{Var}[\theta] = \frac{\alpha_1 \beta_1}{(\alpha_1 + \beta_1 + 1)(\alpha_1 + \beta_1)^2}.$$

We can now compute the average sample size from (9.2), by writing

$$\mathbf{E}[N] = \sum_{\theta,\Delta} g(\theta,\Delta)\pi(\theta,\Delta) = \sum_{\theta,\Delta} g(\theta)\pi(\theta)$$

$$= \sum_{\theta} \frac{\theta(1-\theta)(Z_{1-\alpha/2} - Z_{\beta})^2}{\Delta^2} \frac{\Gamma(\alpha_1 + \beta_1)}{\Gamma(\alpha_1)\Gamma(\beta_1)} \theta^{\alpha_1 - 1}(1-\theta)^{\beta_1 - 1}$$

$$= \frac{(Z_{1-\alpha/2} - Z_{\beta})^2}{\Delta^2} \frac{\Gamma(\alpha_1 + \beta_1)}{\Gamma(\alpha_1)\Gamma(\beta_1)} \sum_{\theta} \theta(1-\theta)\theta^{\alpha_1 - 1}(1-\theta)^{\beta_1 - 1}$$

$$= \frac{(Z_{1-\alpha/2} - Z_{\beta})^2}{\Delta^2} \frac{\Gamma(\alpha_1 + \beta_1)}{\Gamma(\alpha_1)\Gamma(\beta_1)} \sum_{\theta} \theta^{\alpha_1}(1-\theta)^{\beta_1}.$$

From Appendix B, we know $\sum_{\theta} \theta^{\alpha_1}(1-\theta)^{\beta_1}$ for $0 \le \theta \le 1$ is an integral whose value

is $\dfrac{\Gamma(\alpha_1 + 1)\Gamma(\beta_1 + 1)}{\Gamma(\alpha_1 + \beta_1 + 2)}$. Thus

$$\mathbf{E}[N] = \frac{(Z_{1-\alpha/2} - Z_{\beta})^2}{\Delta^2} \frac{\Gamma(\alpha_1 + \beta_1)}{\Gamma(\alpha_1)\Gamma(\beta_1)} \frac{\Gamma(\alpha_1 + 1)\Gamma(\beta_1 + 1)}{\Gamma(\alpha_1 + \beta_1 + 2)}$$

$$= \left[\frac{(Z_{1-\alpha/2} - Z_{\beta})^2}{\Delta^2}\right]\left[\frac{\alpha_1\beta_1}{(\alpha_1 + \beta_1 + 1)(\alpha_1 + \beta_1)}\right].$$

(9.4)

We see that the expected sample size is the product of two terms each of which is easier to evaluate. The first, with its incorporation of type I and type II error rates reflects frequentist concerns while the second resides in the Bayesian domain.

Example 9.1: Leg Amputations in Diabetes Mellitus

One of the consequences of diabetes mellitus is peripheral vascular disease, leading to reduced blood circulation in the arms and legs. The increase in prevalence in diabetes in the United States has been so great that it is now the single largest cause of nontraumatic limb amputations.[*]

In this example, diabetologists wish to learn about the prevalence of diabetes induced limb amputations in the poor. Reasoning that the incidence of this terrible consequence is smaller for patients who are better able to monitor control of their diabetes, and that monitoring ability is hampered by economic hardship, they deduce that the prevalence rate in the poor should be greater than those unimpoverished.

The investigators believe that the diabetic poor will experience a rate that is 10% greater in absolute percentage points than the background rate of limb am-

---

[*] It is not uncommon for diabetic patients in kidney failure, having suffered through multiple amputations of their feet, ankles, fingers and hands, and facing yet more anquishing amputative surgery, to simply discontinue their renal dialysis, an action that kills them in less than two weeks.

putation θ. They wish to detect this increase with a two-sided type I error of 0.025 and 90% power. In this circumstance, although Δ, $Z_{1-\alpha/2}$, and Z_β are known, the investigators are uncertain about the value of θ.

In the frequentist circumstance, these investigators would discuss among themselves the possible values of θ, and settle on one, basing their sample size on that consensus determination. However, in this setting, they discuss not values of θ, but alternative values of its prior distribution, $\pi(\theta)$. There are three investigators, each of whom has a different sense of the distribution of the event rate (Figure 9.1).

The first investigator's experience suggests that the distribution of θ is clustered around relatively small values, suggesting that the proportion of diabetic patients with leg amputations is small. This is consistent with a beta distribution with parameter $\alpha_1 = 2$ and $\beta_1 = 50$. It is important to note that the investigator does not and should not be expected to justify the selection of the probability distribution or the selection of parameters. The distribution serves only as a vehicle to capture the investigator's prior knowledge and belief. In this case, the scientist posits his belief first, thereby providing the statistician the direction he or she needs to select the value of α_1 and β_1 that best depict this conviction.

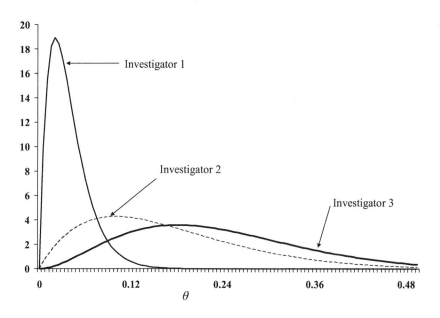

Figure 9.1. Each of three investigators has a different prior distribution for the value of θ, the proportion of diabetic patients with leg amputations in their state.

Investigator 2's experience suggests a shift in the distribution of θ to the right, reflected by a beta distribution with parameters $\alpha_2 = 2$ and $\beta_2 = 10$. The third investigator, influenced by both her experience and the sense that the reporting of amputation rates among the indigent are artificially low because of underreporting of the procedure, has a distribution of θ in mind best depicted by the selection of α_3 = 3 and β_3 = 10.

The investigators discuss among themselves the relative merits of their positions, being open to the influences of each other as they attempt to persuade their colleagues of the strength of their own position. Let p_1, p_2, and p_3 be the mixture probabilities for these three separate opinions, such that $p_1 + p_2 + p_3 = 1$.

The possible mixtures of these opinions have a remarkable variety of shapes (Figure 9.2). The shapes of these distributions can make us uneasy. Certainly, the true distribution of θ does not have the fluctuations such as when p_1 = 0.20, p_2 = 0.40, and p_3 = 0.40. Yet, we must keep in mind, that in the absence of clear information to the contrary, this is the best that the investigators disparate opinions can generate.

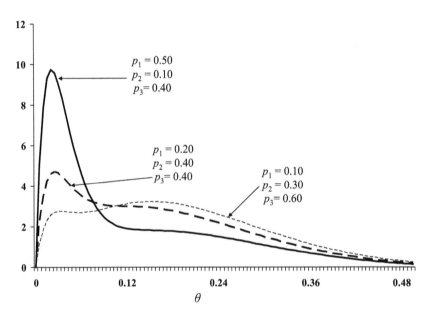

Figure 9.2. Three possible mixture distribution as the investigators labor toward consensus for the distribution of the diabetic patients with leg amputations in their state.

Now it remains to compute the sample size. We have shown that

$$E[N] = \left[\frac{\left(Z_{1-\alpha/2} - Z_\beta\right)^2}{\Delta^2} \right] \left[\frac{\alpha_1 \beta_1}{(\alpha_1 + \beta_1 + 1)(\alpha_1 + \beta_1)} \right], \tag{9.5}$$

but this formula applies only when one investigator's prior is being considered. In this we have the mixture of three investigators' opinions, and the priors must be mixed. Following our demonstrations in Chapter Two, we write

$$E[N] = \left[\frac{\left(Z_{1-\alpha/2} - Z_{\beta}\right)^2}{\Delta^2} \right] \left[\frac{p_1\alpha_1\beta_1}{(\alpha_1+\beta_1+1)(\alpha_1+\beta_1)} + \frac{p_2\alpha_2\beta_2}{(\alpha_2+\beta_2+1)(\alpha_2+\beta_2)} + \frac{p_3\alpha_3\beta_3}{(\alpha_3+\beta_3+1)(\alpha_3+\beta_3)} \right], \quad (9.6)$$

$p_{i,}$ is the mixture probability for the ith investigator, whose prior is reflected by a beta distribution with parameters α_i and β_i.

The investigators settle on the choices $p_1 = 0.20$, $p_2 = 0.40$, and $p_3 = 0.40$. Recall that the investigators wish to be able to detect a 10% greater rate of limb amputations in the poor (absolute percentage points) with a two-sided type I error of 0.025 and 90% power. Thus, they compute

$$E[N] = \left[\frac{\left(2.242 - (-1.28)\right)^2}{(0.10)^2} \right] (0.0078 + 0.0513 + 0.0659) = 155$$

or 155 diabetic patients in the urban poor must be identified.

9.3.2 Two Sample Computation

The previous section demonstrated the utility of a prior distribution on the event rate θ in a one sample test of proportions. In the two-sample scenario, the investigators are interested in comparing the proportions of events (called primary endpoint events[*]) that occur in each of two treatment groups. Let θ_c be the cumulative incidence rate of the primary endpoint in the control group and let θ_t be the cumulative incidence rate of the primary endpoint in the treatment group. The classical hypothesis test for the primary endpoint in this clinical trial is

$$H_0 : \theta_c = \theta_t \quad \text{versus} \quad H_a : \theta_c \neq \theta_t.$$

Let Z_c be the cth percentile from the standard normal distribution. The investigators have chosen an *a priori* test-specific type I error level α, and the power of the statistical hypothesis test is $1 - \beta$. The hypothesis test will be two-sided. Let p_c be the cumulative incidence rate of the primary endpoint in the control group of the research sample, and let p_t be the cumulative incidence rate of the active group in the research sample. Then, from Appendix M, we may write the trial size, or the sample size of the clinical trial, N as

---

[*] The primary endpoint is the single measure of effectiveness that the clinical trial was designed to test. The trial will be positive (if there is a treatment benefit) or not based on the findings for the primary endpoint.

$$N = \frac{2\left[\theta_c\left(1-\theta_c\right)+\theta_t\left(1-\theta_t\right)\right]\left[Z_{1-\alpha/2}-Z_\beta\right]^2}{\left(\theta_c - \theta_t\right)^2}. \tag{9.7}$$

Both values for θ_c and θ_t are required here. However, neither may be known with certainty. Typically, investigators write the treatment group event rate as a function of the control group rate and the efficacy, or percent reduction in the control group rate that is produced by the intervention. If ϕ is the efficacy, then $\theta_t = \theta_c\left(1-\phi\right)$. We may therefore write the sample size formula not as function of the control group and treatment group rates but instead in terms of the control group rate and the efficacy. Dropping the subscript θ in the sample size formula, we rewrite (9.7) as

$$N = \frac{2\left[\theta(1-\theta)+\theta(1-\phi)\left(1-\theta(1-\phi)\right)\right]\left[Z_{1-\alpha/2}-Z_\beta\right]^2}{\theta^2\phi^2},$$

using $\theta_c - \theta_t = \theta_c - (1-\phi)\theta_c = \theta_c\phi = \theta\phi$.

　　With this reformulation of the sample size, our goal is to assign a probability distribution for both parameters θ and ϕ, then identify the expected value of the sample size.

　　Thus, if $\pi(\theta,\phi)$ is the joint prior distribution of θ and ϕ, then we can write $N = g(\theta,\phi)$,

$$\mathbf{E}[N] = \sum_{\theta,\phi} g(\theta,\phi)\pi(\theta,\phi), \tag{9.8}$$

in which

$$g(\theta,\phi) = \frac{2\left[\theta(1-\theta)+\theta(1-\phi)\left(1-\theta(1-\phi)\right)\right]\left[Z_{1-\alpha/2}+Z_\beta\right]^2}{\left(\theta\phi\right)^2}.$$

Now, assume that θ and ϕ each have independent beta distributions. Then

$$\pi(\theta,\phi) = \frac{\Gamma(\alpha_1+\beta_1)}{\Gamma(\alpha_1)\Gamma(\beta_1)}\theta^{\alpha_1-1}(1-\theta)^{\beta_1-1}\frac{\Gamma(\alpha_2+\beta_2)}{\Gamma(\alpha_2)\Gamma(\beta_2)}\phi^{\alpha_2-1}(1-\phi)^{\beta_2-1}, \tag{9.9}$$

and our goal is to identify $\mathbf{E}[N]$ from equation (9.8). In Appendix K, we show that

$$E[N] =$$

$$2\left[Z_{1-\alpha/2} + Z_\beta\right]^2 \left[\frac{\beta_1}{\alpha_1 - 1} \frac{(\alpha_2 + \beta_2 - 1)(\alpha_2 + \beta_2 - 2)}{(\alpha_2 - 1)(\alpha_2 - 2)} + \frac{(\alpha_1 + \beta_1 - 1)}{(\alpha_1 - 1)} \frac{\beta_2(\alpha_2 + \beta_2 - 1)}{(\alpha_2 - 1)(\alpha_2 - 2)} - \frac{(\beta_2 + 1)\beta_2}{(\alpha_2 - 1)(\alpha_2 - 2)}\right]$$

an easily manipulated formula which, is a function of only the percentile values of the normal distribution and the parameters of the prior distributions of both the control group event rate θ and the efficacy ϕ. Aspects of this approach have been adopted in the literature [8], and we adopt it for our use in the hybrid sample size construction.

Example 9.2: Clinical Trial Sample Size

Investigators, intrigued by the assertions that many cases of congestive heart failure may be the result of an uncontrolled infection-like effect on the heart muscle focus their attention on the use of anti-inflammatory medications to prevent the progression of heart failure. Their goal is to examine patients with mild to moderate heart failure (New York Heart Association Class II or III), and then randomize them to receive either several injections of either an anti-inflammatory medicine, or inactive placebo.

They wish to compute the sample size for this clinical trial whose primary endpoint is the cumulative total mortality rate. For this seven year study, previous studies suggest that the mean total mortality rate will be 20%. The investigators select a beta distribution for the prior distribution of cumulative mortality rate θ (Figure 9.3). The selection of $\alpha = 20$ and $\beta = 80$ not only ensures that the mean value of the control group event rate will be 0.20, but also produces the concentration of probability around the mean, a clear expression of the investigator's confidence that the mean value will be 0.20.

However, this tight distribution, a manifestation of the investigators "unshakable" opinion of the future total mortality rate of their control cohort, ignores other factors that require consideration. The use of new, effective medications for the treatment of heart failure during the study will most likely decrease the cumulative total mortality rate. In addition, the volunteer effect[*] will depress the control group event rate further. Alternatively, these influences will be counterbalanced by the investigators insistence in recruiting from an immigrant population. These patients will have more severe disease and experience higher death rates because of their lifelong limited access to care.

---

[*] The volunteer effect is the influence of patients who choose to participate in clinical trials. Their possession of the physical, mental, and emotional qualities to hold themselves out (and are sometimes eager) for the experimentation experience produces lower than anticipated event rates. This observation, in combination with the fact that they have none of the diseases commonly used to exclude patients from clinical trial produces a stronger health profile, leading to depressed control group event rates.

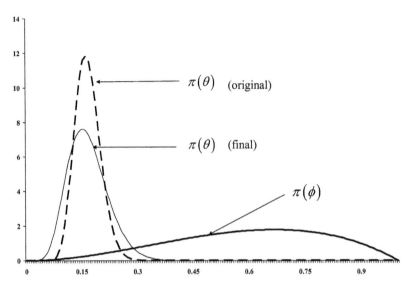

Figure 9.3. Prior distributions of the control group event rate, θ and the efficacy φ for a clinical trial.

After consideration of these factors, the investigators modify their selection of the beta prior distribution for the control group total mortality rate, now selecting $\alpha_1 = 8$ and $\beta_1 = 40$. This produces a smaller mean value of 0.167 with substantially more weight placed on the lower event rates.

These difficult conversations are likely to be much tougher if the sample size computation resided entirely in the frequentist domain. There, the requirement that they settle on a single cumulative total mortality would seem an impossible goal given the strongly held opinions of vehement investigators with diverse backgrounds. In the Bayesian domain, the choice of a distribution is made easier by the fact that there is built-in variance for the cumulative total mortality rate. This variance measures not just true variability of θ in the community but also incorporates the uncertainty in the scientists' opinions.

Similarly, the selection of efficacy is also problematic. The choice of a single value for the intervention-induced percent reduction in the cumulative mortality rate is much less data based than that for the underlying control group event rate. The investigators have little to guide them, given the small number of preliminary human studies available. In addition, the scientists must also consider the expectation of the cardiovascular community; a small intervention induced percent reduction in the cumulative mortality rate will not persuade wary cardiologists concerned about the possibility of adverse effects [9]. In the end, the investigators settle on a beta prior with $\alpha_2 = 3$ and $\beta_2 = 8$. The mean $\pi(\phi)$ is 0.27, and its wide dispersion (Figure 9.3) indicates the investigators' own uncertainty about the magnitude of the compound's effectiveness.

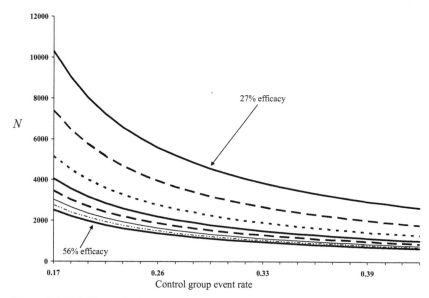

Figure 9.4. Hybrid sample size computation for a clinical trial in heart failure patients as a function of control group mortality rate and efficacy.

This is all we need for the sample size computation. Using

$$E[N] =$$
$$2\left[Z_{1-\alpha/2}+Z_{\beta}\right]^2\left[\frac{\beta_1}{\alpha_1-1}\frac{(\alpha_2+\beta_2-1)(\alpha_2+\beta_2-2)}{(\alpha_2-1)(\alpha_2-2)}+\frac{(\alpha_1+\beta_1-1)}{(\alpha_1-1)}\frac{\beta_2(\alpha_2+\beta_2-1)}{(\alpha_2-1)(\alpha_2-2)}-\frac{(\beta_2+1)\beta_2}{(\alpha_2-1)(\alpha_2-2)}\right] \tag{9.10}$$

we can quickly compute the minimal sample size for $\alpha_1 = 8$, $\beta_1 = 40$, $\alpha_2 = 3$ and $\beta_2 = 8$ is 10,291. Equation (9.10) can be used to assess the relationship between this hybrid computation, the mean control group event rate, and the mean efficacy of the compound (Figure 9.4).

Figure 9.4 demonstrates the anticipated relationships between sample size, efficacy and control group event, with larger mean event rates and greater efficacy producing smaller sample sizes.

9.4 Complete Bayesian Sample Size Computations

Our previous discussion mixed both the Bayesian and frequentist themes within a single sample size calculation. It is a useful device, since many clinical studies whose analysis is executed in the frequentist domain of hypothesis testing, requiring explicit statements about type I and type II error levels, are carried out in an environment of uncertainty about parameter estimates such as event rates [10]. These hybrid calculations have the added benefit of being straightforward.

Nevertheless, the blending of the frequentist and the Bayesian perspective is not a satisfying one to those wishing to encompass the sample size calculation entirely within the Bayesian point of view. A decision theoretic approach that actually applies a loss function to N, selecting an N that minimizes the risk [11] has the usual appeal of the Bayesian point of view. However, to be successful, the loss function must be accurate in order to accurately compute the sample size. In addition, there must be a prior distribution for N. These approach, completely devoid of frequentist concerns can be quite complex [12,13].

An adaptation of this procedure would be to keep the Bayesian framework focused on θ, and then choose a value of N that maximizes the occurrence of a desirable feature of the posterior distribution of θ. We will develop an adaptation of these more complex processes.

Example 9.3: Parkinson's Disease

Parkinson's disease is a motor symptom disorder. Voluntary muscle movement and coordination is managed in the brain, and, in order to generate coherent and purposeful movement, brain cells or neurons must interact with each other. These communications are mediated by electrical-chemical communications, and one of the necessary chemicals is the amino acid dopamine. Many of the cells that produce dopamine can be found in the region of the brain known as the striata nigra. In Parkinson's disease, these cells lose their ability to produce dopamine.

The four primary symptoms of Parkinson's Disease are trembling (primarily in the hands, arms, legs, jaw, and face), stiffness in the arms, legs, and trunk, slow movement, and impaired balance. The symptoms generally have a gradual onset. There is currently no cure for this disorder.

Consider a researcher interested in estimating the proportion of patients who have Parkinson's disease among patients who are greater than sixty years old. Although she must select a sample of N patients to screen for this disease she recognizes that it would be easier to select the sample size N if she knew the proportion of patients with the disease, but of course that is the purpose of the research effort. She therefore allows the probability distribution to govern the proportion's value.

The investigator assigns θ to the proportion of patients with Parkinson's disease. However, rather than choose the type I and type II error rates and compute a value of N as we did in equation (9.4), we will instead develop the posterior distribution of θ as a function of N and then examine the effect of N on the posterior distribution's shape and characteristics.

Let x be the number of patients in the sample of N patients screened for Parkinson's disease. Then, if the investigator knows both N and θ, the distribution of x will be binomial, i.e.,

$$f\left(x \mid N, \theta\right) = \binom{N}{x} \theta^x \left(1 - \theta\right)^{N-x}. \tag{9.11}$$

Let the prior distribution of θ follow a beta distribution with parameters α and β. The investigator selected $\alpha = 10$ and $\beta = 100$ consistent with a mean of 0.091, producing

$$\frac{\Gamma(\alpha+\beta)}{\Gamma(\alpha)\Gamma(\beta)}\theta^{\alpha-1}(1-\theta)^{\beta-1}\mathbf{1}_{0\le\theta\le1}$$

Appendix K demonstrates that the posterior distribution of θ is itself a beta distribution, i.e.,

$$\frac{\Gamma(N+\alpha+\beta)}{\Gamma(\alpha+x)\Gamma(N-x+\beta)}\theta^{\alpha+x-1}(1-\theta)^{N-x+\beta-1}\mathbf{1}_{0\le\theta\le1} \qquad (9.12)$$

which we recognize as a beta distribution with parameters $\alpha+x$ and $N-x+\beta$. The investigator's task is now to simply evaluate this distribution as a function of N. Note however, that the posterior distribution is also a function of x, the number of patients with Parkinson's disease that the investigator identifies in her sample. Thus, we would expect that as N increases, in the face of a fixed number of Parkinson patients, the location of the distribution would shift to the left as the proportion of patients with Parkinson's disease is progressively reduced by the larger sample size. In this case, the investigator assumes that she would identify 3 patients with Parkinson's disease (Figure 9.5).

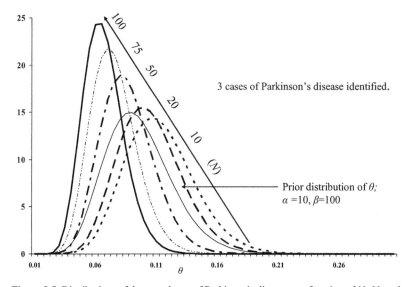

Figure 9.5. Distributions of the prevalence of Parkinson's disease as a function of N. Note that both the location and the variance of the distribution changes as a function of N.

Figure 9.5 depicts the prior distribution for θ and several posterior distributions for θ as a function of N.

Now that the investigator has identified α, β, and x, she examines the form of the posterior distribution as a function of N. As N increases from 10 to 100, the posterior distribution shifts to the left, all the while decreasing its variance. This same behavior is observed if the assumption for the number of cases observed is altered from $x = 3$ to $x = 10$ (Figure 9.6). Again, both the location and the dispersion of the posterior distribution change as a function of the sample size.

In determining the criteria for the sample size N, effort has focused on the smallest range of θ that produces the highest posterior probability. This is known as the *highest posterior density* (HPD) region. For example, if the posterior distribution follows a normal distribution, then the 95% HPD is simply the standard (i.e., frequentist derived) 95% confidence interval. For more complicated posterior probability functions the identification of this region can be complex [14].

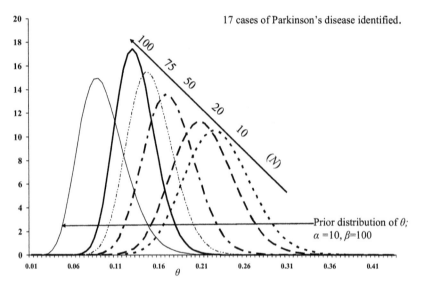

Figure 9.6. Distributions of the prevalence of Parkinson's disease as a function of N. The larger number of observed cases of Parkinson's disease shifts the distribution to the right.

However, this is not the only criteria that one can select for optimizing the sample size. For example, assume that the investigator chooses a beta prior distribution with a mean of 0.118. She is most interested in the best estimate of the probability that the proportion of patients with Parkinson's disease is between 0.05 and 0.10. She notes that, to be the most useful, this posterior probability should either be very large or very small. Using equation (9.12) she is able to examine the posterior probability of this region as a function of the sample size and the number of patients that she identifies as having Parkinson's disease (Figure 9.7).

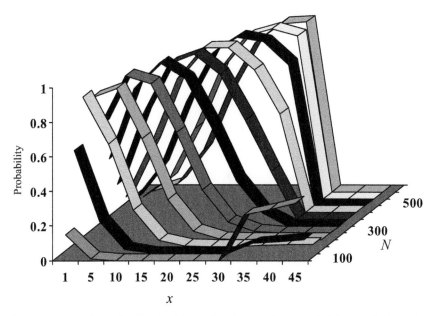

Figure 9.7. Posterior probability that $0.05 <= \theta <= 0.20$ as a function of N, the sample size and x, the number of Parkinson's disease patients when the mean of the prior distribution is 0.118.

The probability portrayed in Figure 9.7 is the posterior probability that $0.05 \leq \theta \leq 0.10$. For the smallest values of N, the posterior probability remains relatively low regardless of the number of Parkinson's disease patients observed in the sample. This observation nicely aligns with our intuition that small values of N will provide little insight into the value of $P[0.05 \leq \theta \leq 0.10]$. However, for larger values of N, the investigator notes the change in the posterior probability as a function of the number of patients with Parkinson's disease. When small numbers of patients with Parkinson's disease are identified, the posterior probability that $P[0.05 \leq \theta \leq 0.10]$ is low. As x increases, and as the proportion of identified Parkinsonian patients first approaches from below, then moves through the interval $0.05 \leq \theta \leq 0.10$, the posterior probability $P[0.05 \leq \theta \leq 0.10]$ increases. As x continues to increase, the proportion of patients with Parkinson's disease patients increases beyond 0.10, and the posterior probability decreases (Figure 9.8). This behavior satisfies our intuition about the relationship between the proportion of identified Parkinson patients and the posterior $P[0.05 \leq \theta \leq 0.10]$. However, what additional advantage do larger values of N offer?

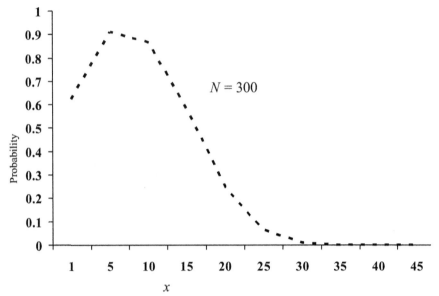

Figure 9.8. Posterior probability that $0.05 <= \theta <= 0.20$ for $N = 300$ as a function of x, the number of Parkinson's disease patients when the mean of the prior distribution is 0.118.

An examination of the rate of rise and decline of the posterior probability, suggests one (Figure 9.9). Here, the posterior probability as a function of the number of Parkinson's patients is displayed for the two cases of $N = 300$ and $N = 500$. Note that not only has the curve shifted to the right for the larger sample size, but the rate of decline of the probability $P[0.05 \leq \theta \leq 0.10]$ is much greater for the larger sample size. For the larger sample size, the range of x for which the $P[0.05 \leq \theta \leq 0.10]$ has intermediate values is much smaller. This smaller range makes it less likely that the probability will fall in this range, producing an experience that is more likely to generate extremely high or extremely low values of $P[0.05 \leq \theta \leq 0.10]$. The larger sample size sharpens the utility of this tool, and further sharpening is provided for even larger sample sizes (Figure 9.10). A value of $N = 550$ nicely generates a sharp boundary for the posterior probability that $P[0.05 \leq \theta \leq 0.10]$.

9.5 Conclusions

The sample size computation remains a staple of applied statistics in each of the frequentist and Bayesian paradigms. Pure Bayes computations, while elegant, can be fraught with computational complexity. Nevertheless, diligent workers have

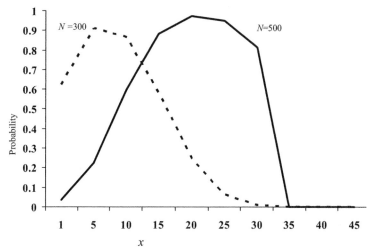

Figure 9.9. Posterior probability that $0.05 <= \theta <= 0.20$ for $N = 300$ and $N=500$ as a function of x, the number of Parkinson's disease patients when the mean of the prior distribution is 0.118.

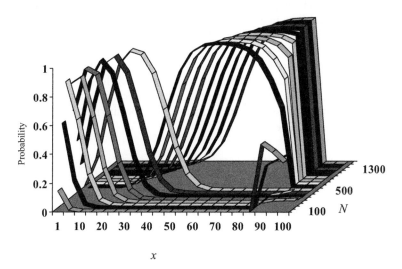

Figure 9.10. Posterior probability that $0.05 <= \theta <= 0.20$ as a function of N, the sample size and x, the number of Parkinson's disease patients when the mean of the prior distribution is 0.118.

persevered, producing illustrative Bayesian sample size calculations using the binomial distribution [15], and case control studies [16]. This perspective has been particularly useful when working with dichotomous endpoints in the presence of misclassification [17,18], when one is carefully justifying the model's parameters [19].

However, sample size computations must be practical and efficient in a research-resource starved environment. For clinical trial workers, the hybrid computation may offer the best of both worlds. It brings the familiar concepts of type I and type II errors that are commonly invoked in the assessment of the effect size observed at the study's conclusions. In addition, these calculations allow researchers to acknowledge that they may have only inexact knowledge of the parameters on which the sample size is constructed, giving them the option of placing a probability distribution on these unknown quantities. The resulting sample size is an average over the range of possible values of the unknown parameters.

Ultimately, sample size computations be they Bayesian, frequentist, or a mixture, must bow to reality. These calculations are unhelpful if they ignore the scarcity of patients, the high cost of the intervention, or the low funding level of the study. These latter, pragmatic considerations are just as important as the erudite statistical thought process for useful sample size computations.

Problems

1.   Assume a clinical trial is carried out designed to reduce the blood pressure by an amount Δ. Assume that Δ has a 30% chance of being 5 mm Hg, a 60% chance of being 11 mm Hg, and a 10% chance of bring 15 mm Hg. Compute the sample size for the clinical trial to assess the effect of the therapy on blood pressure reduction for $\sigma = 3.5$ assuming a two-sided type I error level of 0.05 and 95% power.

2.   Two investigators are interested in carrying out a one sample test on the proportion of patients who have influenza. Each has two different senses of the proportion of events as reflected in their prior distribution. Assume p is the weight placed on investigator 1's prior distribution. Then the prior distribution can be written as

$$\pi(\theta) = p\frac{\Gamma(\alpha_1 + \beta_1)}{\Gamma(\alpha_1)\Gamma(\beta_1)}\theta^{\alpha_1 - 1}(1-\theta)^{\beta_1 - 1} + (1-p)\frac{\Gamma(\alpha_2 + \beta_2)}{\Gamma(\alpha_2)\Gamma(\beta_2)}\theta^{\alpha_2 - 1}(1-\theta)^{\beta_2 - 1}.$$

Graph the prior probability when $\beta_1 = \beta_2 = 40$, $\alpha_1 = 1$, $\alpha_2 = 1000$, and $p = 0.5$. Compare the sample size for the study based on $\pi(\theta)$, adapting equation (9.5).

3.   Find the variance of the sample size derived from the normal approximation of the binomial distribution, $N = \dfrac{\theta(1-\theta)\left(Z_{1-\alpha/2} - Z_\beta\right)^2}{\Delta^2}$, where the $\pi(\theta)$ follows a beta distribution with parameters α_1 and β_1. Combine this result with equation (9.4) to identify a 95% confidence interval for the sample size.

References

1. Moore A., Joseph L. (1999). Sample size considerations for superiority trials in Systemic Lupus Erythematosus (SLE). *Lupus*. **8**:612–619.
2. Lachim J.M. (1981). Introduction to sample size determinations and power analyses for clinical trials. *Controlled Clinical Trial* **2**:93–114.
3. Sahai H. Khurshid, A. (1996). Formulae and tables for determination of sample size and power in clinical trials for testing differences in proportions for the two sample design. *Statistics in Medicine*. **15**:1–21.
4. Davy S.J., Graham, O.T. (1991). Sample size estimation for comparing two or more treatment groups in clinical trials. *Statistics in Medicine*. **10**:3–43.
5. Donner A. (1984) Approach to sample size estimation in the design of clinical trials – a review.*Statistics in Medicine*. **3**:199–214.
6. George S.L., Desue M.M. (1974). Planning the size and duration of a clinical trial studying the time to some critical event. *Journal of Chronic Disease* **27**:15–24.
7. Moyé L.A. (2006). Statistical Reasoning in Medicine. The Intuitive *P*-Value Primer. New York. Springer. Chapter Six.
8. Joseph L., du Berger R., and Bélisle P. (1997). Bayesian and mixed Bayesian/likelihood criteria for sample size determination *Statistics in Medicine*;16(7):769–781.
9. Moyé L.A. (2003). *Multiple Analyses in Clinical Trials* New York. Springer. pp 324–332.
10. Joseph L., Wolfson D. (1997). Interval-based versus decision theoretic criteria for the choice of sample size *The Statistician* **46**(2):145–149.
11. Lindley DV. (1997). The choice of sample size. *The Statistician* **46**:129–138.
12. Joseph L., Wolfson D., and du Berger R. (1995). Sample size calculations for binomial proportions via highest posterior density intervals *The Statistician*: **44**(2):143–154.
13. Joseph L., Wolfson D., and du Berger R. (1995). Some comments on Bayesian sample size determination *The Statistician* **44**:167–171.
14. Wei G.C.G., Tanner M.A. (1990). Calculating the content and boundaryof the highest posterior density region via data augmentation. *Biometrika* **77**:649–652.
15. Rahme E., Joseph L. (1998). Exact sample size determination for binomial experiments. *Journal of Statistical Planning and Inference* **66**:83–93.
16. M'Lan E., Joseph L., Wolfson D. (2006) Bayesian sample size determination for case-control studies. *Journal of the American Statistical Association* **101**:(474):760–772.
17. Dendukuri N., Rahme E., Bélisle P., Joseph L. (2004). Bayesian sample size determination for prevalence and diagnostic studies in the absence of a gold standard test *Biometrics* **60**:388–397.

18. Rahme E., Joseph L., and Gyorkos T. (2000). Bayesian sample size determination for estimating binomial parameters from data subject to misclassification. *Applied Statistics* **49**(1):119–228.

19. Joseph L., Bélisle P. (1997). Bayesian sample size determination for Normal means and differences between Normal means *The Statistician* **46**(2):209–226.

10
Predictive Power and Adaptive Proced res

10.1 Introduction

The Bayesian philosophy is building important new inroads in applied biostatistics. Two of the most exciting arenas involve clinical trials. Adaptive Bayes procedures focus on how patients are accrued, and predictive power focuses on the ending of these research endeavors. Each is an active field of investigation holding great promise for the future. This chapter serves as a basic introduction to these noteworthy areas.

10.2 Predictive Power

Predictive power is the application of Bayes procedures to the critical process of clinical research monitoring. Much like the hybrid Bayes sample size procedures we discussed in the previous chapter, predictive power adds a unique Bayesian component to a traditional frequentist perspective. After motivating the need to monitor a research effort on an ongoing basis, we will demonstrate how a Bayesian perspective can favorably influence the ability to precisely monitor ongoing clinical research.

10.2.1 The Importance of Monitoring Clinical Trials

While the implementation of the random allocation of therapy, in combination with the technique of "double-blinding," permits a clear attribution of therapy effect in a clinical trial, these procedures pose a new problem for the study's ethical execution. Shielding investigators from the therapy assignment during the course of the study ensures that the researchers will not bias their assessment of any particular patient's performance by knowledge of that patient's therapy medication. However, it also implies that the investigators will be unable to assess how effective the therapy is during the course of the study. Specifically, blinding the investigators to knowledge of therapy assignment until the conclusion of the study ensures the researchers will not know of unanticipated important early evidence of benefit or risk attributable to the therapy.

The Data Monitoring Committee (DMC) was created to correct this research blind spot. Composed of a small number of distinguish scientists with the relevant clinical and epidemiologic/biostatistical expertise to evaluate the ongoing clinical trial, the DMC reviews all of the data in an unblinded fashion, determining whether an early therapeutic triumph (or catastrophe) has occurred.[*] The DMC observes the effect of therapy that may appear early in the trial, while at the same time ensuring the double-blind property remains intact.

To aid in this review, methodologists have developed statistical monitoring rules that provide an assessment of the early effect of therapy, while simultaneously incorporating the considerable variability associated with the estimate of this early therapy effect. Established before the trial begins recruiting patients, the monitoring rule specifies how large the test statistic will be allowed to become before the trial is stopped. For this reason, these rules are commonly referred to as stopping rules.

However, since there are many other considerations that the DMC must evaluate before the clinical trial is discontinued prematurely (e.g., the availability of alternative treatments, the treated condition's severity, the clinical importance of the observed difference, and the consistency of the results with the findings of other researchers), the monitoring rule is not necessarily a signal that the trial must be stopped. It instead cues the DMC to consider whether the study should be discontinued. These other influences are the motivation for the more appropriate term *monitoring procedure*, rather than stopping rule [1].

10.2.2 Test Statistic Trajectories

These statistical guidelines used to monitor the importance of therapy effect magnitudes in clinical trials examine cohorts of patients that increase in size over time. At the first evaluation, n_1 patients are evaluated. At the second interim analysis executed some months later, the first n_1 patients are reevaluated in addition to an additional set of n_2 patients for which new data is collected. These growing cohorts or groups of patients are evaluated sequentially during the course of the study, leading to the moniker *group sequential procedure.* The three specific steps are

Step 1: Calculate the test statistic at this point in the study.

Step 2: If the test statistic is too large, then stop the trial in favor of treatment 1. If the test statistic is too small, then stop the trial in favor of the other treatment.

Step 3: If the test statistic is not in these regions, continue the trial until the next testing period.

Group sequential procedures are a mixture of trajectory analysis (i.e., they compute the likelihood that the test statistic would have followed the path it did if there was no treatment effect), and classical statistics (the answer is in terms of type I error rates). Thus, group sequential procedures construct a boundary for the test statistic at each monitoring point in the clinical trial. If the test statistic at any of these points is larger than the boundary at that point in time, we say that the monitoring

---

[*] That material has been very nicely developed in *Data Monitoring Committees in Clinical Trials: A Practical Perspective* by Susan Ellenberg, Thomas Fleming, and David DeMets (John Wiley & Sons, Ltd., West Sussex, 2002). Their text is very broad in scope, focusing on the DMC's evolution and contemporary operation.

rule suggests that early termination be considered. Rules such as those of Lans–DeMets are very popular group sequential procedures [2,3].

One group sequential approach is *stochastic curtailment* or *conditional power* [4,5]. One of the important questions DMCs commonly ask concerns the future trajectory of a test statistic i.e., "what is the likely result of the clinical trial had it been permitted to continue with the current information in hand?" This path evaluation is of course based on assumptions about the treatment effect. Assuming no additional treatment effect for the unexpired duration of the study is a useful conservative tack. This is termed conditional power under the null hypothesis. If, on the other hand, the investigators assume that an additional treatment effect will be seen for the remainder of the study, other test statistic paths become more likely. These procedures have also become valuable in the interim monitoring of clinical trials. The incorporation of some elementary concepts of Brownian motion simplify these computations immensely.

10.2.3 Brownian Motion and Conditional Power

Let I be the proportion of expected results observed in a clinical trial. Then we may index the progress of the trial not just by the passage of time, but also by the value I where $0 \leq I \leq 1$. The measure I is known as the *information time* of the study.

Straightforward computations can generate the probability of future test statistic trajectories. As an illustration, assume that an investigator in a clinical research effort has a test statistic of 2.95 at the $I = 0.60$ interim time point in the study (i.e., the endpoint events that have occurred at this point in the study comprise 60% of the events anticipated to occur by the study's end). She would like to compute the probability that the test statistic TS will be at least as large as 1.96 at the 90% information time point. This probability is the conditional power, or CP. She begins the computation with the statement

$$CP = P\big[TS(0.90) \geq 1.96 \,|\, TS(0.60) = 2.95\big]. \tag{10.13}$$

where $TS(I)$ simply denotes the value of the test statistic at information time I. The conditional probability in terms of the test statistic is difficult to solve, so we first convert this to Brownian motion, multiplying each event in the expression by $\sqrt{I}$. Thus

$$\begin{aligned} CP &= P\Big[\sqrt{0.90}\,TS(0.90) \geq \sqrt{0.90}\,1.96 \,|\, \sqrt{0.60}\,TS(0.60) = \sqrt{0.60}\,2.95\Big] \\ &= P\Big[\sqrt{0.90}\,TS(0.90) \geq 1.86 \,|\, \sqrt{0.60}\,TS(0.60) = 2.29\Big]. \end{aligned} \tag{10.14}$$

Denote $B(I) = \sqrt{I}\,TS(I)$. In the contemporary monitoring of clinical trials, the measure of the effectiveness of therapy is approximated by Brownian motion (Figure 10.1).

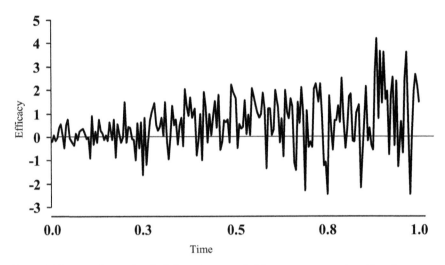

Figure 10.1. Brownian motion depiction of a test statistic's movement over time. Note the increasing variance the test statistic as information time increases. This movement is approximated by Brownian motion.

From Figure 10.1, we observe that the magnitude of therapy efficacy is not constant over time but instead develops over time, exhibiting a jerky movement with increasingly larger deviations from zero as the trial progresses. These properties of the efficacy's measure correspond to those of Brownian motion. Thus, we may rewrite the last line of expression (10.14) as

$$P\left[B(0.90) \geq 1.86 \mid B(0.60) = 2.29\right]. \tag{10.15}$$

Although Brownian motion is a complicated topic, we only need to draw on two useful features.[*] The first property is that for time t_1 and t_2 where $t_2 > t_1$, then, $P\left[B(t_2) > b \mid B(t_1) = a\right] = P\left[B(t_2 - t_1) > b - a\right]$. Applying that result here reveals that our probability of interest becomes

$$P\left[B(0.90 - 0.60) \geq 1.86 - 2.29\right] = P\left[B(0.30) \geq -0.43\right].$$

The second useful property of standard Brownian motion is that $B(t)$ follows a standard normal distribution. Its mean of zero is consistent with carrying out the analysis under the assumption of no treatment effect for the remainder of the study. Using this assumption, we write

---

[*] A useful introduction to Brownian motion is Moyé L.A. (2006). *Statistical Monitoring for Clinical Trials*: *Fundamentals for Investigators*. New York. Springer.

$$P\left[B(0.30) \geq -0.43\right] = P\left[N(0,0.30) \geq -0.43\right]$$

$$= P\left[N(0,1) \geq \frac{-0.43}{\sqrt{0.30}}\right] = 1 - F_Z\left(-0.786\right) = 0.784.$$

Thus, this evaluation of the future trajectory of the test statistic reveals that there is a 78% chance that the test statistic will be greater than 1.96 when 90% of the information time has elapsed, given the value of the test statistic is 2.95 at $I = 0.60$.

The forgoing computation is a "forward look procedure" since it focuses on events of interest in the future. First known as stochastic curtailment[*][6], it is now recognized by the more helpful term *conditional power* [7].

The prior computation was executed under the null hypothesis of no future treatment effect, an assumption tantamount to assuming that any therapy effect in the research effort has already been seen. This is known as conditional power computed under the null hypothesis, or $C_P(H_0)$. Conditional power may also be computed under the alternative hypothesis, $C_P(H_a)$. Under this alternative hypothesis, we no longer have the assumption $B(t)$ follows a normal distribution with mean 0 and variance t, but that $B(t)$ follows a normal distribution with mean μt and variance t. In traditional Brownian motion discussions, the parameter μ is known as the drift parameter. However, in the context of these discussions it is a measure of the treatment effect. When μ is not zero, we can follow the reasoning of the previous example to show that if $TS(I_1) = s_1$ and $TS(I_2) = s_2$, for information times I_1 and I_2 in a study were $0 \leq I_1 \leq I_2 \leq 1$, then

$$C_P(H_a) = P\left[TS(I_2) \geq s_2 \mid TS(I_1) = s_1\right] = 1 - F_Z\left[\frac{s_2 - \sqrt{I_1}s_1 - \mu(1-I_1)}{\sqrt{1-I_1}}\right]. \quad (10.16)$$

This style of computation was popularized by Lan and Wittes [8].

---

[*] The philosophy first appeared in industry as quality control specialists turned their attention to screening a lot of n manufactured items for acceptability. The decision rule used at the time claimed that the lot was acceptable if it contained less than c defectives; that is, brand the lot as unacceptable if it contained c or more defective items. However, the lot must be acceptable if there are $n - (c - 1)$ nondefects, and so it was suggested that by monitoring the number of nondefectives, the sample of tested items could be reduced. This reduction is described as curtailment. One could curtail the examination by scanning for nondefectives.

In this industrial circumstance, the scanning ceased as soon as the result became inevitable. However, why wait for inevitability? Interim probability computations would allow one to compute how likely it is that the lot would be acceptable based on the results of the lot's partial scan. This modification was termed *stochastic curtailment*. It is this expression that was transferred to the clinical trial arena and is now used as a moniker for the look forward procedure.

10.2.4 An Example of a Bayes Monitoring Rule

The work of Spiegelhalter et al. [9] depicts a useful Bayes contribution to the concept of monitoring rules in clinical research. Beginning with a conditional power argument, a prior distribution is placed on the anticipated research endeavor's treatment effect.

Consider an experiment on senility as an example. In this research effort, patients who are believed to be at high risk from Alzheimer's disease will receive a new therapy. Previous experimental history suggests that the new therapy will profoundly reduce the occurrence of this disease.

The investigators anticipate that, in this patient population at high risk of Alzheimer's disease, the five year incidence rate is 35%. The researchers are interested in producing a risk reduction of 30%, i.e., they expect that the active group will experience only 70% of the control group's rate of Alzheimer's disease. Assuming 90% power, and a two-sided type I error rate of 0.05, the investigators require 788 total patients, 394 in each of the two groups. Based on this information, we can compute the total number of pateints with newly diagnosed Alzheimer cases is anticipated to be $(394)(0.35) + (394)(0.35)(0.70) = 235$.

The investigators are interested in carrying out a conditional power computation during the course of the study. However, using the Bayesian perspective, they incorporate prior information about the effect size (expressed as the relative risk of the therapy for Alzheimer's diseases) associated with therapy. For this they use the log-normal distribution, i.e., the log of the relative risk θ follows a normal distribution. Thus $\pi(\theta)$ is expressed as

$$\pi(\theta) = \frac{a}{\theta\sqrt{2\pi}} e^{-(a\ln\theta+b)^2/2}. \tag{10.17}$$

where a and b are parameters selected by the investigators. The investigators have the freedom to calibrate $\pi(\theta)$ with their sense about the possible values of the relative risks (Figure 10.2).

This distribution of the values of the relative risk θ in Figure 10.2 expresses the prior knowledge and beliefs of the investigators for the location of the relative risk associated with the new therapy. In two of these three candidate prior distributions, most of the distribution of probability is amassed over values of the relative risk that are less than one, suggesting that the intervention will be effective. The remaining distribution, however, places substantial probability on the possibility of a harmful effect.

Several of the researchers believe the preliminary data available suggests the therapy will be quite successful, whereas others, less convinced by this assessment, expect the data will have no beneficial effect, and perhaps a harmful one. After much discussion among themselves, these researchers decide to divide the prior probability between two of these functions, selecting, $\pi(\theta)$ as

$$\pi(\theta) = 0.25 \frac{10}{\theta\sqrt{2\pi}} e^{-(10\ln\theta)^2/2} + 0.75 \frac{10}{\theta\sqrt{2\pi}} e^{-(10\ln\theta+2)^2/2} \qquad (10.18)$$

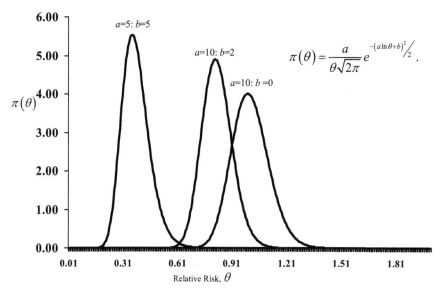

Figure 10.2. Three possible prior distributions for the effect size (relative risk) .

This final evaluation reflects their concern about the possibility that harm can occur as a result of the intervention (Figure 10.3).

The investigators wish to compute the conditional power given the test statistic is equal to some value s, i.e., $P\left[TS(1) \geq Z_{1-\alpha/2} \mid TS(I_1) = s\right]$. However, now we compute the predictive power, P_P, or the expected value of this conditional probability with respect to the prior distribution of the relative risk. From Appendix N, we find the predictive power is

$$P_P = 1 - F_Z\left[\frac{1.96 - s\sqrt{I} - \sqrt{\frac{E}{4a^2}}b(1-I)}{\sqrt{\frac{E}{4a^2} + (1-I)^4}}\right].$$

Note that this is a function of not only the value of the test statistic s at information time I, but also requires the parameters from the prior distribution a and b, as well. Since the prior distribution for this example is a mixture of two different log-normal distributions, we compute

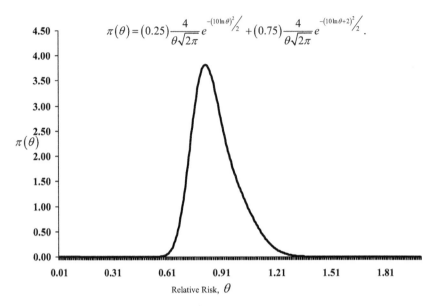

$$\pi(\theta) = (0.25)\frac{4}{\theta\sqrt{2\pi}}e^{-(10\ln\theta)^2/2} + (0.75)\frac{4}{\theta\sqrt{2\pi}}e^{-(10\ln\theta+2)^2/2}.$$

Figure 10.3. Prior distribution of relative risk of an intervention for total mortality. Note the region under prior distribution that is associated with hazard (shaded arrow).

$$P_p = 0.25\left[1 - F_Z\left[\frac{1.96 - s\sqrt{I}}{\sqrt{5.88 + (1-I)^4}}\right]\right] + 0.75\left[1 - F_Z\left[\frac{1.96 - s\sqrt{I} - 4.85(1-I)}{\sqrt{5.88 + (1-I)^4}}\right]\right].$$

Figure 10.4 demonstrates the relationship between the predictive power for the investigators based on their mixture prior as a function of both the test statistic and the information time, or the point in the study at which the test statistic is to be evaluated. Predictive power is the probability that the test statistic falls in the critical region given the value of the test statistic at a given point during the execution of the trial, I where $0 \le I \le 1$. Thus, the larger the test statistic is at the information time I, the greater this probability will be.

The relationship between the test statistic and the predictive power can also be assessed as a function of the mixture probability p of the prior distribution for the effect of therapy (Figure 10.5). In this case, we express the prior distribution as

$$\pi(\theta) = (1-p)\frac{10}{\theta\sqrt{2\pi}}e^{-(10\ln\theta+2)^2/2} + p\frac{10}{\theta\sqrt{2\pi}}e^{-(10\ln\theta)^2/2}$$

where $0 \le p \le 1$.

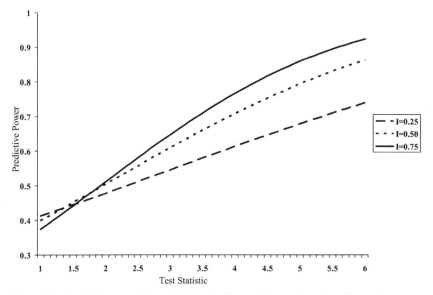

Figure 10.4. Predictive power for an Alzheimer's disease study as a function of the test statistic and the information time.

10.2.5 Comments on Predictive Value

Bayes procedures are an important new contribution to the statistical monitoring of clinical research. The incorporation of prior information provides flexibility to the investigator and a smooth, defensible, and reproducible way to incorporate the prior information into the monitoring procedure.

However, the requirement of the explicit specification of the prior distribution can be problematic if there is not much good information about the parameter to be estimated. In general, in order to be useful, prior distributions must reflect the state of information about the level of efficacy while simultaneously avoiding unnecessary mathematical complexity. Like other design parameters, this should be completely prespecified before the trial commences.

Each of the Bayes and frequentist perspectives' are useful, and one should not always be considered preferable to the other. If there is good prior information, the Bayes approach is a natural alternative. However, if there is little or no prior information, the researcher might be best served by staying with the classical perspective.

10.3 Adaptive Bayes Procedures

A second innovative application of the Bayesian philosophy in biostatistics is the field of adaptive Bayes procedures. This attractive recruitment strategy has been implemented in Phase II clinical trial methodology [10,11], and is credited with aiding drug discovery [12].

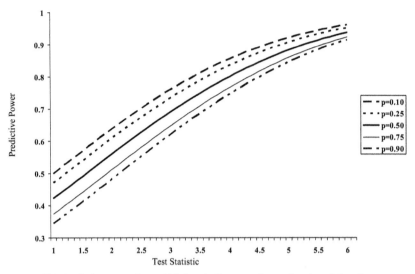

Figure 10.5. Predictive power for an Alzheimer's disease study as a function of the mixture probability *p* for the prior distribution.

10.3.1 Introduction
The idea behind the adaptive Bayes approach is simple; allow the therapy's effect to modify the recruitment algorithm for subjects into the treatment arms of the clinical trials.

Assume that investigators intend to carry out a small clinical trial with a control and an active treatment group. The researchers use the traditional 1:1 randomization procedure. Randomization is the process by which treatment group assignment is carried out without regard to the patient's characteristics. This procedure helps to ensure that the only difference between those patients assigned to active treatment and those assigned to the control group is the active therapy itself. Thus, differences in the endpoint of the study that appear between the control group and therapy group at the end of the study (assuming that they are not due to sampling error) must be created by the treatment because there are no other differences between the two groups.[*]

In addition, the recruitment strategy remains in force throughout the duration of the study. Whether the therapy has no effect, or a directional one, patients continued to be assigned in a 1:1 manner. Therapy assignment is not just independent of patient characteristics, it is also separate and apart from the therapy's emerging effect.

It is this second feature of the random allocation of therapy on which Bayesians have focused. The trial may begin with a randomization strategy that

---

[*] For an example of how dismantling randomization can affect a trial's results, see Moyé LA. (2006). *Statistical Monitoring of Clinical Trials: Fundamentals for Investigators.* New York, Springer. 9–10.

equally allocates patients to either the active or the control group. However, it needn't remain that way (Figure 10.6).

Bayesians argue that the treatment allocation ratio can change with the evolving treatment effect magnitude. Thus, when an interim evaluation of the data reveals that the therapy is producing a benefit, the adaptive Bayes procedure permits altering the treatment allocation ratio, adding more patients to the treatment group. Alternatively, additional patients would be placed in the control group if the risk-benefit assessment suggested that the treatment was beginning to produce harm.

Figure 10.6 demonstrates the overall strategy of the adaptive Bayes procedure in a clinical trial with two arms (treatment versus control). As recruitment commences, patients are allocated in a 1:1 ratio to the study. At the first interim evaluation time point A, the treatment is observed to have demonstrated an early benefit. At this point, the treatment allocation ratio is adjusted to permit twice as many patients in the active group as in the control group. At the next interim evaluation time point B, observers note the even greater benefit of the active group therapy. This leads to a further increase in the therapy assignment ratio to 3:1 until the end of recruitment.

The observation that the sum of the lengths of the duration of the lines under the various treatment allocation ratios is less than the duration of the study if it continued to recruit patients at the 1:1 ratio until the end demonstrates another hallmark of adaptive Bayes; they can (although they are not guaranteed to) reduce the number of patients required in the study. This can reduce the study's duration, and the influence of both of these factors can reduce the overall study cost. This is another attractive feature of adaptive Bayes procedures.

10.3.2 Acute Pancreatitis

Consider the design and execution of a small clinical trial to assess the effect of a therapy for the treatment of acute pancreatitis. This condition, in which the destruction of the pancreas causes that organ's caustic digestive enzymes to be released not just on the intraluminal food bolus, but also outside the digestive tract on the surface of the surrounding organs, produces ravaging internal organ damage and unbearable pain.[*] The therapy is believed to act quickly, producing its effect within the first hour after treatment.

The control group rate of the repeated use of morphine in this study is 90%. This randomized study was designed to detect a 30% reduction in patients experiencing pain that requires repeated morphine injections. Assuming a two-sided type I error rate of 0.05 and 90% power, the study requires ninety patients, 45 in each of the active and control group. The investigators begin recruiting immediately, anticipating that the trial will last for two years.

---

[*] An adage in emergency room care is that acute pancreatitis is one of the three emergency conditions that can make a grown man cry. The other two are renal colic (kidney stones) and dissecting aortic aneurism.

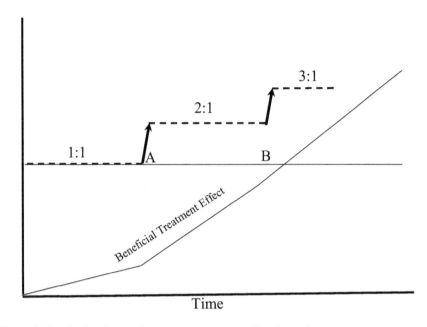

Figure 10.6. Adaptive Bayes adjustments to treatment allocation ratio.

However, after only the first 30 patients are recruited in the study the investigators discover the early emergence of a treatment effect. Fourteen of the 15 patients recruited to the control group experience enough pain to reach the study's endpoint. However, of the 15 patients recruited to the active group, only 10 patients reached this pain endpoint. These results while promising, are moderate. Not only are they not statistically significant (application of the *t*-test reveals a test statistic of 1.83; two sided *p*-value = 0.068 (Table 10.1), but they are well below the magnitude required for an early study termination.

Nevertheless, although the investigators must continue the study, they can fold the early treatment effect into their recruitment strategy. They have already recruited 30 of the 90 required patients, allocating half to each therapy group. They now alter this strategy for the next 30 patients in the study, randomizing 17 to the active group and 13 to the control group. With this new strategy in place, they aggressively recruit their study's next 30 patients.

The next interim analysis occurs after the evaluation of the second cohort of 30 new patients, at which time the investigators learn that 13 active group patients and 12 control group patients reached the endpoint. Thus, of the 60 patients recruited in the trial thus far, 23 of 32 active group patients and 26 of 28 control group patients reached the endpoint. These results are statistically significant, fueling the discussion of whether the study should be discontinued early.

Table 10.1 Effect of Adaptive Randomization on Study Conduct

| | Active Group | | Control Group | | | |
	n	patients with endpoints	n	patients with endpoints	test statistic	p-value
First Cohort	15	10	15	14	1.83	0.068
Second Cohort	17	13	13	12		
Total	36	23	28	26	2.10	0.036

10.3.3 Some Implications of Adaptive Bayes Procedures

The investigator's alteration of their randomization allocation raises a number of issues. One is, of course, that the investigators may have been misled in their evaluation of the first thirty patients. There are two forces that could have produced the early treatment effect: 1) the treatment itself, generating an effect that could be accurately generalized to the population at large, or 2) sampling error. The investigators altered their recruitment strategy based on the assumption that the early beneficial effect was genuine, reproducible, and would likely continue to be seen in subsequent patients. However, it might very well have been produced by the random play of chance. If so, the investigators would have increased recruitment in the active group only to have that undone by a diminution or an outright reversal of the finding in the next cohort. In this case, the investigators could argue that they could change the randomization allocation again, but the process begins to resemble jigging madly on the head of a pin.

There are also ethical considerations the investigators must address. Based on the substantial pain relief attributed to the first cohort of 30 patients in the study, one might argue that it is no longer acceptable to recruit the same proportion of patients to the (now seen as inferior) control group arm in the face of an emerging treatment benefit. The natural, human tendency is to recruit more patients into the therapy arm that provides the greatest benefit. Following this line of reasoning to the end, the investigators would recruit an even greater proportion of patients into the active group in the final cohort of thirty patients required for the study, should the study be permitted to continue.

However, the ethical considerations require consideration of a less attractive possibility. If, for example, the therapy has real risk associated with it (e.g., the likelihood of pulmonary emboli) then patients in the active group assume not just additional benefit but substantial risk of harm as well. Increasing the number of patients in the active group is best justified if a global assessment of the risk-benefit equation demonstrates the therapy is (based on the data so far) in the patient's best interest. Thus, as was the case with monitoring guidelines for clinical trials, while discussion to change the allocation ratio may be triggered by an emerging treatment effect, the actual decision to change this important ratio requires a more complete assessment of all the potential benefits and risks of the intervention.

In addition, there must be a tight temporal link between the therapy effect and recruitment. If an intervention does not produce a therapy effect until years after randomization e.g., the demonstration of the mortality benefit associated with "statin" therapy [13], this gradually appearing treatment effect will be unable to affect the randomization allocation ratio. Thus, this adaptive procedure is most useful when the therapy effect is observed shortly after the intervention's administration.

10.3.4 Setting the Allocation Ratio

A remaining question is how to determine the randomization allocation ratio in this process. It is this specific procedure that incorporates the formal Bayesian approach.

The approach is theoretically simple. Every clinical trial is designed to produce and assess the intervention's effect when compared to the result observed in the control group. If one can place a probability distribution on this treatment effect, then the magnitude of this probability for a given effect size can be used to determine the allocation ratio. The greater the probability of a large beneficial treatment effect, the greater the allocation of patients to the treatment group.

This approach is tailored to the Bayesian, who already has established a prior distribution for the treatment effect. This would itself allow an assessment of the treatment effect magnitude. However, the Bayesian is not satisfied with the prior probability distribution, devoid of the trials data itself. Thus, the trial's interim results will be used to update these prior probabilities. These updated posterior probabilities are the basis of the treatment allocation ratio.

10.3.5. Anti-Obesity Therapy

A clinical trial is designed to assess the effect of a new anti-obesity medication. Overweight patients will first be weighed, then placed on a program of diet and exercise. Immediately thereafter, these patients will be randomly allocated to either active therapy (the anti-obesity medication) or placebo. After six weeks of continuous therapy, patients will have their weights measured again. The endpoint of the study is the weight change experienced in the active group when compared to the control group. The study is expected to last one year.

In this study, let $y_1, y_2, y_3, \ldots y_n$ be the weight changes in the active group, and $x_1, x_2, x_3, \ldots x_n$ be the weight changes in the control group.[*] Patients are independent of one another, and within each treatment group, have a common distribution. We assume that the weight change in the active group for the ith patient y_i follows a normal distribution with mean θ_a and variance σ_a^2. However, θ_a itself has its own prior distribution; normal with mean $_a$ and variance τ_a^2.

Analogously, the weight change for the ith patient in the control group x_i follows a normal distribution with mean θ_c and variance σ_c^2. In this case, the prior distribution for θ_c has a normal prior distribution with mean $_c$ and variance τ_c^2.

Thus, the prior distribution of the change in weight between the two groups θ_a and θ_c itself follows a normal distribution with mean $u_a - u_c$ and variance

---

[*] For this exercise, assume that baseline and follow-up weights are available for all patients.

$\tau_a^2 + \tau_c^2$. Under the null hypothesis that the anti-obesity medication has no effect, then $u_a - u_c = 0$, and the symmetry of the normal distribution tells us $P[\theta_a \geq \theta_c] = P[\theta_a \leq \theta_c] = 0.50$, providing a justification for the 1:1 allocation ratio.

However, after n patients have been observed, we now have the mean change in weight for the active group $\overline{Y}_n$, and the analogous weight change for the control group patients $\overline{X}_n$. The investigators are interested in the posterior probability distribution of $P\left[\theta_a - \theta_c \mid \overline{Y}_n - \overline{X}_n\right]$. Adapting the results from Appendix I, this probability can be identified from invoking a normal distribution with mean ω and variance v where

$$\omega = \frac{\tau_a^2 + \tau_c^2}{\tau_a^2 + \tau_c^2 + n^{-1}\left(\sigma_a^2 + \sigma_c^2\right)}\left(\overline{Y}_n - \overline{X}_n\right) + \frac{n^{-1}\left(\sigma_a^2 + \sigma_c^2\right)}{\tau_a^2 + \tau_c^2 + n^{-1}\left(\sigma_a^2 + \sigma_c^2\right)}\left(\mu_a - \mu_c\right)$$

(10.19)

$$v = \frac{n^{-1}\left(\sigma_a^2 + \sigma_c^2\right)\left(\tau_a^2 + \tau_c^2\right)}{\tau_a^2 + \tau_c^2 + n^{-1}\left(\sigma_a^2 + \sigma_c^2\right)}.$$

In this research effort the investigator selects the parameters (in lbs) for the prior distribution (Table 10.2).

The prior information suggests a three pound weight loss in the control group can be attributable to their use of diet and exercise. A six pound weight loss is expected in the active group, the additional weight change due to the intervention. The standard deviation of the active group weight loss is slightly larger than the control group weight loss. The investigators begin with 1:1 treatment group to control group recruitment allocation.

Why? The investigators possess prior information suggesting a greater weight loss in the active group. Why settle for equal recruitment allocation ratio? The clearest explanation is that the collision of Bayesian and traditional frequentist philosophy commonly produces an unpredictable, fractional product containing elements of both philosophies. A purely Bayesian perspective would allow the prior information to generate differential recruitment into the active group from the very beginning of the study. However, to the frequentist (and, in fact much of the medical community) permitting this presumption of a greater treatment effect to affect the conduct of the study is a built-in bias.

Table 10.2 Assumptions Used in Weight Loss Clinical Trial

	Control	Active
Prior Distribution		
Mean	3	9
Standard Deviation	4	5
Conditional Distribution		
n		15
Mean	4	10
Standard Deviation	4	5
Posterior Distribution of Difference		
Mean		6
Standard Deviation		1.60

Thus, the current research culture suggests that there must be an early appearance of a treatment effect during the study itself to alter the treatment allocation ratio. Thus, adaptive randomization procedures in their current implementation are hybrid processes, borrowing from the frequentist domain in their application.

However, once the study commences, how does one translate the observed treatment effect to an adjusted treatment allocation ratio? Assume the investigators wish to demonstrate a five pound greater weight loss in the active group than in the control group. They use the probability of this event to determine the treatment allocation ratio. For example, after fifteen patients have been examined in the control group, the mean weight loss in the control group was 4 pounds, while the fifteen patients in the active group experienced a 10 pound weight loss. The investigators need to compute $P\left[\theta_a - \theta_c \geq 5 \mid \overline{Y}_n - \overline{X}_n = 6\right]$. From the contents of expression (10.19) they compute

$$P\left[\theta_a - \theta_c \geq 5 \mid \overline{Y}_n - \overline{X}_n = 6\right]$$

$$= 1 - F_Z\left[\frac{5 - \dfrac{\tau_a^2 + \tau_c^2}{\tau_a^2 + \tau_c^2 + n^{-1}\left(\sigma_a^2 + \sigma_c^2\right)}\left(\overline{Y}_n - \overline{X}_n\right) + \dfrac{n^{-1}\left(\sigma_a^2 + \sigma_c^2\right)}{\tau_a^2 + \tau_c^2 + n^{-1}\left(\sigma_a^2 + \sigma_c^2\right)}\left(\mu_a - \mu_c\right)}{\sqrt{\dfrac{n^{-1}\left(\sigma_a^2 + \sigma_c^2\right)\left(\tau_a^2 + \tau_c^2\right)}{\tau_a^2 + \tau_c^2 + n^{-1}\left(\sigma_a^2 + \sigma_c^2\right)}}}\right]$$

which from the values in Table 10.2 is 0.69. Thus, they would allocate 69 percent of future randomizations to the active group, and 31 percent of patients to the treatment group. This probability is clearly a function of the prior information $\mu_a - \mu_c$ (Figure 10.7).

Figure 10.7 confirms our intuition. The probability of a small difference in $\theta_a - \theta_c$ is large, and this probability decreases as $\theta_a - \theta_c$ increases. Further evaluation reveals that this curve is relatively robust with regard to the mean of the prior distribution for the difference in weight change for the two groups. For example, in the current example where we assumed that $u_a - \mu_c = 3$, we know that $P\left[\theta_a - \theta_c \geq 5 \mid \overline{Y}_n - \overline{X}_n = 6\right] = 0.69$. However, if the information from the prior distribution was more definitive suggesting a greater treatment effect, e.g., $u_a - \mu_c = 4$, then $P\left[\theta_a - \theta_c \geq 5 \mid \overline{Y}_n - \overline{X}_n = 6\right] = 0.71$, reflecting a very small increase in the treatment allocation ratio. Continuing, if the difference in the prior means increases to 6 lbs, the posterior probability only increases to 0.73. Thus the treatment allocation ratio in this scenario is protected from large differences in the prior distribution. Of course, treatment allocation ratios can be computed in the circumstance of mixture probabilities, i.e., where the prior distribution is a mixture of normal distributions with different parameters.

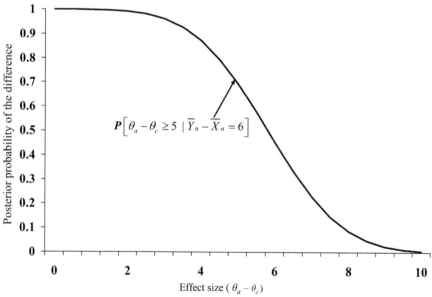

Figure 10.7. Posterior probability of the change in weight between active and control group (effect) size as a function of the effect size.

However, what guarantee do the investigators have that this strategy would reduce the expected sample size of the study over commonly used frequentist designs? We have seen earlier that assumptions concerning the future effect size can produce smaller sample sizes, however, these assumptions may be incorrect. At this stage in the development of adaptive procedures the best assessment comes from simulation, which is used to identify both false positive rates as well as conditional and predictive power assessments.

10.4 Conclusions

Bayesian procedures make important new inroads into clinical biostatistics. The ethical oversight of a trial and the recruitment allocation of a clinical research effort, historically well entrenched in the frequentist domain are being first dissected and injected with Bayesian perspective. Predictive power calculations produce an easily understood adaptation of conditional power. Adaptive Bayes procedures offer an exciting alternative to the static randomization process, a staple of clinical trials for over sixty years.

Both procedures are adaptations of research design methodology, and retain a frequentist component. The resulting hybrid procedures may make passionate Bayesians and vehement frequentists uncomfortable, but they are tailor-made for clinical investigators who are interested in choosing the best of both approaches for their contemporary research.

References

1. Moyé L.A. (2003). *Multiple Analyses in Clinical Trials*. New York. Springer.
2. Lan, K.K.G., DeMets, D.L. (1983). Discrete sequential boundaries for clinical trials. *Biometrika* **70**:659–663.
3. DeMets, D., Lan, G. (1984). An overview of sequential methods and their application in clinical trials. *Communications in Statistics* **13**:2315–38.
4. Lan K.K.G., Wittes J. (1988). The B-value: A tool for monitoring data. *Biometrics* **44**:579–685.
5. Davis, B.R., Hardy, R.T. (1990). Upper Bounds for type I and type II error rates in conditional power calculations. *Communications in Statistics* **19**:3571–3584.
6. Alling D.W. (1966). Closed sequential testing for binomial probabilities. *Biometrika* **53**:73–84.
7. Halperin M., Lan K.K.G., Ware J.H., Johnson N.J., DeMets D.L. (1982). An aid to data monitoring in long-term clinical trials. *Controlled Clinical Trials* **3**:311–323.
8. Lan K.K. and Wittes J. (1988). The B-value. A tool for monitoring data. *Biometrics* **44**:579–585.
9. Speigelhalter D.J., Freedman L.S, Blackburn P.R. (1986). Monitoring clinical trials: conditional or predictive power. *Controlled Clinical Trials* **7**:8–17.
10. Berry D.A., Eick S.G. (1995). Adapative assignment versus balanced randomization in clinical trials — a decision analysis. *Statistics in Medicine* **14** :231–246.
11. Berry D.A., Müller P., Grieve A.P., Smith M., Parke T., Blazek R., Mitchard N. and Krams M. (2002). *Adaptive Bayesian designs for dose-ranging drug trials*

In Case Studies in Bayesian Statistics V. Lecture Notes in Statist. **162**:99–181. New York, Springer.

12. Berry D. (2006). A guide to drug discovery; Bayesian clinical trials. *Nature Reviews Drug Discovery* **5**:27–36.

13. Sacks F.M., Pfeffer M.A., Moyé L.A., Rouleau J.L., Rutherford J.D., Cole T.G., Brown L., Warnica J.W., Arnold J.M.O., Wun C.C. Davis B.R., Braunwald E. for the Cholestrol and recurrent Events Trial Investigators. (1996). The effect of pravastatin on coronary events after myocardial infarction in patients with average cholesterol levels. *New England Journal of Medicine* **335**:1001–9.

11

Is My Problem a Bayes Problem?

11.1 Introduction

Whatever we may think of the Bayes approach to biostatistics, it is undeniable that this Bayes perspective provides us with an alternative solution to biostatistical problems.

Alternative points of view are critical to a field required to address complex issues. Mapping the human genome, a Herculean task of the 1990s, now pales in significance to understanding the gene-environment interaction affecting human health and behavior. Viral therapy and myocardial stem cell implantation have multifaceted implications, often requiring new thoughtful methodology for its assessment.

In addition, populations the world over are vulnerable to new threats whose measurement requires precision. Dangerous adverse effects linked to the use of approved medications (e.g., the relationship between the first generation thiodolizenediones and liver failure, or the use of cyclooyenase-2 (Cox-2) inhibitors and thromboembolic phenomena) require rapid assessment for protective population health measures to be taken. On a larger scale, the lives and livelihoods of millions rely on the rapid and accurate computation of hurricane strength and landfall probabilities. Finally, both the magnitude of (and the role mankind plays in) global warming, perhaps the ultimate public health problem, requires the best biostatistical and computing tools that we as a species can produce.

Each of these problems is complicated, controversial, and has critical implications. Constrained by imperfect knowledge, our initial ideas for solutions almost assuredly miss the mark. Seeing children, neighbors, and communities in peril drives our desire to quickly find a cure or policy that will stave off disaster. However as scientists we are self-disciplined by a cold, unforgiving reality; lasting solutions come only from complete understanding, and complete understanding comes only from slow, painstaking work.

This chapter focuses on how to determine whether the Bayesian or frequentist light provides the clearest illumination of the possible solutions to difficult biostatistical problems.

11.2 Unidimensional versus Multidimensional Problems

Only theoretical treatments can defensibly present a modern applied biostatistical problem as wholly frequentist, or wholly Bayesian. The fact is that in the contemporary scientific world, intelligent, defensible solutions are available using each perspective. It is hard to imagine looking at a complex problem such as whether antipsychotic medications produce diabetes mellitus separate and apart from the weight gain these medicines induce, from a wholly frequentist, or wholly Bayesian perspective.

Fortunately, the problem requires neither a frequentist nor a Bayesian solution; it simply requires a correct one. Investigators can use each of these perspectives to more completely inform themselves about the nature of the problem, e.g., the state of the problem's background information, and the losses sustained should they grasp at an incorrect solution. Problems are multidimensional. Looking at them as though they are entirely frequentist or entirely Bayesian is like viewing a charging bear in only the x-plane or the y-plane. Both provide information, but the force and complexity of the issue can be missed.

In this matter, we can be instructed by human disease. The contemporary study of medicine divides the body into neat organizational compartments. Students study diseases of the heart, illnesses of the pancreas, blood dyscrasias, and brain maladies. The cause, pathophysiology, natural history, and treatment of these diseases is presented in great detail, and it is not uncommon for students completing two years of didactic medical training to overestimate the worth of this compartmentalized knowledge.

However the practice of clinical medicine requires treating patients who commonly have a combination of diseases. An accident victim suffering intense blood loss suddenly sustains a massive stroke. A patient with chronic asthma goes into heart failure. A mother presents not just with intractable stomach ulcers, but from the unbearable stress of learning that her 13 year-old daughter is pregnant. The effect of disease combinations on an individual and their family comprise the complex illness that befuddles the medical student.

Wise clinicians choose not merely to find the best therapy for the disease, but to seek out the best treatment for the patient. Tools that were developed to solve isolated problems are used in combinations, providing a global solution to a multidimensional problem.

It is in this hybrid environment in which the Bayesian must work. The pressing problems mentioned in this chapter's first section are examples of contemporary multidimensional problems that biostatisticians confront. Their complexity forces us to discard the notion that the best approach resides in only the frequentist domain or solely the Bayesian realm. For example, in the complex clinical trial environment, we should not be surprised to find a Bayesian sample size estimation and a Bayesian interim monitoring rule, combined with a frequentist-based final analysis. Complicated problems require a variety of approaches.

While it is possible that a problem can be entirely Bayes, or entirely frequentist, they will have elements of both. Thus, taking our cue from this discussion, we will not ask about whether a problem should be a frequentist or Bayesian solution, we will ask what are the best tools to solve the problem. This revolves around the availability of prior information, the presence of an acceptable loss function, and the receptivity of the medical and scientific community. The following is an example of this approach.

11.3 Ovulation Timing

11.3.1 Introduction

Women desiring to become pregnant quickly learn about the complexities of conception. In order to successively conceive, her egg (the ovum) must break free from the ovary, navigating the short, dangerous gap between the ovary itself and the irregular, fimbriated edge of the fallopian tubes. After entering one of these tubes, the ovum is available for fertilization by the sperm. Although the average woman's cycle is 28 days long, the egg is only available for conception for approximately two of those days, typically occurring around the middle of the cycle. If the egg is fertilized, the embryo must successfully implant in the uterus. When no fertilization takes place, the ovum makes its way though the uterus and is expelled at the end of the cycle.

While mid-cycle fertility has been recognized for centuries, many women commonly need more than knowledge of this cycle for an accurate determination of exactly what day during the cycle initiates their fertility period. The body does undergo several temporary changes during the ovulation period that are signs of fertility. Cervical mucous changes in consistency, and the cervix alters its texture. Some women actually experience pain.[*] However, the most reliable fertility indicator is the change in their internal temperature, known as basal body temperature (BBT).

The daily measure of BBT has come to be relied upon by women and fertility experts in determining when a women's fertile period begins.[†] In general a woman will have an increase of 0.4 to 1 degree Fahrenheit in BBT when she ovulates. These temperatures are easily plotted, permitting the observer to, looking back over the month, determine when ovulation commenced (Figure 11.1). In Figure 11.1 the increase in temperature beginning on day 13–14 of the cycle most likely indicates ovulation has taken place.

The determination of ovulation by following BBT can actually be straightforward. However, there are two complications with this approach. The first is that clearest picture of ovulation occurs retrospectively. Once the cycle is over and the graph is complete, it can be relatively easy to determine the day of ovulation. However, women need real time information. Specifically they need to know whether they are ovulating today, or whether they ovulated yesterday. For example, for a particulary cycle, with only BBT measurements through day 8 of the cycle it is difficult to know whether ovulation was commencing on day 7–8 (Figure 11.1).

---

[*] Women can sometimes experience one-sided low abdominal pain during ovulation, known as mittelschmerz. Some estimate that 20% of women endure mittelschmerz during some of their reproductive periods.

[†] To reduce variability, women are encouraged to take three consecutive measurments each day during the same time, using the same thermometer after at least five hours of sleep.

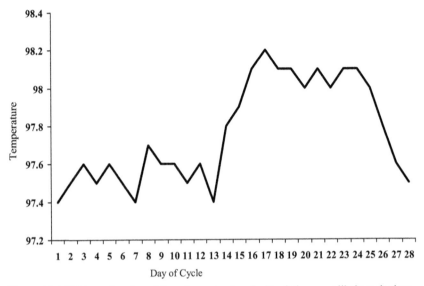

Figure 11.1 BBT as a function of day of menstrual cycle. Ovulation most likely took place on day 13–14.

Another problem is that not all cycles provide a clear depiction of the ovulation day (Figure 11.2).

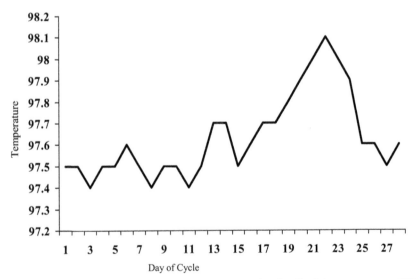

Figure 11.2 BBT cycle with ambiguous temperature acceleration. Real-time assessment of BBT on day 12 and 13 suggest ovulation has commenced. However, the time of ovulation is actually day 15–16 of the cycle.

In this case, the woman at day 12–13 of her cycle, based on BBT might believe she had ovulated. However, ovulation did not take place until day 15–16 , a fact that was not clear until the cycle was complete.

A useful tool in the prediction of ovulatory time would permit accurate real time assessments. The question before us is whether a Bayes tool would be useful in this setting.

In addition, in order to be accepted by reproductive specialists, the device should build on their understanding and intuition about the process. In addition, it must be relatively easy for a non-mathematician (e.g., a fertility expert or a patient) to use.

11.3.2 Framework of the Problem

The goal is to provide an estimate of the ovulation day of a particular women, given her ovulatory and temperature patterns in previous cycles. Ultimately, the investigators need an assessment that any day in the cycle (including future days in the same cycle) will be the ovulation day. This is in distinction to the task of estimating an "average ovulation day" in a sample of women.

Let θ be the day of ovulation. Then θ is an integer from 1 to the duration of the cycle (most commonly but not always 28 days). Our ultimate goal is to estimate θ, an estimate that we will label δ_B. Let t_k be the temperature (in Fahrenheit) on the kth day. Then our Bayes estimator will be a function of the posterior distribution of $\pi(\theta|t_k)$, or $P[\theta = j|t_k]$. This is the probability that the jth day of the cycle is the ovulation day, given the BBT on day k is t_k. From Bayes theorem, we can write this as.

$$\pi(\theta|t_k) = P[\theta = j|t_k] = \frac{f(t_k|\theta)\pi(\theta)}{\sum_j f(t_k|\theta)\pi(\theta)}. \tag{11.1}$$

However, this formulation is not sufficient for us to conclude that a Bayes approach will work. The investigators require a realistic and useful parameterization of the prior distribution $\pi(\theta)$, the conditional distribution $f(t_k|\theta)$, and the loss function $L(\theta, \delta_B)$. In addition, the posterior distribution must be computed in real time, i.e., the posterior probability $P[\theta = j|t_k]$ will be based only on one temperature obtained on a single day. It cannot be based on future values of k, i.e., waiting until the cycle is complete to assess the most likely day of ovulation.

11.3.3 Setting the Loss Function

Setting the loss function requires us to estimate the risk of underestimating or overestimating θ.

If $\delta_B < \theta$, we are saying that the ovulation day has arrived too early, and the reverse inequality concludes that ovulation has occurred later than it actually has. We must return to the original problem to assess the magnitude of these errors. Assume the purpose of the procedure is to maximize the likelihood of pregnancy, i.e., timing intercourse so that the probability of pregnancy is maximized. Wilcox et al. [1] determined that conception is most likely when intercourse occurs during the six–day period ending on the day of ovulation. Thus values of δ_B greater than θ (e.g., prediction $\theta = 18$ when in fact $\theta = 16$, incur great loss, because the opportunity for conception is most likely to be missed. A reasonable loss function in this circumstance is weighted linear loss, i.e.,

$$L(\theta, \delta_B) = K_1(\theta - \delta_B)\mathbf{1}_{\theta > \delta_B} + K_2(\delta_B - \theta)\mathbf{1}_{\theta \leq \delta_B}. \tag{11.2}$$

where K_1 and K_2 are the penalties for a prediction of θ that is too early, or too late, respectively. We know from Chapter Seven that the Bayes predictor, δ_B in this case is the r^{th*} percentile of the posterior distribution, where

$$r = \frac{K_1}{K_1 + K_2}. \tag{11.3}$$

At this point we will simply say that since overestimation produces the greater penalty, $K_2 > K_1$ the value of Bayes procedure will be one of the lower percentile values of the posterior distribution.

11.3.4 Prior Probabilities of θ

The fertility experts and statisticians who jointly worked to estimate ovulation timing all agreed that prior information for a woman's ovulation cycle was critical in making future predictions. However, important disagreements soon emerged about the format of this information.

Statisticians were interested in a parametric approach to the characterization of a woman's prior ovulation history. Parametric distributions avoided making day by day decisions about the probability that θ would be a particular value, instead focusing on a smooth reproducible form of the probability over the entire cycle. In addition, the assumption that $\pi(\theta)$ followed a well-known distribution permitted them the instant ability to apply all that they knew about the distribution (e.g., mean and variance) to the distribution of the mean ovulation time. A popular distribution was the conditional chi-square distribution, stated as $P[d_1 < \theta < d_2 \mid \theta \leq 28]$ where θ represents the ovulation day in a 28–day cycle and $0 \leq d_1 < d_2 \leq 28$ (Figure 11.3). The statisticians believed that the chi-square distribution was flexible enough to handle different shapes for the ovulation pattern of a woman's previous cycles, $\pi(\theta)$.

---

[*] Refer to Chapter Seven, Figure 7.8.

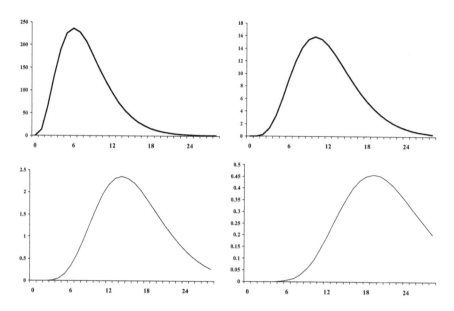

Figure 11.3 Different chi-square distributions to capture the prior information about ovulation timing.

However, the investigators were unconvinced by the statisticians' arguments. The doctors, with little formal statistical training, did not see the advantage of applying what to them was a complex, arbitrary, and nonintuitive mathematical formulation for the prior distribution of the ovulation day. In addition, the fertility experts were quite concerned that these parametric distributions placed too much probability on days they believed were unlikely to signal ovulation. Finally, they were uncomfortable with exactly how these probabilities would be updated. In the end, it was believed that the assumption of the chi-square distribution essentially detached the physicians from the prior building process, and unless replaced would disconnect them from the problem.

The fertility doctors were more comfortable with placing discrete probability mass on particular cycle days. This information was readily obtained from a woman's prior ovulatory patterns. It was these probabilities that they wished to update using the Bayes procedure, hoping that the process would take only a small number of consecutive cycles of a woman to obtain reliable estimates of the ovulation day θ (Figure 11.4).

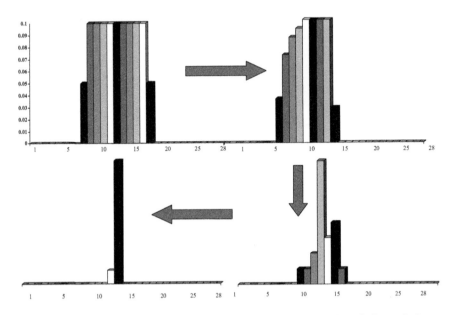

Figure 11.4 Desired improvement in ovulation timing prediction. With each cycle the prediction focuses on a small number of days which can be identified before that cycle ends.

In the end, the statisticians accepted the fertility specialists arguments, accepting $\pi(\theta)$ in the format $\pi(\theta) = \sum_{k=1}^{L} P[\theta = k]$ for an L day length cycle.

11.3.5 Conditional Distribution

Discussions concerning the conditional distribution of BBT t on day k given the value of θ were much less contentious. All parties agreed that t should follow a normal distribution. The variance of this distribution σ^2 was assumed to be fixed. If the woman followed instructions for the measurement of BBT (i.e., measuring it at the same time of the day, following the same daily procedure and used the same thermometer σ^2 was anticipated to be small.

Conversation focused on the mean BBT as a function of the day of ovulation. The cycle was divided into two regions, pre-ovulatory and post-ovulatory. All acknowledged that the greater the distance between the current day of the cycle k and θ, the closer the temperature would be to base temperature, $t(L)$. As the ovulation day approached, the temperature would increase, finally reaching the maximum temperature $t(H)$. Once ovulation occurred, the mean temperature would decrease again to $t(L)$. However, the rate of rise of the temperature must be faster than the rate of decline. The investigators agreed on the following formulation for the mean temperature on the kth day of the cycle, given θ, the day of ovulation;

$$\mu(k \mid \theta) = \frac{(\theta-k)t(L)+\left(\dfrac{1}{\theta-k+c}\right)t(H)}{\theta-k+\dfrac{1}{\theta-k+c}}1_{k\le\theta} + \frac{(S-k)t(H)+(k-\theta)t(L)}{S-\theta}1_{k>\theta} \quad (11.4)$$

Since it is not uncommon for women to have unusually short or long ovulatory cycles, the variable S was selected as the cycle length in days.

This mean function for the normal distribution is simply a combination of two functions. Early in the woman's cycle before ovulation takes place, $k < \theta$, and

$$\mu(k \mid \theta) = \frac{(\theta-k)t(L)+\left(\dfrac{1}{\theta-k+c}\right)t(H)}{\theta-k+\dfrac{1}{\theta-k+c}}. \quad (11.5)$$

Equation (11.5) is simply a weighted average of $t(L)$ and $t(H)$. The rapid rise of $\mu(k \mid \theta)$ as k gets close to θ approximates the sudden increase in BBT that women experience at or near the day of ovulation. The term c is simply a correction that avoids a denominator of 0 when $k = \theta$, and also determines the rate of rise of the BBT at or near the ovulation time.

The term $\dfrac{(S-k)t(H)+(k-\theta)t(L)}{S-\theta}$ characterizes the mean temperature in the post-ovulatory phase of the cycle. This is simply a linear function of k, assuring that as the woman progresses to the end of her cycle, the BBT decreases from t_H to t_L.

This mean function $\mu(k \mid \theta)$ can be evaluated for any cycle. One only need have a measure of the BBT during the non-ovulatory phase, an idea of the peak temperature during ovulation, the duration of the cycle, and the ovulation day, Knowledge of these parameters allows one to configure $\mu(k \mid \theta)$ for individual women (Figure 11.5). In this example, the non-ovulatory basal body temperature is 97.5. The investigators expect the peak ovulatory temperature to be 98.1, and ovulation occurs on day 14 of a 28-day cycle. Other ovulatory patterns can also be configured. (Figure 11.6).

Here, both $t(H)$ and $t(L)$ are different from their values in the previous examples. Ovulation occurs on day 10 in a 22-day cycle. In addition, the rate of rise of the temperature is more gradual than in the example of Figure 11.5. This slope is governed by the parameter c in equation (11.4).

Thus, $f(t \mid \theta)$ can be precisely specified; small values of σ^2 further amplify this precision.

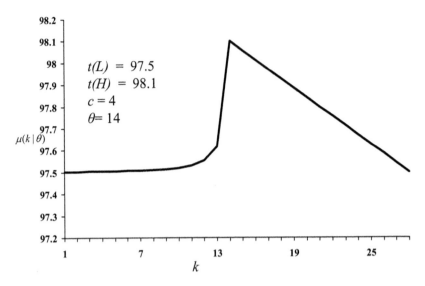

Figure 11.5 Modeled mean basal body temperature as a function of θ for a 28-day cycle length when the ovulation day is day 14.

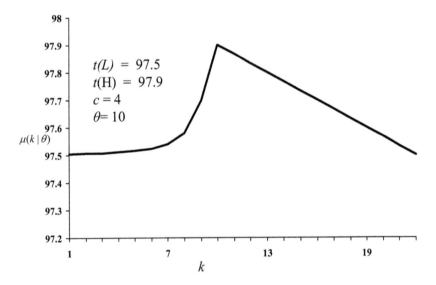

Figure 11.6 Modeled mean basal body temperature as a function of θ for a 22-day cycle length when the ovulation day is day 10.

11.3.6 Building the Posterior Distribution

Our goal is to compute the posterior probability distribution of the day of ovulation θ based on the BBT t on day k. This is a simple application of Bayes Theorem.

$$\pi(\theta \mid t) = \frac{f(t \mid \theta)\pi(\theta)}{\sum_{\theta} f(t \mid \theta)\pi(\theta)}.$$

Our work from the previous two sections allows us to write this as

$$P[\theta = j \mid t_k] = \frac{\dfrac{1}{\sqrt{2\pi\sigma^2}} e^{-\left(\frac{t_k - \mu(k\mid\theta=j)}{2}\right)^2} P[\theta = j]}{\sum_{j=1}^{S} \dfrac{1}{\sqrt{2\pi\sigma^2}} e^{-\left(\frac{t_k - \mu(k\mid\theta=j)}{2}\right)^2} P[\theta = j]}$$

$$\qquad\qquad\qquad\qquad (11.6)$$

$$= \frac{e^{-\left(\frac{t_k - \mu(k\mid\theta=j)}{2}\right)^2} P[\theta = j]}{\sum_{j=1}^{S} e^{-\left(\frac{t_k - \mu(k\mid\theta=j)}{2}\right)^2} P[\theta = j]}.$$

This is all we need do to identify the posterior distribution. This function can be easily examined as a function of the woman's prior information, and her current temperature.

11.3.7 Results

We can apply this evaluation system to the particular situation of a women who requests help in predicting her ovulation day. As requested, she provides an assessment of her previous ovulation pattern. This history was obtained from a collection of prior monthly BBT measurements that permitted the patient and investigators to jointly assess which day was her ovulation day in each of these previous months. From these retrospective evaluations, the investigators constructed a histogram of the frequency that any given day was the ovulation day. This is precisely what it requires for $\pi(\theta)$ (Figure 11.6).

The investigators note that while the most likely days of ovulation are the twelfth and thirteenth day of her cycle, the patient has experienced months in which ovulation has been very early (day 10) and quite late (day 16). Since the previous history demonstrates that ovulation only occurs in this range of days, the posterior distribution will be focused on this interval as well.

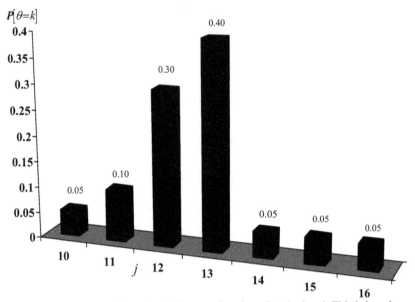

Figure 11.7 Prior probability of ovulation as a function of cycle day, j. This is based only a collection of the patient's previous cycle history.

The investigators learn that the patient's BBT's typically varied from 97.5 to 98.1 during her 28-day cycle. However, since the patient has not been sufficiently trained in measuring BBT, the quality of the temperatures measurements is relatively low, and the estimate of σ was 0.5.

      Letting $j = 12$ in formulation (11.7), allows us to compute the probability that ovulation occurs today. The mean function $\mu(k\,|\,12)$ as a function of k can be computed and examined (Figure 11.8).

      This information is sufficient to provide a posterior estimate of the probability of ovulation. Assuming that today is the 12th day of the cycle, and this morning's BBT is 98, we can compute $P\left[\theta = j\,|\,t_{12} = 98\right]$ from equation (11.6)

$$P\left[\theta = j\,|\,t_{k} = 98\right] = \frac{e^{-\left(\frac{98-\mu(k\,|\,\theta=j)}{2}\right)^{2}}\,P\left[\theta = j\right]}{\sum\limits_{j=1}^{28} e^{-\left(\frac{98-\mu(k\,|\,\theta=j)}{2}\right)^{2}}\,P\left[\theta = j\right]}. \qquad (11.7)$$

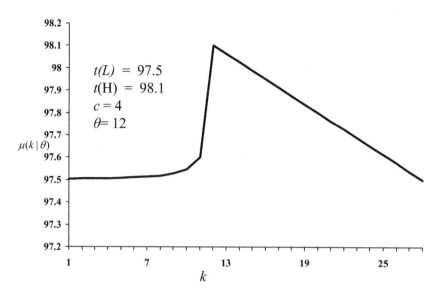

Figure 11.8 Modeled mean basal body temperature as a function of θ for a this woman's 28-day cycle assuming day 12 is the ovulation day.

From equation (11.7) we can compute $P[\theta = 12 \mid t = 98] = 0.291$. There is a 29% chance that the 12th day of the cycle will be the ovulation day, given the temperature is 98.

However, equation (11.7) permits us to compute additional probabilities as well. For example, by setting $j = 11$, we can compute the probability that ovulation occurred yesterday, given today's BBT is 98 (i.e., the patient missed ovulation by one day). In fact, this equation permits a complete elaboration of the ovulation day distribution as a function of θ given that the 12th day's BBT is 98 (Figure 11.9). Figure 11.9 provides ovulation probabilities for days 10 through 16, which was the only range of days that had nonzero prior probability. For example the probability that ovulation occurred yesterday is $P[\theta = 11 \mid t_{12} = 98] = 0.143$, where as the prior probability that ovulation occurred on day 11 was 0.10.

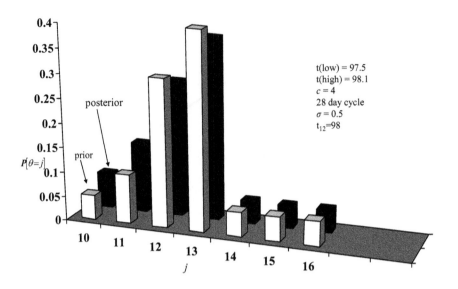

Figure 11.9 Comparison of prior and posterior probability of ovulation as a function of cycle day, j when the basal body temperature on day 12 is 98.

A closer examination of Figure 11.9 reveals the close correspondence between the prior and posterior probabilities of the ovulation throughout the distribution of candidate days, suggesting that the posterior distribution does not contribute substantial new information to the posterior probability. One reason for the similarity of these two probability distributions is the value of σ. The standard deviation temperature value of 0.5 is quite large, given the range of BBT is itself less than one degree for this patient. If, for example, the patient measures her BBT using the same thermometer at the same time of the day and following the same insertion procedure, σ can be reduced from 0.5 to 0.2 producing a more illuminating probability distribution (Figure 11.10). The more precise estimate of the temperature has sharpened the distinction between the prior and posterior distributions, with ovulation seen as much likely to have occurred on the eleventh and twelfth days of the cycle.

Since equation (11.7) permits predictions of the ovulation day as a function of the BBT and the day the BBT was measured, the posterior distribution of θ can be computed and displayed as a measure of these two variables. The depiction of this relationship allows the patient to visualize the temperature she must have on a given day to be reasonably assured that she is ovulating during that time in her cycle.

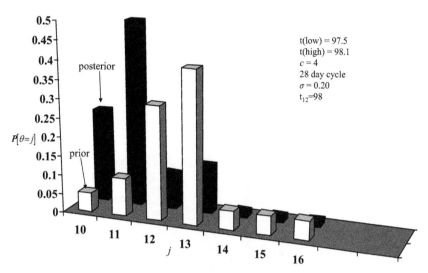

Figure 11.10 Comparison of prior and posterior probability of ovulation as a function of cycle day, j when the basal body temperature on day 12 is 98 and $\sigma = 0.20$.

For this examination, we focus on a particular women whose ovulation day lies between day 10 and day 16 of her cycle. This patient measures her BBT consistently, using the same technique, generating a relatively small standard deviation for BBT ($\sigma = 0.20$). In general her BBT when she is in the non-ovulatory phase of her cycle is 97.3. The maximum temperature she usually sustains during ovulation is 98.4. Her cycle is 28 days long. An examination of her prior cycle history reveals that she typically ovulates on day 13 of her cycle. Today is the 11th day of her cycle. From this information we can examine the distribution of ovulation day as a function of the BBT (Figure 11.11).

Figure 11.11 provides the posterior probability distribution of the ovulation day, $P[\theta = j]$, as a function of the BBT. The first row of this figure provides the prior distribution of θ. Each subsequent row depicts the posterior distribution as a function of the BBT obtained on day 11. We see that for relatively low BBTs, the posterior distribution of θ closely matches the prior distribution. In this case, low BBT's early in the cycle suggest the woman has not yet ovulated, a finding consistent with the prior distribution. However, for higher BBTs on day 11, the posterior probability shifts to the left, favoring early ovulation days.

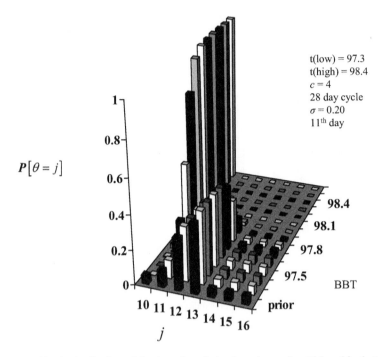

Figure 11.11 Distribution of the day of ovulation based on a day 11 basal body temperature.

The higher BBTs on day 11 suggests that the patient has already started her ovulation cycle. Even though this is an unlikely occurrence under the prior distribution, the high precision of the temperature estimates places greater emphasis on the information provided by temperature.

If for the same women the BBT was obtained on day 16 of her cycle, a different relationship is observed (Figure 11.12). In this case the temperature is obtained on day 16 of the cycle. We observe that the distribution of θ is markedly dependent on the BBT. For lower BBT, θ follows a bimodal distribution with probability divided between the ovulation day being very late, and much earlier day of ovulation. However, for larger temperatures, the likelihood of ovulation shifts to earlier in the cycle.

Recall that the investigators formulated a loss function for the estimation of θ based on weighted linear loss. Equation (11.3) reflects the investigators' decision to place a greater loss on estimates of the ovulation day that were too late rather than two early. From our discussions about loss function in Chapter Seven, we know that the Bayes procedure δ_B will be a percentile of the posterior distribution.

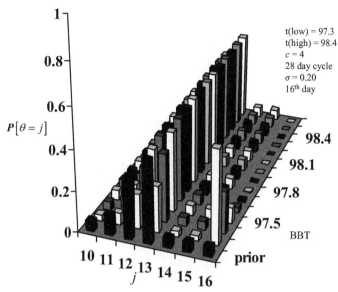

Figure 11.12 Distribution of the day of ovulation based on a day 16 basal body temperature.

If we assume that it is three times more costly to have missed the day of ovulation than to precede, it, the investigators calculate that δ_B is the 25th percentile of the posterior distribution.

We can compute the Bayes procedure in another scenario, where the temperature is obtained on day 12 of the woman's cycle. The prior distribution of θ is equally distributed from days ten through nineteen, and unfortunately, her BBT estimates are relatively imprecise ($\sigma = 0.60$). The influence of temperature on predictions on the date of ovulation are quite revealing (Figure 11.13). Only when temperatures are high does the posterior estimate of the ovulation day provide information different than that of the prior. We define the Bayes estimate $\delta_B(t_k)$ as the predicted ovulation day when the BBT on day k is t_k. For example, $\delta_B(t_{12} = 97.6)$ is 11. The relationship between $\delta_B(t_{12})$ and t_{12} reveals the relative robustness of the Bayes procedure for different temperature (Figure 11.14).

11.3.8 Commentary
The remarkable observation about this Bayes procedure was the relatively small contribution of advanced mathematics, a factor that was adumbrated by the critical requirement for clear discussions between physicians and statisticians. The major construction effort during this work was not building the procedure but building the relationship with the fertility experts. They knew little about Bayes procedures, but were immediately attracted to the idea of using prior information to predict ovulation days.

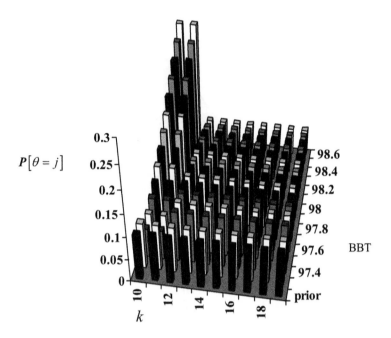

$P[\theta = j]$

Figure 11.13 Distribution of the day of ovulation based on a day 12 basal body temperature.

Most of the mathematical work was based on building the conditional distribution's mean value. The investigators were perfectly willing to permit this construction in all of its mathematical complexity. This was perhaps for two reasons: 1) the relationship between ovulation and BBT has been well established, and 2) the investigators already bought into the need to combine information about the patient's prior cycles with current information about the BBT on a particular day. In essence the statistician's job was facilitated by the history of the investigators who, unbeknownst to themselves, had been trying to build mental Bayes procedures on their own.

11.4 Building Community Intuition

Applied biostatisticians and ultimately, clinical investigators, must have useful intuition about the performance of Bayes procedures if these methods are to become generally accepted. After all, like all biostatistical methods of estimation and inference, Bayes procedures can mislead when used inappropriately. In science, we learn by doing.

For example, it has taken clinical trialists several generations of experience to understand the appropriate role of subgroup analyses in clinical trials. Subgroup analysis is the evaluation of a clinical trial's tested intervention in a subcohort (e.g., men, or people of Hispanic descent less than 50 years of age) of the entire randomized collection of patients.

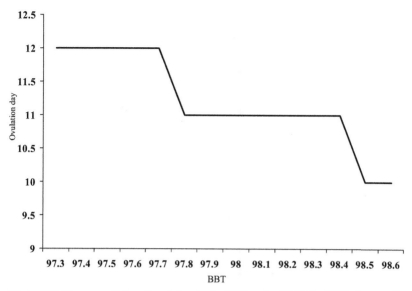

Figure 11.14 Bayes prediction of ovulation day by BBT on day 12. Higher BBTs favor earlier ovulation days.

When first elaborated, these subgroup analyses were seen as important investigational tools, strengthening the penetrating ability of clinical trial to illuminate many of the nuances of an intervention's effect. Thus investigators believed that clinical trials could provide not just the effect of therapy on the entire randomized cohort, but also the different effects in groups of patients of clinical interest (e.g., women, or patients who were compliant with therapy).

However, prominent examples of the failure of subgroup analysis arose [2], leading to influential criticism of subgroup analyses as confirmatory [3], culminating with Yusuf's incisive review [4]. The perils and consequences of subgroup analyses with international consequences were elaborated [5], and additional examples of their misleading propensity appeared [6, 7] . However, more recently, a specific set of conditions have been elaborated in which subgroup analyses in clinical trials can be confirmatory [8].

Thus, over forty years, the clinical trial community has, through hard work and bitter disappointment, learned the appropriate use of subgroup analyses in clinical trials. In retrospect this effort could not have been reduced. There is no useful shortcut over the rough terrain of experience if the goal is the solution of a complex problem.

This is likely to be the path of over which Bayes procedures will be mastered. However, the most illumination is provided if the motivation for the Bayes procedures are clear and its impact can be directly assessed, separate and apart from the other aspects of the research effort.

Consider a well designed, well executed clinical trial whose primary endpoint is well established and accepted by the research community. In this stable research environment, a Bayesian analysis can be quite illuminating. The community, already comfortable with the design and endpoint of the study, can readily build on this intuition to understand the unique contribution the Bayesian perspective adds.

Suppose investigators are interested in studying the effect of a new medication on the cumulative mortality rate of patients with hypertension. Following their sample size computations, they recruit 4500 patients into their study and randomly allocate 2250 to each group. Patients will be followed for four years. In this case, the intervention is well understood, and the design of this clinical trial in hypertension is well accepted by the cardiovascular community. Thus, a Bayesian analysis, using prior information to develop a posterior distribution for the mortality effect is an analysis that the community, although perhaps a bit disoriented at first, can come to appreciate. Intuition develops naturally as the scientists rely on their insight about the intervention and research design to appreciate what the Bayesian approach has to offer. Educated by a long experience with the classical frequentist-style analyses, they can compare the traditional solution with the Bayes result, permitting a clear view of the new contribution the Bayesian analysis provides.

However, consider a study in patients with diabetes mellitus. Even in the early 21st century, physicians do not yet know the best way to reduce the sequela of diabetes mellitus (including, but not limited to fatal and nonfatal heart attacks, fatal and nonfatal strokes, kidney disease, blindness, and nontraumatic amputations). Assume investigators wish to study a new intervention to reduce the terrible outcomes of this disease. With no experiences with this or other related interventions, the medical community has little intuition about the intervention's mechanism of action, or its panoply of effects.

In addition, assume that the investigators introduce a novel surrogate for the endpoint (e.g., serum cytokine levels). They believe these levels are useful intermediate measures of the previously mentioned clinical consequences of diabetes mellitus. However, again, the clinical community has little experience with this new endpoint.

In this complex trial that develops an alien, surrogate endpoint in an unfamiliar intervention for a disease that is not well understood, a Bayesian analysis would most likely blunt, rather than sharpen the clinical trial's assessment. It will already be difficult for the medical community to understand the new intervention's effect on a novel endpoint in a complex and incompletely understood disease. There is little familiar about the study to them, and with few recognizable features, the medical community is easily confused. In this setting, the Bayesian approach makes a bad situation worse by adding yet one more complicated and unfamiliar tool to the assessment process. More innovation is the last thing the research community needs in this research. They need well-recognized, time-tested standards that can be relied upon to assess the effect of the therapy.

Admitted these are two extremes, designed merely to make a point. The Bayesian perspective, in order to be contributory needs to be integrated in such a way that the consumer clearly understands the contribution it is making. The less familiar the disease-intervention complex, the less a new and unfamiliar procedure (be it a Bayes procedure or another tool) will be helpful (Figure 11.15).

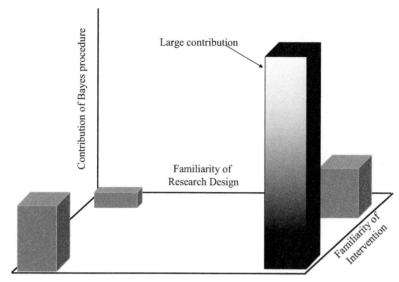

Figure 11.15 Utility of Bayes procedures. When the intervention, and research design are familiar, Bayes procedures are the most useful. However, when the research community has little insight into the intervention or the research design, Bayes procedures can add to the confusion.

References

1. Wilcox A.J., Weinber C.R., Baird D.D. (1995). Timing of sexual intercourse in relation to ovulation. Effects on the probability of conception, survival of the pregnancy, and sex of the baby. *New England Journal of Medicine* **333**:1517–1521.
2. MRFIT Investigators. (1982). Multiple risk factor intervention trial. *Journal of the American Medical Association* **248**:1465–77.
3. Bulpitt C. (1988). Subgroup Analysis. *Lancet*: 31–34 .
4. Yusuf S., Wittes J., Probstfield J., Tyroler H.A. (1991). Analysis and interpretation of treatment effects in subgroups of patients in randomized clinical trials. *Journal of the American Medical Association* **266**:93–8.
5. Moyé L.A. (2003). *Multiple Analysis in Clinical Trials. Fundamentals for Investigators* New York, Springer. Chapter 10.
6. Packer M., O'Connor C.M., Ghali J.K., et. al for the Prospective Randomized Amlodipine Survival Evaluation Study Group (1996). Effect of amlodipine on morbidity and mortality in severe chronic heart failure. *New England Journal of Medicine* **335**:1107–14.

7. Packer M. (2000). Presentation of the results of the Prospective Randomized Amlodipine Survival Evaluation-2 Trial (PRAISE-2) at the American College of Cardiology Scientific Sessions, Anaheim, CA, March 15, 2000.

8. Moyé L.A., Deswal A. (2001). Trials within trials; confirmatory subgroup analyses in controlled clinical experiments. *Control Clinical Trials* **22**:605–619.

12
Concl sions and Commentary

Even its critics must admit that the Bayesian point of view with its new and refreshing perspective for biostatistics can, like the first spring breeze blowing through a musty room, be energizing.[*] Allowing the scientist to focus on the hypothesis that he or she actually believes (rather than being forced to disprove what they don't believe) is a powerful idea, and the facility to formally incorporate relevant preliminary information is invigorating.

When first exposed to the Bayesian perspective, physician-scientists commonly react like weary travelers who, after a long and perilous journey through alien lands, have finally come home. The notion that prior impressions and information, almost always in full supply, can now be formally incorporated in an analysis is not just intuitive — its order shattering thought process is liberating. In fact, audience members wonder aloud how the field of statistics ever allowed itself to wander away from this intuitive Bayesian point of view, available for hundreds of years.

Bayesians are now breaking down traditional barriers in clinical trials. The possibility of including them was tentatively raised fifteen years ago [1,2]; now they boldly stake a claim on the clinical trial landscape. Flexing their computational muscles, Bayesians demonstrate undeniably impressive abilities in sample size computations [3,4,5,6,7,8,9,10]. Bayesian workers focus on the implementation of Bayesian procedures in assessing the causal nature of the exposure-disease relationship when clinical preference drives the exposure [11]. The ethics of the use of Bayes procedures have been discussed [12], and monitoring procedures from a Bayes perspective have been formulated and adopted [13,14,15,16]. Bayes procedures are also being applied to observational studies [17,18], and a particular series of useful analyses on missing data is now available [19]. The role of adaptive randomization in clinical trials, i.e., permitting the trends in treatment effect within the trial itself to influence the proportion of patients who are allocated to a particular therapy is steadily expanding into Phase II clinical trial methodology [20,21], aid-

---

[*] This is taken from Moyé L. (2007) Bayesians in clinical trials. Asleep at the switch. *Statistics in Medicine* In press.

ing drug discovery [22]. And, while several textbooks on Bayes procedures have been available [23,24,25], there is now a textbook devoted solely to the application of Bayes procedures in clinical trials [26].

In addition, the Bayesian approach is being absorbed by the pharmaceutical review and approval process, attracting new attention from the U.S. Food and Drug Administration (FDA). The Center for Devices and Radiological Health (CDRH) accepts Bayesian procedures as a standard statistical approach. Approximately 10% of FDA approvals for medical and radiological devices (e.g., spinal implants and cardiovascular stents) are based on Bayesian analysis. If required to go through traditionally designed Phase III trials, these medical implements may have taken longer to become available.

In fact, the tide of Bayesian procedures is rising so rapidly that the uninitiated may be forgiven for reacting like the newcomer to a beach during high tide. The onlooker concludes that, since the water level is high now, it must always be so. Yet the experienced observer appreciates tidal ebb and flow, and the established clinical trial methodologist, disciplined by a long, bitter experience with methodologic and clinical "breakthroughs" that promised much but delivered little of practical consequence, understands that the most useful perspective when assessing a new tool's utility is time and practice, followed by calm assessment.

While relatively new to biostatistics, the Bayesian perspective has existed for over 225 years, almost three times longer than the Fisherian hypothesis testing perspective, and four times longer than the clinical trial mind-set. It is useful to stop for a moment to see where the Bayesian perspective has been before biostatistics takes the path it has chosen for our future.

12.1 Validity of the Key Ingredients
As it was at the beginning of the 19th century, Bayesians are again poised to make rapid progress in statistical sciences. This time biostatistics is the target. However, they cannot decisively take this ground until they demonstrate how to *constructively* apply the three innovations their philosophy generates: 1) the likelihood principle, 2) the prior distribution, and 3) the loss function, to a field that poses unique and sometimes treacherous dilemmas. Unfortunately, the challenges clinical investigation holds for the application of these precepts may be just as daunting as the obstructions that stunted the growth of the applied Bayesian biostatistics 100 years ago.

12.1.1 The Likelihood Principle
The likelihood principle is one of the cornerstones on which the modern Bayes edifice now rests. It stands for the elegant proposition that the only relevant part of an experiment is, in the end, what has actually occurred [23]. While this simple statement may appear self-evident, Bayesians, quite perceptively fault frequentists in their standard violation of this foundational principle. The frequentist argues that unobserved data can be just as influential as the observations that have occurred. An illustration of the conundrum frequentists find themselves in when caught in a likelihood principle violation was first developed by Pratt as an engineering problem [27], and later adopted for the health care research field [28]. follows:

"I was just interested in producing a confidence interval for diastolic blood pressures in my clinic," one physician exclaimed to another at a clinical trial meeting. "That's all I wanted to do! I had an automated device that would read blood pressure very accurately and produce data that appeared to be normally distributed with a mean of 87 and a standard deviation of 5. I turned the data over to a statistician for a simple analysis.

"When the statistician came to my clinic to share his findings, he had a conversation with the staff nurse who told him that the automated blood-pressure-measuring device did not read above 100 mm Hg. When I confirmed this, the statistician said that he now had to do a new analysis, removing the underlying assumption of a normal distribution, since the blood pressure cuff would read any diastolic blood pressures greater than 100 mm Hg as only 100 mm Hg. I understood his point, but assured him that in my data, no patient had a diastolic blood pressure greater than 97 mm Hg. Also, if there had been one, I would have called another clinic for a backup automated device, equally sensitive to BP readings greater than 100 mm Hg.

"The statistician was relieved, thanked me, and returned to his office. However, after he left, I noticed that my backup unit was broken, and e-mailed this circumstance to him. He e-mailed me back, saying that he would have to redo the analysis after all! I was astonished and called him immediately. Why should the analysis be redone? No blood pressure was greater than 100 mm Hg, so the broken backup device would not have had to be used. My measurements were just as precise and accurate as they would have been if all instruments were working fine. The results would have been no different. Soon he would be asking me about my stethoscope!"

To the Bayesian, the statistician's fixation on the availability of a confirmatory sphygmomanometer is nonsensical. Since the data never required it, they ask, why be concerned about its presence? At first glance, one can only be amused (or angered) by the feckless frequentist as portrayed.

However, the statistician depicted in the example is quite right in his demand to learn of the availability of the backup meter, if his concern is generalizing to the population at large.[*] The raison d'être of clinical trials is precisely this type of generalization.

---

[*] Clearly, no backup unit is required in the sample, since every subject's blood pressure was less than 100mm Hg. However, if the statistician is no longer concerned about what occurs in the sample, but in the population at large, his concern about the backup meter is central. In order to generalize the findings to the population at large, specifically in patients who have DBP > 100 mm. Hg. they must have had the opportunity to be admitted to the sample and had their blood pressure meaured. If their blood pressure was > 100 mm Hg, their BP would

The likelihood principle also suggests the inadvisability of the two-tailed hypothesis test. Two-tailed testing ensures that there is adequate protection for the finding that a therapeutic intervention may produce harm. The investigator creates their critical region so that the null hypothesis is rejected for hazard as well as for benefit. However, at the study's conclusion, the test statistic can only fall on one side of the distribution – it can't be in both. Physician-scientists are commonly confused about this, asking "Why, when we now know what side of the distribution the test statistic is on, must we bother with the type I error allocated in the other tail?" but frequentists have successfully argued that since they said prospectively that they would divide the type I error in two, they should then follow through on their original plan. Bayesians argue that since the data do not identify harm, then regardless of what they stated prospectively, the investigator can focus all of their concern to the benefit side. This is a central, clarifying difference. The likelihood principle permits the Bayesian to divorce him or herself from the prospectively declared methodology. The frequentist would not.

In all fairness, one cannot fault this conclusion of Bayesian deductions without faulting the logic of the frequentists as well. The theoretical optimality of the one-tailed test to the two-tailed test has been established for many years. However, frequentists have learned to disregard such artificial optimality in clinical trials where two-tailed testing appropriately predominates.

Will Bayesians use the likelihood principle to dismantle a foundation tenet of clinical trial methodology – the importance of a prospective plan separate and apart from the data? Frequentists insist that if a sample's results are to be extended to the population, then there must be in place a population-derived methodology (i.e., a methodology that will apply to all members of the population) for the evaluation of the sample results. However, the likelihood principle asserts that the only methodology that should be used is a sample-based one. This is a tremendous paradigm shift.

12.1.2 Prior Information

In medicine, "prior belief" is an amorphous mixture of fact-based knowledge with subjective impressions. Acting on prior belief and its important subjective component is unavoidable in clinical medicine simply because we as physicians are required to treat diseases that we only incompletely understand.

The challenge facing Bayesians in this arena are nothing short of monumental. Although we desire a degree of belief of "1" in all true propositions, and "0" in all false propositions, this lofty standard rises above what is achievable in clinical science [29]. Bayesians must therefore fall back to the best, most accurate prior information available, but here lies the trap — in medicine, the best, most accurate prior information is 1) frequently difficult to quantify, and 2) commonly inaccurate if not outright wrong.

Clinical trial investigators are among the world's greatest and saddest authorities in being led astray by false leads and unreliable prior information. The

---

remain unknown and hence the blood pressure distribution would have to be censored. Generalization from the sample to the population requires a violation of the likelihood principle.

Cardiac Arrhythmia Suppression Trial (CAST), a one-sided (benefit-only) clinical trial designed to detect a beneficial effect of ecanide, flecanide, and moritzacine was prematurely ended in the face of overwhelming evidence that two of these drugs (and eventually the third) generated excess mortality [30]. This study revealed the difficulties that occur when research design is based on strong but incorrect physician belief [31].[*] Yet the clinical trial permitted the true nature of the effect size to be revealed precisely because the methodology utilized to measure the effect size was segregated from the prior belief. This is not the case in Bayesian analysis, and a Bayesian approach to CAST in which the prior belief influences the effect size estimator would have deepened the interpretational conundrum. Other examples, e.g., the United Kingdom Prospective Diabetes Trial (UKPDS) [32,33,34,35] abound.

One useful device that we researchers use on our quest for truth is the measuring rod of consistency. The observation that a set of different experiments, carried out by different investigators, in different patients, using different study designs produce similar results, bolsters our belief in the truth of the findings. In this circumstance, our prior belief is smoothly updated and refined through the cascade of consistency. This circumstance is tailored made for the Bayesian statistician who requires reliable prior information.

Yet even consistency can be a difficult track record to sustain in clinical research. The suggestion that the anticholinesterase inhibitor vesnarione was first helpful [36] and then harmful [37] in patients with congestive heart failure (CHF) flummoxed the cardiology community, wreaking havoc with its "priors". The collection of Evaluation of Losartan in the Elderly Study ELITE [38,39,40] trials and Prospective Randomized Amlodipine Survival Evaluation (PRAISE) [41,42], each conducted to identify a beneficial effect of a medication, both demonstrate the wild ride prior information can take. In each study, the investigators were surprised by a finding of benefit, leading them to conduct a second a study to confirm the promising finding. Both second studies reversed the findings of the first study, bringing the investigators back to their original prior. One can be forgiven a sense of vertigo as one ponders the reaction of Bayesian trialists who must update their prior repeatedly with information that suggests not just different magnitudes of effects but different directional effects.

It is difficult to create a consensus on prior information when different experiments purporting to study the same problem produce conclusions that are mirror images of each other. While frequentists are also troubled by this conflicting information, they can be comforted by the fact that the estimate of effect size is not affected by the prior information. This is inefficient when the prior information is accurate, but a useful buffer in the face of inaccurate prior "knowledge."

There may be some small solace in the use of meta-analyses in developing prior belief. The literature contains useful discussions of the strengths and weaknesses of meta-analyses [43]. The controversies they can produce are commonly focused on the studies included in the analyses, e.g., when an analysis of corticosteroid use for brain injury [44] was believed to be flawed based on the ex-

---

[*] Much of the discussion is taken from Thomas Moore's book entitled *Deadly Medicine*.

clusion of an influential study that demonstrated a benefit [45]. Thus, while a small oasis in this desert of prior information may appear as meta-analyses, the Bayesian must be especially cautious that it is not a mirage.

Both Bayesians and frequentists alike lament the unreliability of prior information in many clinical trials. However, only Bayesians are required to formally incorporate it into their measure of efficacy. Even though frequentists must also build an effect size in, it does not affect the estimate itself. Yet prior information for the Bayesian directly affects the estimate. There are many tools at their disposal permitting them to distance themselves from faulty prior information, for example the use of vague, uninformative priors. However, the degree to which Bayesians distance themselves from prior information is the degree to which they enter the land of the frequentist; there, the strict rule is to completely separate *a priori* belief from the evidence-based product of the research effort.

12.1.3 Loss Function
The third contribution of Bayesian procedures to clinical trials is the loss function. This function guides the Bayesian trialist in interpreting the posterior distribution, essentially telling the Bayesian how they should use the posterior distribution to come to a decision.

Bayesians have great flexibility in choosing the loss function for the circumstance. However, in clinical medicine, real life loss functions are rarely accurately represented by dichotomous loss, absolute error loss, or squared error loss, and these useful didactic tools have little relevance in clinical trials. For example, a patient's blood sugar assessment must be accurate, but the loss function varies with whether the patient is hypoglycemic (and overestimations may be lethal) or hyperglycemic (where underestimates are intolerable). The overall loss function will be complicated. Yet it is incumbent upon the Bayesian who insists that the clinical research world is ready for Bayesian methods, to construct realist loss functions. We required that they depict the true risk – benefit calculus the physician and their patient must work through as they ponder whether a therapy's salubrious effects are with its adverse ones.

12.2 Dark Clouds
Clearly Bayesians have much good work before them as their reputation as clinical trialists moves through its nascent period. Few doubt that the technical obstacles in computing, and assembling helpful loss functions will block Bayesian progress for much longer. Bayesians will continue to overcome computing obstacles as they have in the past, and their insight into the intricacies of the complicated cost-benefit loss functions will only deepen over time.

Nevertheless, there are several dark clouds under which Bayesian biostatisticians labor. Among the most threatening is the nagging suspicion that, while the Bayesian philosophy may be a giant leap forward for other applied sciences, it represents a step backward in clinical research. Specifically, the embrace of prior, untested and subjective information, in combination with the likelihood principle's implications will create a chaotic research environment in which, once again it will be difficult to disentangle fact-based result from expert but misleading opinion.

Clinical medicine is overwhelmed with prior belief and opinion which is many times both honest and inaccurate. Without specific safeguards, use of Bayesian procedures will set the stage for the entry of nonfact-based information that, unable to make it through the "evidence-based" front door, will sneak in through the back door of "prior distributions." There it will wield its influence, perhaps wreaking havoc on the research's interpretation.

In addition, the likelihood principle, with its insistence on making decisions based only on observations that have occurred and not those that haven't, reduces the moderating influence of established methodology that was put in place to curb the inappropriate generation of sampling error-generated results.

Frequentists have argued for years that clinical trial researchers must begin with not what they believe, but what has been established as the standard. They then build a fact-based case against this null hypothesis, and the research community requires the clinical trial to affirmatively and decisively reject the current community standard of care. This time-tested frequentist approach makes clinical investigators uncomfortable precisely because it so completely protects us from our own natural weakness – our need to believe that the therapy that we are advocating will work!

We physicians are devoted, intelligent, and driven specialists; we are also quite human. We care about the patients we see with a compassion that is uniquely ours, personified in the oath that we take. As one of the first responders to the Hurricane Katrina debacle, my colleagues and I did not function as dispassionate observers of a human tragedy, we continuously consoled, actively treated, and were deeply affected by the patients so desperate for attention and good medical care [46]. Physicians just don't look for cures, we ache for them! So, when we learn of a potential new treatment, our natural tendency is to give it the benefit of the doubt. It is difficult for physicians to keep in mind how bad things may be with an untested intervention in the face of the reality of how bad things are without it. The frequentist approach plays the critical role of protecting us from our own strong convictions about the effects of untested therapy.

This edifice separating the physician-scientist's research from his or her own beliefs was not easily built. It was assembled brick by brick through uncountable many debates, discussions and arguments over the 60 year history of clinical trials. Yet Bayesians, although supported by a doctrine that has been existence for over 225 years, did not participate in these pivotal discussions during the formative years of clinical trial development. Bayesians were relatively unavailable as frequentists argued repeatedly and heatedly with physicians that clinical research methodology should be structured, that research questions should be stated objectively, that null findings be as easily interpretable as positive ones, and that we physicians must be concerned about the possibility of therapy-induced harm even when we "believe" that no harm will occur. Bayesians were curiously absent for the five decades that these arguments raged furiously.

Yet now, when the investigator-community finally understands the problems that stem from relying on their own untested assumptions, and appreciates that the research benefits of a disciplined methodology outweigh its risks, Bayesians burst onto the scene with a mathematical justification for the use of prior information. The havoc from this confusion is something that the iconoclast Reverend Price may have delighted in, but neither Bayesians nor their frequentist counterparts can afford this now.

Frequentists have shed their intellectual and emotional blood building a wall that separates the clinical investigator's research execution and analysis from their prior belief. It may be that General George S. Patton was right when he said that "fixed fortifications are monuments to the stupidty of man," but, nevertheless disaster strikes in clinical trials when the wall is breached. If Bayesian trialists are not vigilant, the work that they have started to break this wall down will be used to their own undoing, and we may very well have to wait to the beginning of the 22nd century for the next Bayesian wave.

12.3 Recommendations

The following represent seven steps Bayesians can take to improve their standing in the community as rigorous clinical trialists.

Step 1. Take a strong stand for disciplined research methodology.

Frequentists in clinical trials have a well-enunciated perspective on research discipline. The perspective of the Bayesian community has not been articulated, and their omnipresent likelihood principle opens the door to the possibility that Bayesians believe in "letting the data decide" in clinical trials.

Bayesians must send an unmistakably clear message through the clinical trial research community about the importance of methodologic rigor in clinical research. They cannot afford to stand idly by while loosely trained clinical investigators convert the impassioned Bayesian argument for prior information inclusion into a lever to pry open the entire case of disciplined research methodology. Bayesians stand to lose all they have worked so hard for by being asleep at the switch at this important junction. Bayesian methodologists must act at once to ensure the scientific community that Bayes clinical trials must be expertly designed and concordantly executed.

Step 2. Fix the miss-translation.

While Bayesians have made an elegant and mathematically persuasive argument for the incorporation of prior information into clinical research, they have not sufficiently differentiated between prior information and prior belief. Thus, clinical investigators commonly think that their untested and sometimes wild opinions can be formally incorporated into research as "prior knowledge." This is certainly not the message Bayesians mean to transmit, yet it is the message many clinical investigators manage to receive. In this regard, Bayesians stand to make the same mistake that frequentists made with the p-value. It was never the intent of the field of frequentist biostatistics to allow a small p-value to "cover a host of methodologic sins", e.g., small sample size and data-driven protocol deviation. Yet, because frequentists were asleep at the switch during that critical junction, the clinical research community must still pay the price for a re-search climate contaminated by the "0.05 culture." By remaining mute, Bayesians run the risk of making an equally catastrophic error.

Step 3. Show us something new.

The research paradigm should offer an illumination of biologic processes and therapy-human interaction. For example, it was the clinical trial para-digm that revealed the "placebo effect." What such revelation will come from the application of Bayesian processes? If there are none, then the Bayesian approach will simply be a tepid alternative to the frequentist per-spective, much of whose own luster has been rubbed away by years of dif-ficult clinical trial experience.

Step 4. Develop realistic prior distributions and loss functions.

Many didactic tools begin with simple priors and loss functions which il-luminate Bayesian principles. However, the real clinical world is a messy place. In order to be truly illuminating, Bayesians need to move away from the safe haven of uniform prior probabilities, conjugate distributions, and squared error loss. Very few results can be as impressive as a new re-search insight that comes from a Bayesian clinical trial with an illuminat-ing prior distribution and a sensitively constructed loss function. Many scientists would rush to embrace Bayesian procedures if Bayesians would construct helpful loss functions that allow municipal managers to deter-mine when they should call for evacuations in the threat of hurricanes. We need prior distributions and loss functions that don't just support, but illu-minate clinical research.

Step 5. Actively incorporate counterintuitive prior information.

Experienced clinical trial biostatisticians know to follow the peroration of clinical opinion leaders with a healthy dollop of skepticism. These opin-ions of clinical thought leaders must not be allowed to imbalance the prior distributions Bayesian incorporate in clinical trials. To many ill-trained clinical scientists, prior information is an opportunity to infuse nonfact based "information" into a trial to influence the results. A useful rule of thumb might be, the more passionate the investigator, the greater the pro-tection the prior requires from their strongly held opinion. This role would be filled by not simply a non-informative prior, but a counterintuitive prior, to actively counterbalance the strong, frequently wrong opinions of clinical experts.

Step 6. Banish discussion of "improper priors" from clinical research.

Clinical scientists have worked hard to master the concepts of probability sufficient to understand the testing multiplicity dilemma, proportional hazard regression analysis, and the statistical monitoring of clinical trials. Probability that does not sum to one injects tremendous confusion into an environment in which doctors are already struggling with the proper incorporation of prior belief into their research. Improper priors are a mathematical nicety but an unnecessary clinical conundrum and nuisance.

Step 7. Develop good Bayesian primers for clinical investigators.
Bayesian mathematics while elegant, are simply too dense at the level they are commonly taught for many physicians with only a remote exposure to calculus and a one-semester course in statistics. Bayesians need to write clear simple expositions on what they stand for, and how clinical trials conducted under the Bayesian paradigm are different from current state-of-the-art frequentist clinical trial methodology. This can begin during the early basic science years of medical school, when students can learn to segregate belief from knowledge (the first frequentist course in statistics is commonly offered during the first two years of medical school). In addition, the Bayesian paradigm can be demonstrated during a one-semester course in biostatistics that research assistants and clinical trial project managers take. Designing such a curriculum will be daunting but there is much at stake. An early introduction can provide the uninitiated student with a smooth learning curve, easing their way to becoming seasoned Bayes clinical investigators.

References

1. Berry D.A. (1993). A case for Bayesianism in clinical trials (with discussion). *Statistics in Medicine* **12**:1377–1404.
2. Spiegelhalter D.J., Freedman L.S., and Parmar M.K.B. (1994). Bayesian approaches to randomized trials (with discussion). *J. Roy. Statist. Soc. Ser. A* **157**:357–416.
3. Diamond G.A. Kaul S. (2004). Prior convictions: Bayesian approaches to the analysis and interpretation of clinical megatrials. *Journal of the American College of Cardiology* **43**:1929–1939.
4. Spiegelhalter D.J., Freedma L.S., Parmar M.K. (1993). Applying Bayesian ideas in drug development and clinical trials. *Statistics in Medicine* **12**:1501–1511.
5. Cui L., Hung H.M.J., Wang S. (1999). Modification of sample size in group sequential clinical trials. *Biometrics* **55**: 853–857.
6. Lehmacher W., Wassmer G. (1999). Adaptive sample size calculations in group sequential trials. *Biometrics* **55**:1286–1290.
7. Muller H., Schafer H. (2001). Adaptive group sequential designs for clinical trials: combining the advantages of adaptive and of classical group sequential approaches. *Biometrics* **57**: 886–891.
8. Proschan M.A., Hunsberger S.A. (1995). Designed extension of studies based on conditional power. *Biometrics* **51**:1315–1324.
9. Cheng. Y., Su, F. and Berry D.A. (2003). Choosing sample size for a clinical trial using decision analysis. *Biometrika* **90**:923–936.
10. Moyé L.A. (1997). Sizing Clinical Trials with Variable Endpoint Event Rates. *Statistics in Medicine* **16**:2267–2282.

11. Korn E.L., Baumrind S. (1998). Clinician preferences and the estimation of causal treatment differences. *Statistical Sciences* **13**:209–235.

12. Berry D.A. (2004). Bayesian Statistics and the Efficiency and Ethics of Clinical Trials *Statistisical Sciences* **19**:175–187.

13. Speigelhalter D.J., Freedman L.S., Blackburn P.R. (1986). Monitoring clinical trials: conditional or predictive power. *Controlled Clinical Trials* **7**:8–17.

14. Spiegelhalter D.J., Freedman L.S., Balckburn P.R. (1986). Monitoring clinical trials. Conditional or predictive power? *Controlled Clinical Trials* **7**: 8–17.

15. Freedman L.S., Spiegenhalter D.J. (1989). Comparison of Bayesian with group sequential methods for monitoring clinical trials. *Controlled Clinical Trials* **10**:357–367.

16. Freeman L.S., Spoiegelhbalter D.J., Permar M.K. (1994). The what, why, and how of Bayesian clinical trial monitoring. *Statistics in Medicine* **13**:1371–1383.

17. Ashby D., Hutton J., McGee M. (1993). Simple Bayesian analysis for case-control studies in cancer epidemiology. *The Statistician* **42**:385–397.

18. Dunson D.B. (2001). Practical advantages of Bayesian analysis of epidemiologic data. *American Journal of Epidemiology* **153**: 1222–1226.

19. Kmetic A., Joseph L., Berger C., Tenenhouse A. (2002). Multiple imputation to account for missing data in a survey: estimating the prevalence of osteoporosis. *Epidemiology* **13**:437–444.

20. Berrry D.A., Eick S.G. (1995). Adapative assignment versus balanced randomization in clinical trials — a decision analysis. *Statistics in Medicine* **14**: :231–246.

21. Berry, D.A., Müller P., Grieve A. P., Smith M., Parke T., Blazek R., Mitchard N. and Krams M. (2002). Adaptive Bayesian designs for dose-ranging drug trials. *In Case Studies in Bayesian Statistics V. Lecture Notes in Statistics* **162**: 99–181.

22. Berry D. (2006). A guide to drug discovery; Bayesian clinical trials. *Nature Reviews Drug Discovery* **5**:27–36.

23. Berger J.O. (1980). *Statistical Decision Theory. Foundations, Concepts, and Methods*. New York. Springer.

24. Carlin B.P., Louis T.A. (2000). *Bayes and Empiricle Bayes Methods of Data Analysis – Second Edition*. New York. Chapman &, Hall/CRC.

25. Gelman A, Carlin J.B., Stern H.S., Rubin D.B. (2003). *Bayes Data Analysis – Second Edition*. Boca Raton. Chapman & Hall/CRC.

26. Speigelhalter D.J., Abrams K.R., Myles J.P. (2004). *Bayesian Approach to Clinical Trials and Health-Care Evaluation*. New York. Wiley.

27. Pratt J.W. (1962). Discussion of A. Birnbaum's "On the foundations of statistical inference" *Journal of the American Statistical Association* **57**:269–326.

28. Moyé L.A. (2006). *Statistical Reasoning in Medicine: The Intuitive P-value Primer – 2nd Edition*. New York. Springer.

29. Ramsey F. (1926). Truth and Probability in Ramsey 1931 *The Foundations of Mathematics and othr Logical Essays*, Ch VII, p.156–198, edited by R.B.

Braithwaite, London. Degan, Paul, Trench, Trubner & Co., New York: Harcourt, Brace, and Company. (1999 electronic edition).

30. The CAST Investigators. (1989). Preliminary Report: effect of encainide and flecainide on mortalithy in a randomized trial of arrhythmia suppression after myocardial infarction. *New England Journal of Medicine*. **321**:406–412.

31. Moore T. (1995). *Deadly Medicine*. New York Simon and Schuster.

32. UK Prospective Diabetes Study Group. (1991). UK Prospective Diabetes Study (UKPDS) VIII. Study, design, progress and performance. *Diabetologia* **34**:877–890.

33. Moyé L.A. (2003). *Multiple Analyses in Clinical Trials: Fundamentals for Investigators*. New York. Springer. Chapter 8.

34. UKPDS Study Group. (1998). Intensive blood glucose control with sulphonyl-ureas or insulin compared with conventional treatment and risk of complica-tions in patients with type 2 diabetes.*Lancet* **352**: 837–853.

35. Turner R.C., Holman R.R. on behalf of the UK Prospective Diabetes Study Group. (1998). The UK Prospective Diabetes Study. Finnish Medical Society DUOCECIM, *Annals of Medicine* **28**:439–444.

36. Feldman, AM, Bristow MR, Parmley WW Carson PE, Pepine CJ, Gilbert EM, Strobeck, JE, Hendrix, GH, Powers ER, Bain RP, White BG for the Vesnarinone Study (1993). Effects of vesnarinone on morbidity and mortality in patients with heart failure. *New Engand Journal of Medicine* **329**:149–55.

37. Cohn JN, Goldstein SO, Greenberg BH, Lorell BH, Bourge RC, Jaski BE, Gottlieb SO, McGrew F 3rd, DeMets DL, White BG. (1998). A dose dependent increase in mortality seen with vesnarinone among patients with severe heart failure. *New England Journal of Medicine* **339**:1810–16.

38. Pitt B., Segal R., Martinez F.A. et al. on behalf of the ELITE Study Investiga-tors. (1997). Randomized trial of losartan versus captopril in patients over 65 with heart failure. *Lancet* **349**:747–52.

39. Jensen, B.V., Nielsen, S.L. (1997). Correspondence: Losartan versus captopril in elderly patients with heart failure. *Lancet* **349**:1473.

40. Fournier A., Achard J.M., Fernandez L.A. (1997). Correspondence: Losartan versus captopril in elderly patients with heart failure. *Lancet* **349**:1473.

41. Packer M, O'Connor CM, Ghali JK, Pressler ML, Carson PE, Belkin RN, Miller AB, Neuberg GW, Frid D, Wertheimer JH, Cropp AB, DeMets DL. for the Prospective Randomized Amlodipine Survival Evaluation Study Group (1996). Effect of amlodipine on morbidity and mortality in severe chronic heart failure. *New England Journal of Medicine* **335**:1107–14.

42. Packer M. (2000). Presentation of the results of the Prospective Randomized Amlodipine Survival Evaluation-2 Trial (PRAISE-2) at the American College of Cardiology Scientific Sessions, Anaheim, CA, March 15, 2000.

43. Egger M., Smith G.D., Phillips A.N. (1997). Meta-analyses: principles and procedures. *British Medical Journal* **315**:1533–1537.

44. Alderson P., Roberts I. (1997). Corticosteroids in acute traumatic brain injury: systematic review of randomised controlled trials. *British Medical Journal* **314**:1855–1859.

45. Gregson B,. Todd N.V., Crawford D., Gerber C.J., Fulton B., Tacconi L., Crawford P.J., Sengupta R.P. (1999). CRASH trial is based on problematic meta-analysis. *British Medical Journal* **319:** 578.
46. Moyé L. (2006). *Face to Face with Katrina Suvivors: A First Responder's Account*. Greensboro. Open Hand Publishing LLC.

Appendix A
Compo nd Poisson
Distrib tion

A first simple example of "compounding" combines the binomial distribution with the Poisson distribution. Consider an outcome X that follows a binomial distribution where n and θ are fixed. In this example θ will remain a constant. We write the $P[X = k \mid n]$ as

$$P[X = k \mid n] = \binom{n}{k} \theta^k (1-\theta)^{n-k} . \tag{A.1}$$

However, assume that n is not constant, but follows a Poisson distribution with parameter λ. We are interested in computing the unconditional distribution of X.

Using the law of total probability, we write

$$P[X = k] = \sum_{n=0}^{\infty} P[X = k \mid n] P[n],$$

and substitute the binomial distribution for $P[X = k \mid n]$, and the Poisson distribution with parameter λ for $P[n]$.

$$\begin{aligned} P[X = k] &= \sum_{n=0}^{\infty} P[X = k \mid n] P[n] \\ &= \sum_{n=0}^{\infty} \binom{n}{k} \theta^k (1-\theta)^{n-k} \frac{\lambda^n}{n!} e^{-\lambda} . \end{aligned} \tag{A.2}$$

Rewriting this reveals

$$\begin{aligned} P[X = k] &= \sum_{n=0}^{\infty} \binom{n}{k} \theta^k (1-\theta)^{n-k} \frac{\lambda^n}{n!} e^{-\lambda} \\ &= \sum_{n=0}^{\infty} \frac{n!}{k!(n-k)!} \theta^k (1-\theta)^{n-k} \frac{\lambda^n}{n!} e^{-\lambda} \\ &= \frac{\theta^k}{k!} e^{-\lambda} \sum_{n=0}^{\infty} \frac{1}{(n-k)!} (1-\theta)^{n-k} \lambda^n . \end{aligned} \tag{A.3}$$

Rewriting $\lambda^n = \lambda^k \lambda^{n-k}$, we can write the last line of expression (A.3) as

$$\frac{\theta^k}{k!}e^{-\lambda}\sum_{n=0}^{\infty}\frac{1}{(n-k)!}(1-\theta)^{n-k}\,\lambda^k\lambda^{n-k} \;=\; \frac{\theta^k\lambda^k}{k!}e^{-\lambda}\sum_{n=0}^{\infty}\frac{\left(\lambda(1-\theta)\right)^{n-k}}{(n-k)!}$$

Recognizing $\displaystyle\sum_{n=0}^{\infty}\frac{\left(\lambda(1-\theta)\right)^{n-k}}{(n-k)!}=e^{\lambda(1-\theta)}$, we can write

$$P[X=k]=\frac{\theta^k\lambda^k}{k!}e^{-\lambda}e^{\lambda(1-\theta)}=\frac{(\lambda\theta)^k}{k!}e^{-\lambda\theta},\;\; \text{or Poisson with parameter } \lambda\theta.$$

Appendix B
Eval ations Using the Uniform Distrib tion

The uniform distribution will be one of several helpful probability distributions for us. However, some of the fundamental computations that involve it our complicated. The results and their derivation are provided here

Result 1: $\displaystyle\sum_{\theta} \theta^x (1-\theta)^{n-x} \mathbf{1}_{\theta\in[0,1]} = \int_0^1 \theta^x (1-\theta)^{n-x} d\theta = \frac{x!(n-x)!}{(n+1)!} = \frac{1}{(n+1)\binom{n}{x}}$.

In this case, the summation over all values of θ is an integral, and we write

$$\sum_{\theta} \theta^k (1-\theta)^{n-k} \mathbf{1}_{\theta\in[0,1]} = \int_0^1 \theta^k (1-\theta)^{n-k} d\theta. \tag{B.1}$$

Multiplying the right side of equation (B.1) by 1 in the form $\dfrac{\Gamma(j+1)\Gamma(k+1)}{\Gamma(j+k+2)} \dfrac{\Gamma(j+k+2)}{\Gamma(j+1)\Gamma(k+1)}$, we note

$$\int_0^1 \theta^j (1-\theta)^k d\theta = \frac{\Gamma(j+1)\Gamma(k+1)}{\Gamma(j+k+2)} \int_0^1 \frac{\Gamma(j+k+2)}{\Gamma(j+1)\Gamma(k+1)} \theta^j (1-\theta)^k d\theta$$

Since $\displaystyle\int_0^1 \frac{\Gamma(j+k+2)}{\Gamma(j+1)\Gamma(k+1)} \theta^k (1-\theta)^{n-k} d\theta = 1,$

$$\int_0^1 \theta^j (1-\theta)^k d\theta = \frac{\Gamma(j+1)\Gamma(k+1)}{\Gamma(j+k+2)} = \frac{j!k!}{(j+k+1)!} = \frac{j!k!}{(j+k+1)(j+k)!}$$

$$= \frac{1}{(j+k+1)\dfrac{(j+k)!}{j!k!}} = \frac{1}{(j+k+1)\dbinom{j+k}{k}}.$$

(B.2)

Now, let $j = x$ and $k = n - x$ to find

$$\int_0^1 \theta^x (1-\theta)^{n-x} d\theta = \frac{1}{(n+1)\dbinom{n}{x}}.$$

Result 2: $\displaystyle\sum_\theta \theta^x (1-\theta)^{n-x} \mathbf{1}_{\theta\in[c,1]} = \sum_{i=0}^{n-x} \binom{n-x}{i} \frac{(-1)^i}{x+i+1}\left(1-c^{x+i+1}\right)$, where n and x

an integers.

Proceeding as we did for Result 1, write $\displaystyle\sum_\theta \theta^j (1-\theta)^k \mathbf{1}_{\theta\in[c,1]} = \int_c^1 \theta^j (1-\theta)^k \, d\theta$.

We now use the binomial theorem to find

$$(1-\theta)^k = \sum_{i=0}^k \binom{k}{i}(-1)^i \theta^i.$$

(B.3)

The integral now becomes

$$\int_c^1 \theta^j (1-\theta)^k \, d\theta = \int_c^1 \theta^j \sum_{i=0}^k \binom{k}{i}(-1)^i \theta^i d\theta = \sum_{i=0}^k \binom{k}{i}(-1)^i \int_c^1 \theta^{j+i} d\theta$$

$$= \sum_{i=0}^k \binom{k}{i} \frac{(-1)^i}{j+i+1}\left((1)^{j+i} - c^{j+i+1}\right) = \sum_{i=0}^k \binom{k}{i} \frac{(-1)^i}{j+i+1}\left(1-c^{j+i+1}\right).$$

Finally, letting $j = x$ and $k = n - x$, we find

$$\int_c^1 \theta^x (1-\theta)^{n-x} \, d\theta = \sum_{i=0}^{n-x} \binom{n-x}{i} \frac{(-1)^i}{x+i+1}\left(1-c^{x+i+1}\right).$$

(B.4)

Result 3: $\displaystyle\int_0^c \theta^x (1-\theta)^{n-x} \, d\theta = \sum_{i=0}^{n-x} \binom{n-x}{i} \frac{(-1)^i}{x+i+1} c^{x+i+1}.$

Following the line of reasoning used to generate Result 2, we can easily write

$$\int_0^c \theta^j (1-\theta)^k \, d\theta = \int_0^c \theta^j \sum_{i=0}^k \binom{k}{i} (-1)^i \theta^i \, d\theta = \sum_{i=0}^k \binom{k}{i} (-1)^i \int_0^c \theta^{j+i} \, d\theta$$

$$= \sum_{i=0}^k \binom{k}{i} \frac{(-1)^i}{j+i+1} c^{j+i+1}.$$

and letting $j = x$ and $k = n - x$,

$$\int_0^c \theta^x (1-\theta)^{n-x} \, d\theta = \sum_{i=0}^{n-x} \binom{n-x}{i} \frac{(-1)^i}{x+i+1} c^{x+i+1}.$$

Result 4: $\int_a^b \theta^x (1-\theta)^{n-x} \, d\theta = \sum_{i=0}^{n-x} \binom{n-x}{i} (-1)^i \frac{(-1)^i}{x+i+1} \left(b^{x+i+1} - a^{x+i+1}\right)$ for

$0 < a < b < 1.$

We can adapt the demonstration of Result 2 to write

$$\int_a^b \theta^j (1-\theta)^k \, d\theta = \int_a^b \theta^j \sum_{i=0}^k \binom{k}{i} (-1)^i \theta^i \, d\theta = \sum_{i=0}^k \binom{k}{i} (-1)^i \int_a^b \theta^{j+i} \, d\theta$$

$$= \sum_{i=0}^k \binom{k}{i} \frac{(-1)^i}{j+i+1} \left(b^{j+i+1} - a^{j+i+1}\right).$$

So, letting $j = x$ and $k = n - x$,

$$\int_a^b \theta^x (1-\theta)^{n-x} \, d\theta = \sum_{i=0}^{n-x} \binom{n-x}{i} \frac{(-1)^i}{x+i+1} \left(b^{x+i+1} - a^{x+i+1}\right).$$

for $0 < a < b < 1.$

Appendix C
Comp tations for the Binomial-Uniform Distrib tion

Our introduction to the binomial-uniform combination came in Chapter Two, where a probability of interest denoted by θ was unknown. However, we knew the probability of a random variable X given θ to be binomial, $P[X = k] = \binom{n}{k} \theta^k (1-\theta)^{n-k}$. With no additional information about θ, the investigator implements the uniform distribution to express their knowledge about the possible value of θ.

Using the Law of Total Probability,

$$P[X = k] = \sum_{\theta} P[X = k \mid \theta] \pi(\theta) = \sum_{\theta} \binom{n}{k} \theta^k (1-\theta)^{n-k} \mathbf{1}_{\theta \in [0,1]}$$

$$= \binom{n}{k} \sum_{\theta} \theta^k (1-\theta)^{n-k} \mathbf{1}_{\theta \in [0,1]}$$

This appendix tabulates values of this expression, using the results of Appendix B.

Values of $\dfrac{1}{c}\dbinom{n}{k}\sum_{\theta}\theta^k(1-\theta)^{n-k}\mathbf{1}_{\theta\in[0,c]}$ as a function of n, k, and c

n	k	c 0.2	0.4	0.6	0.8	0.9
4	0	0.67232	0.03213	0.25667	0.16513	0.20125
4	1	0.26272	0.24910	0.17780	0.19813	0.19467
4	2	0.05792	0.38099	0.11986	0.21308	0.18956
4	3	0.00672	0.43436	0.09976	0.21769	0.18765
4	4	0.00032	0.46109	0.09273	0.21956	0.18693
5	1	0.28720	0.20208	0.15892	0.16388	0.16358
5	2	0.08240	0.31351	0.11587	0.17451	0.16066
5	3	0.01413	0.36119	0.09810	0.17828	0.15940
5	4	0.00133	0.38418	0.09200	0.17978	0.15894
5	5	0.00005	0.39722	0.08932	0.18054	0.15873
6	0	0.56449	0.03550	0.17735	0.12748	0.14282
6	1	0.30235	0.17031	0.14215	0.14009	0.14085
6	2	0.10574	0.26543	0.10959	0.14781	0.13905
6	3	0.02382	0.30871	0.09389	0.15090	0.13817
6	4	0.00334	0.32918	0.08823	0.15215	0.13783
6	5	0.00027	0.34047	0.08600	0.15276	0.13769
6	6	0.00001	0.34714	0.08485	0.15310	0.13761
7	0	0.52014	0.03626	0.15293	0.11393	0.12479
7	1	0.31043	0.14766	0.12781	0.12253	0.12358
7	2	0.12693	0.22959	0.10281	0.12826	0.12242
7	3	0.03518	0.26921	0.08900	0.13081	0.12177
7	4	0.00650	0.28787	0.08358	0.13187	0.12151
7	5	0.00077	0.29789	0.08155	0.13237	0.12140
7	6	0.00005	0.30375	0.08062	0.13264	0.12135
7	7	0.00000	0.30725	0.08010	0.13280	0.12132
8	0	0.48099	0.03661	0.13414	0.10283	0.11083
8	1	0.31322	0.13084	0.11565	0.10899	0.11004
8	2	0.14545	0.20200	0.09620	0.11333	0.10926
8	3	0.04758	0.23840	0.08412	0.11544	0.10878
8	4	0.01088	0.25568	0.07888	0.11636	0.10856
8	5	0.00170	0.26477	0.07692	0.11679	0.10848
8	6	0.00017	0.27000	0.07611	0.11701	0.10844
8	7	0.00001	0.27311	0.07568	0.11714	0.10842
8	8	0.00000	0.27498	0.07544	0.11722	0.10841

Values of $\dfrac{1}{c}\dbinom{n}{k}\sum_{\theta}\theta^{k}\left(1-\theta\right)^{n-k}\mathbf{1}_{\theta\in[0,c]}$ as a function of n, k, and c

n	k	c				
		0.2	0.4	0.6	0.8	0.9
9	0	0.44631	0.03665	0.11926	0.09363	0.09970
9	1	0.31210	0.11791	0.10531	0.09821	0.09916
9	2	0.16110	0.18020	0.09000	0.10155	0.09862
9	3	0.06044	0.21372	0.07949	0.10331	0.09825
9	4	0.01640	0.22989	0.07444	0.10412	0.09807
9	5	0.00318	0.23825	0.07248	0.10449	0.09800
9	6	0.00043	0.24299	0.07171	0.10468	0.09797
9	7	0.00004	0.24580	0.07135	0.10479	0.09795
9	8	0.00000	0.24748	0.07115	0.10485	0.09794
9	9	0.00000	0.24849	0.07103	0.10489	0.09794
10	0	0.41550	0.03646	0.10722	0.08588	0.09060
10	1	0.30813	0.10767	0.09647	0.08940	0.09023
10	2	0.17391	0.16262	0.08430	0.09203	0.08984
10	3	0.07325	0.19351	0.07519	0.09350	0.08956
10	4	0.02291	0.20874	0.07037	0.09421	0.08941
10	5	0.00530	0.21654	0.06837	0.09454	0.08934
10	6	0.00089	0.22090	0.06761	0.09471	0.08932
10	7	0.00011	0.22345	0.06728	0.09480	0.08930
10	8	0.00001	0.22498	0.06711	0.09485	0.08930
10	9	0.00000	0.22590	0.06701	0.09488	0.08929
10	10	0.00000	0.22645	0.06695	0.09490	0.08929
11	0	0.38803	0.03609	0.09730	0.07929	0.08304
11	1	0.30213	0.09937	0.08885	0.08206	0.08277
11	2	0.18402	0.14820	0.07909	0.08416	0.08248
11	3	0.08560	0.17670	0.07123	0.08540	0.08226
11	4	0.03023	0.19109	0.06666	0.08602	0.08214
11	5	0.00809	0.19844	0.06463	0.08632	0.08208
11	6	0.00163	0.20248	0.06384	0.08647	0.08205
11	7	0.00024	0.20483	0.06352	0.08655	0.08204
11	8	0.00003	0.20623	0.06337	0.08659	0.08204
11	9	0.00000	0.20707	0.06329	0.08662	0.08204
11	10	0.00000	0.20758	0.06324	0.08664	0.08203
11	11	0.00000	0.20788	0.06321	0.08665	0.08203

Appendix D
Binomial-Exponential
Compo nd Distrib tion

Consider an outcome X that follows a binomial distribution where θ is a constant. We write the $P[X = k \,|\, n]$ as

$$P[X = k \,|\, \upsilon] = \binom{n}{k} e^{-k\upsilon t} \left(1 - e^{-\upsilon t}\right)^{n-k}. \tag{D.1}$$

However, assume that v is not constant, but follows an exponential distribution with parameter λ. We are interested in computing the unconditional distribution of X.

Using the law of total probability, we write

$$P[X = k] = \sum_{v=0}^{\infty} P[X = k \,|\, \upsilon] P[v],$$

and substitute the binomial distribution for $P[X = k \,|\, \upsilon]$, and the exponential distribution with parameter λ for $P[v]$.

$$\begin{aligned} P[X = k] &= \int_{\upsilon} P[X = k \,|\, \upsilon] P[\upsilon] \\ &= \int_{\upsilon} \binom{n}{k} e^{-k\upsilon t} \left(1 - e^{-\upsilon t}\right)^{n-k} \lambda e^{-\lambda \upsilon} d\upsilon \end{aligned} \tag{D.2}$$

Since $n - k$ is a non-negative integer, we may write

$$\left(1 - e^{-\upsilon t}\right)^{n-k} = \sum_{i=0}^{n-k} \binom{n-k}{i} (-1)^i e^{-i\upsilon t}.$$

Substituting this expression into the second line of (D.2), we have

$$P[X=k] = \int_\upsilon \binom{n}{k} e^{-k\upsilon t} \sum_{i=0}^{n-k} \binom{n-k}{i} (-1)^i \, e^{-i\upsilon t} \lambda e^{-\lambda \upsilon} d\upsilon$$

$$= \binom{n}{k} \sum_{i=0}^{n-k} \binom{n-k}{i} (-1)^i \int_\upsilon \lambda e^{-((k+i)t+\lambda)\upsilon} d\upsilon \qquad \text{(D.3)}$$

The remaining integral is simply

$$\int_0^\infty \lambda e^{-((k+i)t+\lambda)\upsilon} d\upsilon = \frac{\lambda}{(k+i)t+\lambda}.$$

Thus

$$P[X=k] = \binom{n}{k} \sum_{i=0}^{n-k} \binom{n-k}{i} (-1)^i \frac{\lambda}{(k+i)t+\lambda}, \qquad \text{(D.4)}$$

which is an easily computable simple finite sum.

Appendix E
Poisson-Gamma Processes

Consider an outcome X_t that represents the number of arrivals to an emergency room through time t. If we assume that X_t follows a Poisson distribution with parameter λ, we may write

$$P[X_t = k \mid \lambda] = \frac{(\lambda t)^k}{k!} e^{\lambda t}$$

for $k = 0, 1, 2, 3, \ldots$ Thus X_t is the cumulative number of arrivals from time 0 to time t. We will also assume that the parameter λ is not constant, but follows a gamma distribution with parameters α and r.

$$P[\lambda] = \frac{\alpha^r}{\Gamma(r)} \lambda^{r-1} e^{-\alpha\lambda} 1_{0 \le \lambda \le \infty}.$$

We are interesting in identifying the unconditional probability distribution of X_t. Using the Law of Total Probability, we write

$$P[X_t = k] = \sum_{\lambda=0}^{\infty} P[X_t = k \mid \lambda] P[\lambda]$$

$$= \int_0^\infty \frac{(\lambda t)^k}{k!} e^{\lambda t} \frac{\alpha^r}{\Gamma(r)} \lambda^{r-1} e^{-\alpha\lambda} d\lambda. \qquad (E.1)$$

Removing all terms not involving the variable λ outside the integral, we can rewrite the second line of expression (E.1) as

$$\frac{\alpha^r}{\Gamma(r)k!} t^k \int_0^\infty \lambda^k e^{\lambda t} \lambda^{r-1} e^{-\alpha\lambda} d\lambda \quad = \quad \frac{\alpha^r}{\Gamma(r)k!} t^k \int_0^\infty \lambda^{k+r-1} e^{-(\alpha+t)\lambda} d\lambda. \qquad (E.2)$$

The integral on the right side of equation (E.2) needs only a constant to allow it to be one. We therefore write

$$\frac{\alpha^r}{\Gamma(r)k!}t^k\int_0^\infty \lambda^{k+r-1}e^{-(\alpha+t)\lambda}\,d\lambda$$

$$=\frac{\alpha^r}{\Gamma(r)k!}t^k\frac{\Gamma(k+r)}{(\alpha+t)^{k+r}}\int_0^\infty \frac{(\alpha+t)^{k+r}}{\Gamma(k+r)}\lambda^{k+r-1}e^{-(\alpha+t)\lambda}\,d\lambda. \tag{E.3}$$

The integral on the right-hand side of equation (E.3) is that of a variable that follows a gamma distribution with scale parameter $\alpha + t$ and shape parameter $k + r$. This integrates to one over the entire range of λ. Thus, we are left with

$$P[X_t = k] = \frac{\alpha^r}{\Gamma(r)k!}t^k\frac{\Gamma(k+r)}{(\alpha+t)^{k+r}}$$

$$=\frac{\Gamma(k+r)}{\Gamma(r)k!}\frac{\alpha^r}{(\alpha+t)^r}\frac{t^k}{(\alpha+t)^k} \tag{E.4}$$

$$=\binom{k+r-1}{r-1}\left(\frac{\alpha}{\alpha+t}\right)^r\left(\frac{t}{\alpha+t}\right)^k.$$

We recognize this last expression as the probability of k failures before the rth success when the probability of a success is $\alpha/(\alpha+t)$, and the probability of failure is $t/(\alpha+t)$.

Posterior Distribution of λ given x.

The problem presented in this appendix can be written using Bayesian notation. We are given that $P[X_t = k \mid \lambda] = \frac{(\lambda t)^k}{k!}e^{-\lambda t}$. We may $\pi(\lambda) = \frac{\alpha^r}{\Gamma(r)}\lambda^{r-1}e^{-\alpha\lambda}\mathbf{1}_{0\le\lambda\le\infty}$, which allows us to write the posterior distribution of λ given k, or $\pi(\lambda \mid k)$ as

$$\pi(\lambda \mid k) = \frac{f(k \mid \lambda)\pi(\lambda)}{\sum_\lambda f(k \mid \lambda)\pi(\lambda)} = \frac{\dfrac{(\lambda t)^k}{k!}e^{-\lambda t}\dfrac{\alpha^r}{\Gamma(r)}\lambda^{r-1}e^{-\alpha\lambda}\mathbf{1}_{0\le\lambda\le\infty}}{\displaystyle\int_0^\infty \dfrac{(\lambda t)^k}{k!}e^{-\lambda t}\dfrac{\alpha^r}{\Gamma(r)}\lambda^{r-1}e^{-\alpha\lambda}}. \tag{E.5}$$

We may write the denominator as

$$\int_0^\infty \frac{(\lambda t)^k}{k!} e^{-\lambda t} \frac{\alpha^r}{\Gamma(r)} \lambda^{r-1} e^{-\alpha\lambda} d\lambda = \frac{\alpha^r}{\Gamma(r)k!} t^k \frac{\Gamma(k+r)}{(\alpha+t)^{k+r}},$$

from expression (E.3). The posterior distribution now becomes

$$\pi(\lambda \mid k) = \frac{f(k \mid \lambda)\pi(\lambda)}{\sum_\lambda f(k \mid \lambda)\pi(\lambda)} = \frac{\dfrac{(\lambda t)^k}{k!} e^{-\lambda t} \dfrac{\alpha^r}{\Gamma(r)} \lambda^{r-1} e^{-\alpha\lambda} \mathbf{1}_{0\leq\lambda\leq\infty}}{\displaystyle\int_0^\infty \frac{(\lambda t)^k}{k!} e^{-\lambda t} \frac{\alpha^r}{\Gamma(r)} \lambda^{r-1} e^{-\alpha\lambda}}$$

$$= \frac{\dfrac{(\lambda t)^k}{k!} e^{-\lambda t} \dfrac{\alpha^r}{\Gamma(r)} \lambda^{r-1} e^{-\alpha\lambda} \mathbf{1}_{0\leq\lambda\leq\infty}}{\dfrac{\alpha^r}{\Gamma(r)k!} t^k \dfrac{\Gamma(k+r)}{(\alpha+t)^{k+r}}},$$

which, after cancellation of terms reveals $\pi(\lambda \mid k) = \dfrac{(\alpha+t)^{k+r}}{\Gamma(k+r)} \lambda^{\alpha+r-1} e^{-(\alpha+t)\lambda} \mathbf{1}_{0\leq\lambda\leq\infty}$,

the probability function for a gamma distribution with mean $\dfrac{k+r}{\alpha+t}$, and variance

$\dfrac{k+r}{(\alpha+t)^2}$.

Appendix F
Gamma and Negative Binomial Distrib tion

Consider an outcome x that follows a gamma distribution with parameters α and n where n is an integer. The function that governs its probabilities is

$$f(x) = \frac{\alpha^n}{\Gamma(n)} x^{n-1} e^{-\alpha x} \mathbf{1}_{0 \le x \le \infty}.$$

In this section, we will assume that n itself has a negative binomial distribution. The probability of any value of n, which we write as P_n, is

$$P_n = \binom{n-1}{r-1} p^r (1-p)^{n-r}$$

for $n = r, r+1, r+2, r+3, \ldots, \infty$. We are interested in finding the marginal distribution of x. Using the Law of Total Probability we write

$$f(x) = \sum_n f(x \mid n) P_n$$

$$= \sum_{n=r}^{\infty} \frac{\alpha^n}{\Gamma(n)} x^{n-1} e^{-\alpha x} \binom{n-1}{r-1} p^r (1-p)^{n-r} \qquad \text{(F.1)}$$

$$= e^{-\alpha x} \frac{1}{x} \left(\frac{p}{1-p} \right)^r \sum_{n=r}^{\infty} \frac{\alpha^n}{\Gamma(n)} x^n \binom{n-1}{r-1} (1-p)^n.$$

Recognizing that

$$\binom{n-1}{r-1} = \frac{\Gamma(n)}{\Gamma(r)(n-r)!}$$

permits cancellation of the $\Gamma(n)$ term in the last line of expression (F.1), allowing us to write

$$f(x) = e^{-\alpha x} \frac{1}{\Gamma(r)} \frac{1}{x} \left(\frac{p}{1-p} \right)^r \sum_{n=r}^{\infty} \frac{\alpha^n}{(n-r)!} x^n (1-p)^n. \tag{F.2}$$

The summand in expression (F.2) may be written as

$$\sum_{n=r}^{\infty} \frac{\alpha^n}{(n-r)!} x^n (1-p)^n = \alpha^r x^r (1-p)^r \sum_{n=r}^{\infty} \frac{\left[\alpha x (1-p) \right]^{n-r}}{(n-r)!} \tag{F.3}$$

$$= \alpha^r x^r (1-p)^r e^{\alpha x (1-p)}.$$

Allowing us to write

$$f(x) = e^{-\alpha x} \frac{1}{\Gamma(r)} \frac{1}{x} \left(\frac{p}{1-p} \right)^r \alpha^r x^r (1-p)^r e^{\alpha x (1-p)}$$

$$= \frac{(\alpha p)^r}{\Gamma(r)} x^{r-1} e^{-\alpha px}$$

which is a gamma density with parameters αp and r.

Appendix G
Gamma-Gamma
Compo nding

Consider an outcome x that follows a gamma distribution with parameters α and m where m is an integer greater than zero. The function that governs its probabilities is

$$f(x) = \frac{\lambda^m}{\Gamma(m)} x^{m-1} e^{-\lambda x} \mathbf{1}_{0 \le x \le \infty}.$$

In this situation the parameter λ has its own probability distribution

$$f(\lambda) = \frac{\alpha^r}{\Gamma(r)} \lambda^{r-1} e^{-\alpha\lambda} \mathbf{1}_{0 \le \lambda \le \infty},$$

where we will assume that r is also a positive integer. We are interested in finding the marginal distribution of x. Using the Law of Total Probability we write

$$f(x) = \sum_\lambda f(x \mid \lambda) f(\lambda)$$
$$= \int_0^\infty \frac{\lambda^m}{\Gamma(m)} x^{m-1} e^{-\lambda x} \frac{\alpha^r}{\Gamma(r)} \lambda^{r-1} e^{-\alpha\lambda} d\lambda. \tag{G.1}$$

Removing terms involving λ, the second line of expression (F.1) becomes

$$f(x) = \frac{\alpha^r}{\Gamma(m)\Gamma(r)} x^{m-1} \int_0^\infty \lambda^{r+m-1} e^{-(\alpha+x)\lambda} d\lambda. \tag{G.2}$$

Recognizing that the integrand in expression (G.2) is related to that of a variable that follows a gamma distribution, we include the appropriate constant so that this integral's value is one.

$$f(x) = \frac{\alpha^r}{\Gamma(m)\Gamma(r)} x^{m-1} \frac{\Gamma(r+m)}{(\alpha+x)^{r+m}} \int_0^\infty \frac{(\alpha+x)^{r+m}}{\Gamma(r+m)} \lambda^{r+m-1} e^{-(\alpha+x)\lambda} d\lambda$$

$$= \frac{\alpha^r}{\Gamma(m)\Gamma(r)} x^{m-1} \frac{\Gamma(r+m)}{(\alpha+x)^{r+m}}.$$

We arranging terms, this becomes

$$f(x) = \frac{\Gamma(r+m)}{\Gamma(m)\Gamma(r)} \frac{\alpha^r}{(\alpha+x)^{r+m}} x^{m-1} = \frac{(r+m-1)!}{(m-1)!(r-1)!} \frac{\alpha^r}{(\alpha+x)^{r+1}} \left(\frac{x}{\alpha+x}\right)^{m-1}$$

$$= \frac{1}{\alpha} \frac{(r+1)r}{r+m} \frac{(r+m)(r+m-1)!}{(m-1)!(r+1)(r)(r-1)!} \left(\frac{\alpha}{\alpha+x}\right)^{r+1} \left(\frac{x}{\alpha+x}\right)^{m-1}$$

$$= \frac{(r+1)r}{a(r+m)} \left(\frac{r+m}{r+1}\right) \left(\frac{\alpha}{\alpha+x}\right)^{r+1} \left(\frac{x}{\alpha+x}\right)^{m-1}. \tag{G.3}$$

Thus the marginal distribution of x is related to a binomial random variable with parameter $n = r + m$ and $p = \alpha/(\alpha+x)$.

Appendix H
Standard Normal Distrib tion

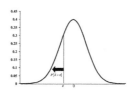

z	P(Z < z)	z	P(Z < z)	z	P(Z < z)	z	P(Z < z)
-3.00	0.001	-1.55	0.061	-0.10	0.460	1.35	0.911
-2.95	0.002	-1.50	0.067	-0.05	0.480	1.40	0.919
-2.90	0.002	-1.45	0.074	0.00	0.500	1.45	0.926
-2.85	0.002	-1.40	0.081	0.05	0.520	1.50	0.933
-2.80	0.003	-1.35	0.089	0.10	0.540	1.55	0.939
-2.75	0.003	-1.30	0.097	0.15	0.560	1.60	0.945
-2.70	0.003	-1.25	0.106	0.20	0.579	1.65	0.951
-2.65	0.004	-1.20	0.115	0.25	0.599	1.70	0.955
-2.60	0.005	-1.15	0.125	0.30	0.618	1.75	0.960
-2.55	0.005	-1.10	0.136	0.35	0.637	1.80	0.964
-2.50	0.006	-1.05	0.147	0.40	0.655	1.85	0.968
-2.45	0.007	-1.00	0.159	0.45	0.674	1.90	0.971
-2.40	0.008	-0.95	0.171	0.50	0.691	1.95	0.974
-2.35	0.009	-0.90	0.184	0.55	0.709	2.00	0.977
-2.30	0.011	-0.85	0.198	0.60	0.726	2.05	0.980
-2.25	0.012	-0.80	0.212	0.65	0.742	2.10	0.982
-2.20	0.014	-0.75	0.227	0.70	0.758	2.15	0.984
-2.15	0.016	-0.70	0.242	0.75	0.773	2.20	0.986
-2.10	0.018	-0.65	0.258	0.80	0.788	2.25	0.988
-2.05	0.020	-0.60	0.274	0.85	0.802	2.30	0.989
-2.00	0.023	-0.55	0.291	0.90	0.816	2.35	0.991
-1.95	0.026	-0.50	0.309	0.95	0.829	2.40	0.992
-1.90	0.029	-0.45	0.326	1.00	0.841	2.45	0.993
-1.85	0.032	-0.40	0.345	1.05	0.853	2.50	0.994
-1.80	0.036	-0.35	0.363	1.10	0.864	2.55	0.995
-1.75	0.040	-0.30	0.382	1.15	0.875	2.60	0.995
-1.70	0.045	-0.25	0.401	1.20	0.885	2.65	0.996
-1.65	0.049	-0.20	0.421	1.25	0.894	2.70	0.997
-1.60	0.055	-0.15	0.440	1.30	0.903	2.75	0.997

Appendix I
Compo nd and Conj gate Normal Distrib tions

Consider an event x that follows a normal distribution with mean θ and variance σ^2. For this demonstration we assume that while σ^2 is known θ follows a normal distribution with known mean μ and known variance v^2. Thus, we have

$$f(x\,|\,\theta) = \frac{1}{\sqrt{2\pi\sigma^2}}e^{-\frac{(x-\theta)^2}{2\sigma^2}} : f(\theta) = \frac{1}{\sqrt{2\pi v^2}}e^{-\frac{(\theta-\mu)^2}{2v^2}}$$

Componding Two Normal Distributions

We are interested in finding the marginal distribution of x. Using the Law of Total Probability we write

$$f(x) = \sum_\theta f(x\,|\,\theta)f(\theta)$$

$$= \int_{-\infty}^{\infty} \frac{1}{\sqrt{2\pi\sigma^2}}e^{-\frac{(x-\theta)^2}{2\sigma^2}}\frac{1}{\sqrt{2\pi v^2}}e^{-\frac{(\theta-\mu)^2}{2v^2}}\,d\theta. \tag{I.4}$$

Our goal is to carry out the integration in the last line of this expression with respect to θ. This expression can be rewritten as

$$\int_{-\infty}^{\infty} \frac{1}{\sqrt{2\pi\sigma^2}}e^{-\frac{(x-\theta)^2}{2\sigma^2}}\frac{1}{\sqrt{2\pi v^2}}e^{-\frac{(\theta-\mu)^2}{2v^2}}\,d\theta$$

$$= \frac{1}{2\pi\sigma v}\int_{-\infty}^{\infty} e^{-\left[\frac{(x-\theta)^2}{2\sigma^2}+\frac{(\theta-\mu)^2}{2v^2}\right]}\,d\theta \tag{I.5}$$

$$= \frac{1}{2\pi\sigma v}\int_{-\infty}^{\infty} e^{-\frac{1}{2}\left[\frac{(x-\theta)^2}{\sigma^2}+\frac{(\theta-\mu)^2}{v^2}\right]}\,d\theta = \frac{1}{2\pi\sigma v}\int_{-\infty}^{\infty} e^{K(x,\theta)}\,d\theta.$$

And our attention turns to simplifying the exponent in this integral. The process we will follow is one of completing the square. Begin by

$$K(x,\theta) = -\frac{1}{2}\left[\frac{(x-\theta)^2}{\sigma^2} + \frac{(\theta-\mu)^2}{\upsilon^2}\right]$$

$$= -\frac{1}{2}\left[\frac{x^2 - 2\theta x + \theta^2}{\sigma^2} + \frac{\theta^2 - 2\theta\mu + \mu^2}{\upsilon^2}\right].$$

Continuing

$$K(x,\theta) = -\frac{1}{2}\left(\left[\frac{1}{\sigma^2} + \frac{1}{\upsilon^2}\right]\theta^2 - 2\left(\frac{x}{\sigma^2} + \frac{\mu}{\upsilon^2}\right)\theta + \frac{x^2}{\sigma^2} + \frac{\mu^2}{\upsilon^2}\right)$$

and if $H(x) = \dfrac{x^2}{\sigma^2} + \dfrac{\mu^2}{\upsilon^2}$, we can write

$$K(x,\theta) = -\frac{1}{2}\left(\left[\frac{\sigma^2+\upsilon^2}{\sigma^2\upsilon^2}\right]\theta^2 - 2\left(\frac{x}{\sigma^2} + \frac{\mu}{\upsilon^2}\right)\theta\right) - \frac{1}{2}H(x).$$

$$= -\frac{\left[\dfrac{\sigma^2+\upsilon^2}{\sigma^2\upsilon^2}\right]}{2}\left(\theta^2 - 2\frac{1}{\left[\dfrac{\sigma^2+\upsilon^2}{\sigma^2\upsilon^2}\right]}\left(\frac{x}{\sigma^2} + \frac{\mu}{\upsilon^2}\right)\theta\right) - \frac{1}{2}H(x) \qquad (I.6)$$

$$= -\frac{1}{2\left[\dfrac{\sigma^2\upsilon^2}{\sigma^2+\upsilon^2}\right]}\left(\theta^2 - \frac{2}{\sigma^2+\upsilon^2}\left(\upsilon^2 x + \sigma^2\mu\right)\theta\right) - \frac{1}{2}H(x)$$

It now remains to complete the square in θ.

$$\theta^2 - \frac{2}{\sigma^2+\upsilon^2}\left(\upsilon^2 x + \sigma^2\mu\right)\theta$$

$$= \theta^2 - \frac{2}{\sigma^2+\upsilon^2}\left(\upsilon^2 x + \sigma^2\mu\right)\theta + \left[\frac{\left(\upsilon^2 x + \sigma^2\mu\right)}{\sigma^2+\upsilon^2}\right]^2 - \left[\frac{\left(\upsilon^2 x + \sigma^2\mu\right)}{\sigma^2+\upsilon^2}\right]^2$$

$$= \left(\theta - \frac{\left(\upsilon^2 x + \sigma^2\mu\right)}{\sigma^2+\upsilon^2}\right)^2 - \left[\frac{\left(\upsilon^2 x + \sigma^2\mu\right)}{\sigma^2+\upsilon^2}\right]^2.$$

We can now incorporate the completed square term in the last line of expression of (I.6).

$$K(x,\theta) = \frac{-1}{2\left[\dfrac{\sigma^2 v^2}{\sigma^2 + v^2}\right]}\left\{\left(\theta - \frac{\left(v^2 x + \sigma^2 \mu\right)}{\sigma^2 + v^2}\right)^2 - \left[\frac{\left(v^2 x + \sigma^2 \mu\right)}{\sigma^2 + v^2}\right]^2\right\} - \frac{1}{2}H(x)$$

$$= \frac{-\left(\theta - \dfrac{\left(v^2 x + \sigma^2 \mu\right)}{\sigma^2 + v^2}\right)^2}{2\left[\dfrac{\sigma^2 v^2}{\sigma^2 + v^2}\right]} + \frac{1}{2}\frac{\left[\dfrac{\left(v^2 x + \sigma^2 \mu\right)}{\sigma^2 + v^2}\right]^2}{\left[\dfrac{\sigma^2 v^2}{\sigma^2 + v^2}\right]} - \frac{1}{2}H(x)$$

$$= \frac{-\left(\theta - \dfrac{\left(v^2 x + \sigma^2 \mu\right)}{\sigma^2 + v^2}\right)^2}{2\left[\dfrac{\sigma^2 v^2}{\sigma^2 + v^2}\right]} - \frac{1}{2}G(x) + \frac{1}{2}H(x)$$

We can return to the last line of expression (I.5) to write

$$f(x) = \frac{1}{2\pi\sigma v}\int_{-\infty}^{\infty} e^{K(x,\theta)}d\theta$$

$$= \frac{\sqrt{\dfrac{\sigma^2 v^2}{\sigma^2 + v^2}}}{\sqrt{2\pi}\sigma v}\int_{-\infty}^{\infty}\frac{1}{\sqrt{2\pi\dfrac{\sigma^2 v^2}{\sigma^2 + v^2}}}e^{-\frac{\left(\theta - \dfrac{\left(v^2 x + \sigma^2 \mu\right)}{\sigma^2 + v^2}\right)^2}{2\left[\dfrac{\sigma^2 v^2}{\sigma^2 + v^2}\right]}}e^{-\frac{1}{2}(-G(x)+H(x))}d\theta \qquad (I.7)$$

$$= \frac{\sqrt{\dfrac{\sigma^2 v^2}{\sigma^2 + v^2}}}{\sqrt{2\pi}\sigma v}e^{-\frac{1}{2}(-G(x)+H(x))}\int_{-\infty}^{\infty}\frac{1}{\sqrt{2\pi\dfrac{\sigma^2 v^2}{\sigma^2 + v^2}}}e^{-\frac{\left(\theta - \dfrac{\left(v^2 x + \sigma^2 \mu\right)}{\sigma^2 + v^2}\right)^2}{2\left[\dfrac{\sigma^2 v^2}{\sigma^2 + v^2}\right]}}d\theta$$

The integral in the last line of expression (I.7) is 1, and we are left with

$$f(x) = \frac{1}{\sqrt{2\pi\left(\sigma^2 + v^2\right)}}e^{-\frac{1}{2}(-G(x)+H(x))} \qquad (I.8)$$

and it remains to simply $\dfrac{1}{2}\left(-G(x)+H(x)\right)$. We begin by writing

$$-G(x)+H(x) = -\dfrac{\left[\dfrac{\left(\upsilon^2 x+\sigma^2\mu\right)}{\sigma^2+\upsilon^2}\right]^2}{\left[\dfrac{\sigma^2\upsilon^2}{\sigma^2+\upsilon^2}\right]} + \dfrac{x^2}{\sigma^2} + \dfrac{\mu^2}{\upsilon^2}$$

$$= -\left(\dfrac{\sigma^2+\upsilon^2}{\sigma^2\upsilon^2}\left[\dfrac{\left(\upsilon^2 x+\sigma^2\mu\right)}{\sigma^2+\upsilon^2}\right]^2\right) + \dfrac{x^2}{\sigma^2} + \dfrac{\mu^2}{\upsilon^2}$$

$$= \dfrac{-\left(\upsilon^2 x+\sigma^2\mu\right)^2}{\sigma^2\upsilon^2\left(\sigma^2+\upsilon^2\right)} + \dfrac{x^2}{\sigma^2} + \dfrac{\mu^2}{\upsilon^2}$$

$$= \dfrac{-\left(\upsilon^2 x+\sigma^2\mu\right)^2 + \upsilon^2\left(\sigma^2+\upsilon^2\right)x^2 + \sigma^2\left(\sigma^2+\upsilon^2\right)\mu^2}{\sigma^2\upsilon^2\left(\sigma^2+\upsilon^2\right)}$$

$$= \dfrac{-\upsilon^4 x^2 - 2\sigma^2\upsilon^2\mu x - \sigma^4\mu^2 + \upsilon^2\sigma^2 x^2 + \upsilon^4 x^2 + \sigma^4\mu^2 + \sigma^2\upsilon^2\mu^2}{\sigma^2\upsilon^2\left(\sigma^2+\upsilon^2\right)}.$$

Cancellation reveals

$$-G(x)+H(x) = \dfrac{-2\sigma^2\upsilon^2\mu x + \upsilon^2\sigma^2 x^2 + \sigma^2\upsilon^2\mu^2}{\sigma^2\upsilon^2\left(\sigma^2+\upsilon^2\right)}$$

$$= \dfrac{\sigma^2\upsilon^2\left(x^2 - 2\mu x + \mu^2\right)}{\sigma^2\upsilon^2\left(\sigma^2+\upsilon^2\right)}$$

$$= \dfrac{1}{\left(\sigma^2+\upsilon^2\right)}\left(x-\mu\right)^2.$$

We can now write $f(x)$ as

$$f(x) = \dfrac{1}{\sqrt{2\pi\left(\sigma^2+\upsilon^2\right)}}\,e^{-\frac{1}{2\left(\sigma^2+\upsilon^2\right)}(x-\mu)^2}$$

which is the function of a normal distribution with mean μ and variance $\sigma^2+\upsilon^2$.

Obtaining the Posterior Distribution

To obtain the posterior distribution of θ, $\pi\left(\theta\,|\,x\right)$ we write

$$\pi(\theta \mid x) = \frac{f(x \mid \theta)\pi(\theta)}{\sum_{\theta} f(x \mid \theta)\pi(\theta)}. \tag{I.9}$$

We already know the denominator of this quantity, so we can write

$$\pi(\theta \mid x) = \frac{\dfrac{1}{\sqrt{2\pi\sigma^2}} e^{-\frac{(x-\theta)^2}{2\sigma^2}} \dfrac{1}{\sqrt{2\pi\upsilon^2}} e^{-\frac{(\theta-\mu)^2}{2\upsilon^2}}}{\dfrac{1}{\sqrt{2\pi(\sigma^2+\upsilon^2)}} e^{-\frac{(x-u)^2}{2(\sigma^2+\upsilon^2)}}}$$

$$= \frac{1}{\sqrt{2\pi \dfrac{(\sigma^2+\upsilon^2)}{\sigma^2\upsilon^2}}} e^{-\left[\frac{(x-\theta)^2}{2\sigma^2}+\frac{(\theta-\mu)^2}{2\upsilon^2}-\frac{(x-u)^2}{2(\sigma^2+\upsilon^2)}\right]}. \tag{I.10}$$

The exponent of this function can be rewritten as

$$-\left[\frac{(x-\theta)^2}{2\sigma^2}+\frac{(\theta-\mu)^2}{2\upsilon^2}\right]+\frac{(x-u)^2}{2(\sigma^2+\upsilon^2)}.$$

However, we know from the first segment of this appendix that

$$-\left[\frac{(x-\theta)^2}{2\sigma^2}+\frac{(\theta-\mu)^2}{2\upsilon^2}\right]=\frac{-\left(\theta-\dfrac{(\upsilon^2 x+\sigma^2\mu)}{\sigma^2+\upsilon^2}\right)^2}{2\left[\dfrac{\sigma^2\upsilon^2}{\sigma^2+\upsilon^2}\right]}-\frac{(x-u)^2}{2(\sigma^2+\upsilon^2)},$$

Thus

$$-\left[\frac{(x-\theta)^2}{2\sigma^2}+\frac{(\theta-\mu)^2}{2\upsilon^2}\right]+\frac{(x-u)^2}{2\left(\sigma^2+\upsilon^2\right)}$$

$$=\frac{-\left(\theta-\frac{\left(\upsilon^2 x+\sigma^2\mu\right)}{\sigma^2+\upsilon^2}\right)^2}{2\left[\frac{\sigma^2\upsilon^2}{\sigma^2+\upsilon^2}\right]}-\frac{(x-u)^2}{2\left(\sigma^2+\upsilon^2\right)}+\frac{(x-u)^2}{2\left(\sigma^2+\upsilon^2\right)}$$

$$=-\frac{1}{2}\frac{\left(\theta-\frac{\left(\upsilon^2 x+\sigma^2\mu\right)}{\sigma^2+\upsilon^2}\right)^2}{\left[\frac{\sigma^2\upsilon^2}{\sigma^2+\upsilon^2}\right]}.$$

Thus, the posterior probability distribution is

$$\pi\left(\theta\mid x\right)=\frac{1}{\sqrt{2\pi\dfrac{\left(\sigma^2+\upsilon^2\right)}{\sigma^2\upsilon^2}}}e^{-\frac{1}{2}\frac{\left(\theta-\frac{\left(\upsilon^2 x+\sigma^2\mu\right)}{\sigma^2+\upsilon^2}\right)^2}{\left[\frac{\sigma^2\upsilon^2}{\sigma^2+\upsilon^2}\right]}},$$

which is a normal distribution with mean $\dfrac{\left(\upsilon^2 x+\sigma^2\mu\right)}{\sigma^2+\upsilon^2}=\dfrac{\upsilon^2}{\sigma^2+\upsilon^2}x+\dfrac{\sigma^2}{\sigma^2+\upsilon^2}\mu,$

and variance $\dfrac{\sigma^2\upsilon^2}{\sigma^2+\upsilon^2}$.

Appendix J

Uniform Prior and Conditional Normal Distrib tion

Consider an event x that follows a normal distribution with mean $\mu\theta$ and variance σ^2 where both μ and σ^2 are known. The parameter θ follows a uniform distribution on the [0,1] interval. Thus, we may write

$$f(x\,|\,\theta) = \frac{1}{\sqrt{2\pi\sigma^2}}e^{-\frac{(x-\mu\theta)^2}{2\sigma^2}} : \pi(\theta) = \mathbf{1}_{\theta\in[0,1]}.$$

To obtain the posterior distribution of θ, $\pi(\theta\,|\,x)$ we begin with

$$\pi(\theta\,|\,x) = \frac{f(x\,|\,\theta)\pi(\theta)}{\sum_{\theta}f(x\,|\,\theta)\pi(\theta)}$$

$$= \frac{\dfrac{1}{\sqrt{2\pi\sigma^2}}e^{-\frac{(x-\mu\theta)^2}{2\sigma^2}}\mathbf{1}_{\theta\in[0,1]}}{\displaystyle\int_{0}\dfrac{1}{\sqrt{2\pi\sigma^2}}e^{-\frac{(x-\mu\theta)^2}{2\sigma^2}}\mathbf{1}_{\theta\in[0,1]}}. \tag{J.1}$$

Since we are interested in the posterior probability that θ is less than some value c where $0 \le c \le 1$, we can write

$$P[0\le\theta\le c] = \frac{\displaystyle\int_{0}^{c}\dfrac{1}{\sqrt{2\pi\sigma^2}}e^{-\frac{(x-\mu\theta)^2}{2\sigma^2}}\,d\theta}{\displaystyle\int_{0}^{1}\dfrac{1}{\sqrt{2\pi\sigma^2}}e^{-\frac{(x-\mu\theta)^2}{2\sigma^2}}\,d\theta}. \tag{J.2}$$

Therefore, if we write $G(b) = \int_0^b \frac{1}{\sqrt{2\pi\sigma^2}} e^{-\frac{(x-\mu\theta)^2}{2\sigma^2}} d\theta$ for $0 \le b \le 1$, we can write

$$P[0 \le \theta \le c] = \frac{G(c)}{G(1)}. \tag{J.3}$$

Begin with

$$G(b) = \int_0^b \frac{1}{\sqrt{2\pi\sigma^2}} e^{-\frac{(x-\mu\theta)^2}{2\sigma^2}} d\theta = \int_0^b \frac{1}{\sqrt{2\pi\sigma^2}} e^{-\frac{(\mu\theta-x)^2}{2\sigma^2}} d\theta.$$

Taking this one step at time, we begin with the substitution $w = u\theta$. Then $\theta = \frac{w}{\mu}$, $d\theta = \frac{dw}{\mu}$, and $0 \le \theta \le b$ translates to $0 \le w \le b\mu$. Thus,

$$G(b) = \frac{1}{\mu} \int_0^{b\mu} \frac{1}{\sqrt{2\pi\sigma^2}} e^{-\frac{(w-x)^2}{2\sigma^2}} dw. \tag{J.4}$$

Now, we let $z = \frac{w-x}{\sigma}$, converting the variable w which is normally distributed with mean x and variance σ^2 to a standard normal variable. We write

$$G(b) = \frac{1}{\mu} \int_{\frac{-x}{\sigma}}^{\frac{b\mu-x}{\sigma}} \frac{1}{\sqrt{2\pi}} e^{-\frac{z^2}{2}} dz = \frac{1}{\mu}\left[\Phi\left(\frac{b\mu-x}{\sigma}\right) - \Phi\left(\frac{-x}{\sigma}\right)\right], \tag{J.5}$$

where $\Phi(z)$ is the cumulative standard normal distribution function. We can now substitute the right-hand side of (J.5) into (J.3) to write

$$P[0 \le \theta \le c] = \frac{\frac{1}{\mu}\left[\Phi\left(\frac{c\mu-x}{\sigma}\right) - \Phi\left(\frac{-x}{\sigma}\right)\right]}{\frac{1}{\mu}\left[\Phi\left(\frac{\mu-x}{\sigma}\right) - \Phi\left(\frac{-x}{\sigma}\right)\right]} = \frac{\left[\Phi\left(\frac{c\mu-x}{\sigma}\right) - \Phi\left(\frac{-x}{\sigma}\right)\right]}{\left[\Phi\left(\frac{u-x}{\sigma}\right) - \Phi\left(\frac{-x}{\sigma}\right)\right]},$$

the desired result.

Appendix K
Beta Distrib tion

K.1 Introduction to the Beta Distribution

The beta distribution is commonly used to model continuous probability variables that are between 0 and 1. In its general form, it is written as

$$\frac{\Gamma(\alpha+\beta)}{\Gamma(\alpha)\Gamma(\beta)}\theta^{\alpha-1}(1-\theta)^{\beta-1}\mathbf{1}_{0\le\theta\le1}. \tag{K.1}$$

We can find the mean of this distribution, $E\left[\theta^{k}\right]$, as

$$
\begin{aligned}
E\left[\theta^{k}\right] &= \int_{0}^{1}\theta^{k}\frac{\Gamma(\alpha+\beta)}{\Gamma(\alpha)\Gamma(\beta)}\theta^{\alpha-1}(1-\theta)^{\beta-1}\,d\theta \\
&= \int_{0}^{1}\frac{\Gamma(\alpha+\beta)}{\Gamma(\alpha)\Gamma(\beta)}\theta^{\alpha+k-1}(1-\theta)^{\beta-1}\,d\theta \\
&= \frac{\Gamma(\alpha+\beta)}{\Gamma(\alpha)\Gamma(\beta)}\int_{0}^{1}\theta^{\alpha+k-1}(1-\theta)^{\beta-1}\,d\theta \\
&= \frac{\Gamma(\alpha+\beta)}{\Gamma(\alpha)\Gamma(\beta)}\int_{0}^{1}\theta^{\alpha+k-1}(1-\theta)^{\beta-1}\,d\theta \\
&= \frac{\Gamma(\alpha+\beta)}{\Gamma(\alpha)\Gamma(\beta)}\frac{\Gamma(\alpha+k)\Gamma(\beta)}{\Gamma(\alpha+\beta+k)}\int_{0}^{1}\frac{\Gamma(\alpha+\beta+k)}{\Gamma(\alpha+k)\Gamma(\beta)}\theta^{\alpha+k-1}(1-\theta)^{\beta-1}\,d\theta \\
&= \frac{\Gamma(\alpha+k)}{\Gamma(\alpha)}\frac{\Gamma(\alpha+\beta)}{\Gamma(\alpha+\beta+k)}.
\end{aligned}
$$

To find the mean and variance, we let $k = 1$ and write

$$E[\theta]=\frac{\Gamma(\alpha+1)}{\Gamma(\alpha)}\frac{\Gamma(\alpha+\beta)}{\Gamma(\alpha+\beta+1)}=\frac{(\alpha)\Gamma(\alpha)}{\Gamma(\alpha)}\frac{\Gamma(\alpha+\beta)}{(\alpha+\beta)\Gamma(\alpha+\beta)}=\frac{\alpha}{\alpha+\beta}.$$

To find the variance, we first compute

$$E\left[\theta^2\right] = \frac{\Gamma(\alpha+2)}{\Gamma(\alpha)}\frac{\Gamma(\alpha+\beta)}{\Gamma(\alpha+\beta+2)} = \frac{(\alpha+1)(\alpha)}{(\alpha+\beta+1)(\alpha+\beta)}.$$

And then write

$$Var\left[\theta\right] = E\left[\theta^2\right] - \left[E\left[\theta\right]\right]^2$$

$$= \frac{(\alpha+1)(\alpha)}{(\alpha+\beta+1)(\alpha+\beta)} - \left[\frac{\alpha}{(\alpha+\beta)}\right]^2$$

$$= \frac{(\alpha+1)(\alpha)(\alpha+\beta)}{(\alpha+\beta)^2(\alpha+\beta+1)} - \frac{\alpha^2(\alpha+\beta+1)}{(\alpha+\beta)^2(\alpha+\beta+1)}$$

$$= \frac{(\alpha+1)(\alpha)(\alpha+\beta)}{(\alpha+\beta)^2(\alpha+\beta+1)} - \frac{\alpha^2(\alpha+\beta+1)}{(\alpha+\beta)^2(\alpha+\beta+1)}$$

$$= \frac{\alpha\beta}{(\alpha+\beta)^2(\alpha+\beta+1)}.$$

The commonality of terms that can be written in the form $\theta^y(1-\theta)^{n-y}$ in both the beta and the binomial distribution suggest that they might be a useful combination in constructing posterior distributions. We let

$$\pi(\theta) = \frac{\Gamma(\alpha+\beta)}{\Gamma(\alpha)\Gamma(\beta)}\theta^{\alpha-1}(1-\theta)^{\beta-1}\mathbf{1}_{0\leq\theta\leq1},$$

and

$$f(x\mid\theta) = \binom{n}{x}\theta^x(1-\theta)^{n-x}.$$

To obtain the posterior distribution of θ, $\pi(\theta\mid x)$ we begin with

$$\pi(\theta\mid x) = \frac{f(x\mid\theta)\pi(\theta)}{\sum_{\theta}f(x\mid\theta)\pi(\theta)}$$

$$= \frac{\binom{n}{x}\frac{\Gamma(\alpha+\beta)}{\Gamma(\alpha)\Gamma(\beta)}\theta^{\alpha+x-1}(1-\theta)^{n-x+\beta-1}\mathbf{1}_{0\leq\theta\leq1}}{\int_{\theta}\binom{n}{x}\frac{\Gamma(\alpha+\beta)}{\Gamma(\alpha)\Gamma(\beta)}\theta^{\alpha+x-1}(1-\theta)^{n-x+\beta-1}}. \qquad (K.2)$$

The denominator of the last line of expression (K.2) becomes

$$\int_\theta \binom{n}{x}\frac{\Gamma(\alpha+\beta)}{\Gamma(\alpha)\Gamma(\beta)}\theta^{\alpha+x-1}(1-\theta)^{n-x+\beta-1}\,d\theta = \binom{n}{x}\frac{\Gamma(\alpha+\beta)}{\Gamma(\alpha)\Gamma(\beta)}\int_0^1\theta^{\alpha+x-1}(1-\theta)^{n-x+\beta-1}\,d\theta$$

$$\binom{n}{x}\frac{\Gamma(\alpha+\beta)}{\Gamma(\alpha)\Gamma(\beta)}\frac{\Gamma(\alpha+x)\Gamma(n-x+\beta)}{\Gamma(n+\alpha+\beta)}\int_0^1\frac{\Gamma(n+\alpha+\beta)}{\Gamma(\alpha+x)\Gamma(n-x+\beta)}\theta^{\alpha+x-1}(1-\theta)^{n-x+\beta-1}\,d\theta$$

$$=\binom{n}{x}\frac{\Gamma(\alpha+\beta)}{\Gamma(\alpha)\Gamma(\beta)}\frac{\Gamma(\alpha+x)\Gamma(n-x+\beta)}{\Gamma(n+\alpha+\beta)}.$$

We may write the posterior distribution as

$$\pi(\theta\,|\,x)=\frac{\binom{n}{x}\dfrac{\Gamma(\alpha+\beta)}{\Gamma(\alpha)\Gamma(\beta)}\theta^{\alpha+x-1}(1-\theta)^{n-x+\beta-1}\mathbf{1}_{0\le\theta\le1}}{\binom{n}{x}\dfrac{\Gamma(\alpha+\beta)}{\Gamma(\alpha)\Gamma(\beta)}\dfrac{\Gamma(\alpha+x)\Gamma(n-x+\beta)}{\Gamma(n+\alpha+\beta)}}$$

$$=\frac{\Gamma(n+\alpha+\beta)}{\Gamma(\alpha+x)\Gamma(n-x+\beta)}\theta^{\alpha+x-1}(1-\theta)^{n-x+\beta-1}\mathbf{1}_{0\le\theta\le1}$$

which is a beta distribution with parameters $\alpha+x$ and $n-x+\beta$.

K.2 Sample Size and Beta Distributions
In the Chapter Nine discussions, we review the sample size computation that requires finding the expected sample size N given the joint distribution of the control group effect size θ and the efficacy ϕ. Thus, if $\pi(\theta,\phi)$ is the joint prior distribution of θ and ϕ, then we can write $N=g(\theta,\phi)$,

$$\mathbf{E}[N]=\sum_{\theta,\phi}g(\theta,\phi)\pi(\theta,\phi),\qquad\text{(K.3)}$$

in which

$$g(\theta,\phi)=\frac{2\big[\theta(1-\theta)+\theta(1-\phi)(1-\theta(1-\phi))\big]\big[Z_{1-\alpha/2}+Z_\beta\big]^2}{(\theta\phi)^2}$$

where Z_c is the cth percentile of the standard normal distribution.

Now, assume that θ and ϕ each have independent beta distributions. Then

$$\pi(\theta,\phi)=\frac{\Gamma(\alpha_1+\beta_1)}{\Gamma(\alpha_1)\Gamma(\beta_1)}\theta^{\alpha_1-1}(1-\theta)^{\beta_1-1}\frac{\Gamma(\alpha_2+\beta_2)}{\Gamma(\alpha_2)\Gamma(\beta_2)}\phi^{\alpha_2-1}(1-\phi)^{\beta_2-1}\quad\text{(K.4)}$$

and we may incorporate (K.4) into the expression for the expected sample size (K.3) to find

$$\mathbf{E}[N] = \sum_{\theta,\phi} g(\theta,\phi)\pi(\theta,\phi)$$

$$= \sum_{\theta,\phi} \frac{2\left[\theta(1-\theta)+\theta(1-\phi)(1-\theta(1-\phi))\right]\left[Z_{1-\alpha/2}+Z_\beta\right]^2}{(\theta\phi)^2} \frac{\Gamma(\alpha_1+\beta_1)}{\Gamma(\alpha_1)\Gamma(\beta_1)}\theta^{\alpha_1-1}(1-\theta)^{\beta_1-1}\frac{\Gamma(\alpha_2+\beta_2)}{\Gamma(\alpha_2)\Gamma(\beta_2)}\phi^{\alpha_2-1}(1-\phi)^{\beta_2-1}$$

$$(K.5)$$

Writing the constant M as $2\dfrac{\Gamma(\alpha_1+\beta_1)}{\Gamma(\alpha_1)\Gamma(\beta_1)}\dfrac{\Gamma(\alpha_2+\beta_2)}{\Gamma(\alpha_2)\Gamma(\beta_2)}\left[Z_{1-\alpha/2}+Z_\beta\right]^2$, we can re-

formulate the expected value of the sample size as

$$\mathbf{E}[N] = M\sum_{\theta,\phi}\frac{\left[\theta(1-\theta)+\theta(1-\phi)\left(1-\theta(1-\phi)\right)\right]}{(\theta\phi)^2}\theta^{\alpha_1-1}(1-\theta)^{\beta_1-1}\phi^{\alpha_2-1}(1-\phi)^{\beta_2-1}.$$

Combining terms, we can simplify to write

$$\mathbf{E}[N] = M\sum_{\theta,\phi}\frac{1}{\theta^2\phi^2}\left[\theta(1-\theta)+\theta(1-\phi)\left(1-\theta(1-\phi)\right)\right]\theta^{\alpha_1-1}(1-\theta)^{\beta_1-1}\phi^{\alpha_2-3}(1-\phi)^{\beta_2-1}$$

$$= M\sum_{\theta,\phi}\theta^{\alpha_1-2}(1-\theta)^{\beta_1}\phi^{\alpha_2-3}(1-\phi)^{\beta_2-1} + \theta^{\alpha_1-2}(1-\theta)^{\beta_1-1}\phi^{\alpha_2-3}(1-\phi)^{\beta_2} - \theta^{\alpha_1-1}(1-\theta)^{\beta_1-1}\phi^{\alpha_2-3}(1-\phi)^{\beta_2+1}.$$

This last formulation consists of the sum and difference of three terms each of which are products of independent beta distributions. These summations are integrals over the [0, 1] real numbers. The first term in the sum may be evaluated as follows.

$$\sum_{\theta,\phi}\theta^{\alpha_1-2}(1-\theta)^{\beta_1}\phi^{\alpha_2-3}(1-\phi)^{\beta_2-1} = \int_0^1\int_0^1\theta^{\alpha_1-2}(1-\theta)^{\beta_1}\phi^{\alpha_2-3}(1-\phi)^{\beta_2-1}d\theta d\phi$$

$$= \int_0^1\theta^{\alpha_1-2}(1-\theta)^{\beta_1}d\theta\int_0^1\phi^{\alpha_2-3}(1-\phi)^{\beta_2-1}d\phi = \frac{\Gamma(\alpha_1-1)\Gamma(\beta_1+1)}{\Gamma(\alpha_1+\beta_1)}\frac{\Gamma(\alpha_2-2)\Gamma(\beta_2)}{\Gamma(\alpha_2+\beta_2-2)}.$$

We may evaluate the other terms similarly

$$\sum_{\theta,\phi}\theta^{\alpha_1-2}(1-\theta)^{\beta_1-1}\phi^{\alpha_2-3}(1-\phi)^{\beta_2} = \frac{\Gamma(\alpha_1-1)\Gamma(\beta_1)}{\Gamma(\alpha_1+\beta_1-1)}\frac{\Gamma(\alpha_2-2)\Gamma(\beta_2+1)}{\Gamma(\alpha_2+\beta_2-1)}$$

$$\sum_{\theta,\phi}\theta^{\alpha_1-1}(1-\theta)^{\beta_1-1}\phi^{\alpha_2-3}(1-\phi)^{\beta_2+1} = \frac{\Gamma(\alpha_1)\Gamma(\beta_1)}{\Gamma(\alpha_1+\beta_1)}\frac{\Gamma(\alpha_2-2)\Gamma(\beta_2+2)}{\Gamma(\alpha_2+\beta_2)}$$

Thus we can write

$$E[N] = 2\frac{\Gamma(\alpha_1+\beta_1)}{\Gamma(\alpha_1)\Gamma(\beta_1)}\frac{\Gamma(\alpha_2+\beta_2)}{\Gamma(\alpha_2)\Gamma(\beta_2)}\left[Z_{1-\alpha/2}+Z_\beta\right]^2$$

$$\left[\frac{\Gamma(\alpha_1-1)\Gamma(\beta_1+1)}{\Gamma(\alpha_1+\beta_1)}\frac{\Gamma(\alpha_2-2)\Gamma(\beta_2)}{\Gamma(\alpha_2+\beta_2-2)}+\frac{\Gamma(\alpha_1-1)\Gamma(\beta_1)}{\Gamma(\alpha_1+\beta_1-1)}\frac{\Gamma(\alpha_2-2)\Gamma(\beta_2+1)}{\Gamma(\alpha_2+\beta_2-1)}-\frac{\Gamma(\alpha_1)\Gamma(\beta_1)}{\Gamma(\alpha_1+\beta_1)}\frac{\Gamma(\alpha_2-2)\Gamma(\beta_2+2)}{\Gamma(\alpha_2+\beta_2)}\right],$$

which simplifies to

$$2\left[Z_{1-\alpha/2}+Z_\beta\right]^2\left[\frac{\beta_1}{\alpha_1-1}\frac{(\alpha_2+\beta_2-1)(\alpha_2+\beta_2-2)}{(\alpha_2-1)(\alpha_2-2)}+\frac{(\alpha_1+\beta_1-1)}{(\alpha_1-1)}\frac{\beta_2(\alpha_2+\beta_2-1)}{(\alpha_2-1)(\alpha_2-2)}-\frac{(\beta_2+1)\beta_2}{(\alpha_2-1)(\alpha_2-2)}\right].$$

Appendix L
Calc lations for Chapter 8

For example one of Chapter Eight, we must evaluate

$$\pi(\theta \mid x) = \frac{\dfrac{(3\theta)^k}{k!}e^{-3\theta}\left[0.30\dfrac{0.40e^{-0.40\theta}}{1-e^{-0.40(3)}}+0.70\dfrac{(0.357)e^{-0.357(3-\theta)}}{1-e^{-0.357(3)}}\right]\mathbf{1}_{\theta\in[0,3]}}{\displaystyle\sum_\theta\dfrac{(3\theta)^k}{k!}e^{-3\theta}\left[0.30\dfrac{0.40e^{-0.40\theta}}{1-e^{-0.40(3)}}+0.70\dfrac{(0.357)e^{-0.357(3-\theta)}}{1-e^{-0.357(3)}}\right]\mathbf{1}_{\theta\in[0,3]}} \qquad (L.1)$$

We evaluate the denominator of the right-hand side of equation (L.1) first, we writing it as

$$\sum_\theta\frac{(3\theta)^k}{k!}e^{-3\theta}0.30\frac{0.40e^{-0.40\theta}}{1-e^{-0.40(3)}}\mathbf{1}_{\theta\in[0,3]} \;+\; \sum_\theta\frac{(3\theta)^k}{k!}e^{-3\theta}0.70\frac{(0.357)e^{-0.357(3-\theta)}}{1-e^{-0.357(3)}}\mathbf{1}_{\theta\in[0,3]}.$$

We will solve this in general

$$p\sum_\theta\frac{(d\theta)^k}{k!}e^{-d\theta}\frac{pe^{-\lambda_1\theta}}{1-e^{-a\lambda_1}}\mathbf{1}_{\theta\in[0,a]} \;+\; (1-p)\sum_\theta\frac{(d\theta)^k}{k!}e^{-d\theta}\frac{\lambda_2 e^{-\lambda_2(3-\theta)}}{1-e^{-a\lambda_2}}\mathbf{1}_{\theta\in[0,a]} \qquad (L.2)$$

where $p = 0.30$, $a = 3$, $d = 3$, $\lambda_1 = 0.40$, and $\lambda_2 = 0.357$. We will take each of the two summands in expression (L.2)

$$p\sum_\theta\frac{(d\theta)^k}{k!}e^{-d\theta}\frac{pe^{-\lambda_1\theta}}{1-e^{-a\lambda_1}}\mathbf{1}_{\theta\in[0,a]} = \frac{pd^k}{k!\left(1-e^{-a\lambda_1}\right)}\int_0^3\theta^k e^{-(d+\lambda_1)\theta}d\theta.$$

For the second term, we find

$$(1-p)\sum_\theta\frac{(d\theta)^k}{k!}e^{-d\theta}\frac{\lambda_2 e^{-\lambda_2(3-\theta)}}{1-e^{-a\lambda_2}}\mathbf{1}_{\theta\in[0,a]} = \frac{(1-p)d^k e^{-a\lambda_2}}{k!\left(1-e^{-a\lambda_2}\right)}\int_0^3\theta^k e^{-(d-\lambda_2)\theta}d\theta$$

Thus the denominator of the posterior distribution is

$$p\sum_{\theta}\frac{(d\theta)^{k}}{k!}e^{-d\theta}\frac{pe^{-\lambda_{1}\theta}}{1-e^{-a\lambda_{1}}}1_{\theta\in[0,a]} + (1-p)\sum_{\theta}\frac{(d\theta)^{k}}{k!}e^{-d\theta}\frac{\lambda_{2}e^{-\lambda_{2}(3-\theta)}}{1-e^{-a\lambda_{2}}}1_{\theta\in[0,a]}$$

$$=\frac{pd^{k}}{k!\left(1-e^{-a\lambda_{1}}\right)}\int_{0}^{3}\theta^{k}e^{-(d+\lambda_{1})\theta}d\theta + \frac{(1-p)d^{k}e^{-a\lambda_{2}}}{k!\left(1-e^{-a\lambda_{2}}\right)}\int_{0}^{3}\theta^{k}e^{-(d-\lambda_{2})\theta}d\theta \qquad (L.3)$$

We now have to address the integral of the form $\int_{0}^{a}\theta^{k}e^{-a\theta}d\theta$. Since

$\int_{0}^{\infty}\frac{\alpha^{k}}{\Gamma(k)}\theta^{k}e^{-a\theta}d\theta = 1$, we can write

$$1 = \int_{0}^{\infty}\frac{\alpha^{k}}{\Gamma(k)}\theta^{k}e^{-a\theta}d\theta = \int_{0}^{a}\frac{\alpha^{k}}{\Gamma(k)}\theta^{k}e^{-a\theta}d\theta + \int_{a}^{\infty}\frac{\alpha^{k}}{\Gamma(k)}\theta^{k}e^{-a\theta}d\theta, \text{ and}$$

$$\int_{0}^{a}\frac{\alpha^{k}}{\Gamma(k)}\theta^{k}e^{-a\theta}d\theta = 1 - \int_{a}^{\infty}\frac{\alpha^{k}}{\Gamma(k)}\theta^{k}e^{-a\theta}d\theta$$

$$\int_{0}^{a}\theta^{k}e^{-a\theta}d\theta = \frac{\Gamma(k)}{\alpha^{k}}\left[1 - \int_{a}^{\infty}\frac{\alpha^{k}}{\Gamma(k)}\theta^{k}e^{-a\theta}d\theta\right].$$

We now evaluate $\int_{a}^{\infty}\frac{\alpha^{k}}{\Gamma(k)}\theta^{k}e^{-a\theta}d\theta$. Begin by writing $w = \theta - a$, then $dw = da$, the range of integration changes from $a \le \theta \le \infty$ to $0 \le w \le \infty$. In addition, since k is an integer, we can write $\theta^{k} = (w+a)^{k} = \sum_{j=0}^{k}\binom{k}{j}w^{j}a^{k=j}$. Thus

$$\int_{a}^{\infty}\frac{\alpha^{k}}{\Gamma(k)}\theta^{k}e^{-a\theta}d\theta = \frac{\alpha^{k}}{\Gamma(k)}\int_{0}^{\infty}\sum_{j=0}^{k}\binom{k}{j}w^{j}a^{k-j}e^{-\alpha(w+a)}d\theta$$

$$= \frac{\alpha^{k}e^{-\alpha a}}{\Gamma(k)}\sum_{j=0}^{k}\binom{k}{j}a^{k-j}\int_{0}^{\infty}w^{j}e^{-\alpha w}d\theta$$

$$= \frac{\alpha^{k}e^{-\alpha a}}{\Gamma(k)}\sum_{j=0}^{k}\binom{k}{j}a^{k-j}\frac{\Gamma(j+1)}{\alpha^{j+1}}\int_{0}^{\infty}\frac{\alpha^{j+1}}{\Gamma(j+1)}w^{j}e^{-\alpha w}d\theta$$

$$= \frac{\alpha^{k}e^{-\alpha a}}{\Gamma(k)}\sum_{j=0}^{k}\binom{k}{j}a^{k-j}\frac{\Gamma(j+1)}{\alpha^{j+1}}.$$

Therefore

$$\int_0^a \theta^k e^{-\alpha\theta}\,d\theta = \frac{\Gamma(k)}{\alpha^k}\left[1 - \int_a^\infty \frac{\alpha^k}{\Gamma(k)}\theta^k e^{-\alpha\theta}\,d\theta\right]$$

$$= \frac{\Gamma(k)}{\alpha^k}\left[1 - \frac{\alpha^k e^{-\alpha a}}{\Gamma(k)}\sum_{j=0}^{k}\binom{k}{j}a^{k-j}\frac{\Gamma(j+1)}{\alpha^{j+1}}\right].$$

Thus the denominator of the posterior distribution is

$$= \frac{pd^k}{k!\left(1-e^{-a\lambda_1}\right)}\int_0^3 \theta^k e^{-(d+\lambda_1)\theta}\,d\theta + \frac{(1-p)d^k e^{-a\lambda_2}}{k!\left(1-e^{-a\lambda_2}\right)}\int_0^3 \theta^k e^{-(d-\lambda_2)\theta}\,d\theta$$

$$= \frac{pd^k}{k!\left(1-e^{-a\lambda_1}\right)}\frac{\Gamma(k)}{(d+\lambda_1)^k}\left[1 - \frac{(d+\lambda_1)^k e^{-3\alpha}}{\Gamma(k)}\sum_{j=0}^{k}\binom{k}{j}a^{k-j}\frac{\Gamma(j+1)}{(d+\lambda_1)^{j+1}}\right]$$

$$+ \frac{(1-p)d^k e^{-a\lambda_2}}{k!\left(1-e^{-a\lambda_2}\right)}\frac{\Gamma(k)}{(d-\lambda_2)^k}\left[1 - \frac{(d-\lambda_2)^k e^{-3\alpha}}{\Gamma(k)}\sum_{j=0}^{k}\binom{k}{j}3^{k-j}\frac{\Gamma(j+1)}{(d-\lambda_2)^{j+1}}\right].$$

The numerator of the posterior distribution (L.1)

$$\frac{(3\theta)^k}{k!}e^{-3\theta}\left[0.30\frac{0.40e^{-0.40\theta}}{1-e^{-0.40(3)}} + 0.70\frac{(0.357)e^{-0.357(3-\theta)}}{1-e^{-0.357(3)}}\right]1_{\theta\in[0,3]}$$

$$= \frac{3^k}{k!}\left[(0.172)\theta^k e^{-3.4\theta} + (0.130)e^{-(1.071+2.964\theta)}\right]1_{\theta\in[0,3]}.$$

Appendix M
Sample Size Primer

M.1 Introduction
The purpose of this appendix is to provide a brief discussion of the underlying principles in sample size computations for a clinical trial from the frequentist perspective. In the process, one of the simplest and most useful formulas for the sample size formulations will be reproduced. These basic formulas are the source of several of the calculations in Chapter Nine. First we will provide the solution and proceed to a discussion that both motivates and derives the sample size and power formulas.

M.2 The One Sample Calculation
Assume that we collect a sample of observations that reflect dichotomous outcomes, e.g. mortality results. We are interested in carrying out a statistical hypothesis test for the value θ, the mortality rate. The hypothesis test is

$$H_0: \theta = \theta_0 \qquad \text{versus} \quad H_a: \theta \neq \theta_0.$$

The investigators have chosen an *a priori* test-specific type I error level α, and the power of the statistical hypothesis test is $1 - \beta$. The hypothesis test will be two-sided, and let Δ be the effect size that the investigators wish to detect, then the minimum sample size N is sample size formula is

$$N = \frac{\theta(1-\theta)\left(Z_{1-\alpha/2} - Z_{\beta}\right)^2}{\Delta^2}. \tag{M.1}$$

The power may be written as

$$1 - \beta = 1 - \Phi_Z\left[Z_{1-\alpha/2} - \frac{\Delta}{\sqrt{\frac{\theta(1-\theta)}{N}}}\right]. \tag{M.2}$$

These computations are the consequences of the hypothesis test construction, as well as the meaning of α and β. It if useful to consider the sample size computation as a three-phased calculation.

Phase 1 :   under the null
Phase 2:   under the alternative
Phase 3:   consolidation

For each demonstration in this appendix, we will step through each of these phases.

M.2.1 Phase 1: Under the Null Hypothesis

We assume that N is large enough for the normal approximation to the binomial distribution to apply. Then, let p be the observed mortality rate and the estimate of θ. Then

$$\frac{p - \theta_0}{\sqrt{Var(p)}} \sim N(0,1), \tag{M.3}$$

If the investigators suspect that the true value of θ is θ_a where $\theta_a \geq \theta_0$ then one the critical region of interest is

$$\frac{p - \theta_0}{\sqrt{Var(p)}} > Z_{1-\alpha/2},$$

or

$$p - \theta_0 > Z_{1-\alpha/2}\sqrt{Var(p)}. \tag{M.4}$$

This is the end of Phase 1.

M.2.2. Phase 2: Under the Alternative Hypothesis

Under the null hypothesis, the true value of θ is not θ_0, but θ_a and we are concerned not about a type I error but about power. We begin with

$$\text{Power} = P[\text{test statistic falls in critical region} \,|\, H_a \text{ is true}].$$

Insert (M.4) into this expression to find

$$1 - \beta = P\left[p - \theta_0 > Z_{1-\alpha/2}\sqrt{Var(p)} \,\mid\, \theta = \theta_a\right]. \tag{M.5}$$

Now we convert the probability event in (M.5) into one involving a standard normal random variable.

$$1-\beta = P\left[\frac{p-\theta_a}{\sqrt{Var(p)}} > \frac{Z_{1-\alpha/2}\sqrt{Var(p)}-(\theta_a-\theta_0)}{\sqrt{Var(p)}}\right]$$

$$= P\left[Z > \frac{Z_{1-\alpha/2}\sqrt{Var(p)}-(\theta_a-\theta_0)}{\sqrt{Var(p)}}\right] \tag{M.6}$$

$$= P\left[Z > Z_{1-\alpha/2} - \frac{(\theta_a-\theta_0)}{\sqrt{Var(p)}}\right],$$

From the definition of percentiles, the probability that a random variable following a standard normal distribution is greater than Z_β is $1-\beta$, we have

$$Z_\beta = Z_{1-\alpha/2} - \frac{(\theta_a-\theta_0)}{\sqrt{Var(p)}}, \tag{M.7}$$

M.2.3. Phase 3: Consolidation

It remains to write the $Var(p)$ as a function of N and solve (M.7) for N. Recall that

$$Var(p) = \frac{\theta(1-\theta)}{N}, \tag{M.8}$$

and, inserting (M.8) into the denominator of (M.7) we write,

$$Z_\beta = Z_{1-\alpha/2} - \frac{(\theta_a-\theta_0)}{\sqrt{\dfrac{\theta(1-\theta)}{N}}},$$

which we easily solve for N to find

$$N = \frac{\theta(1-\theta)\left(Z_{1-\alpha/2}-Z_\beta\right)^2}{(\theta_a-\theta_0)^2} = \frac{\theta(1-\theta)\left(Z_{1-\alpha/2}-Z_\beta\right)^2}{\Delta^2}. \tag{M.9}$$

Note that the sample size is a function of the type I and type II errors, the sidedness of the hypothesis test, and the minimum difference in the value of the parameter θ under the null and alternative hypotheses worth detecting. The power of the hypothesis may be described as

$$1 - \beta = P \left[Z > Z_{1-\alpha/2} - \frac{\Delta}{\sqrt{\theta(1-\theta)/N}} \right]. \tag{M.10}$$

M3. Clinical Trial with a Dichotomous Endpoint

Assume that a clinical trial has been designed to measure the effect of a randomly allocated intervention on a prospectively defined primary endpoint. Let θ_c be the cumulative incidence rate of the primary endpoint in the control group and let θ_t be the cumulative incidence rate of the primary endpoint in the treatment group. Then the statistical hypothesis for the primary endpoint in this clinical trial is

$$H_0 : \theta_c = \theta_t \quad \text{versus} \quad H_a : \theta_c \neq \theta_t. \tag{M.11}$$

Let Z_a be the ath percentile from the standard normal distribution. The investigators have chosen an a priori test-specific type I error level α, and the power of the statistical hypothesis test is $1 - \beta$. The hypothesis test will be two-sided. Let p_c be the cumulative incidence rate of the primary endpoint in the control group of the research sample, and let p_t be the cumulative incidence rate of the active group in the research sample. Then the trial size, or the sample size of the clinical trial,[*] N may be written as

$$N = \frac{2 \left[p_c(1-p_c) + p_t(1-p_t) \right] \left[Z_{1-\alpha/2} - Z_\beta \right]^2}{\left(p_c - p_t \right)^2}. \tag{M.12}$$

Analogously, the power of the study may be calculated as a function of N,

$$1 - \beta = P \left[N(0,1) > Z_{1-\alpha/2} - \frac{p_c - p_t}{\sqrt{\dfrac{p_c(1-p_c)}{N/2} + \dfrac{p_t(1-p_t)}{N/2}}} \right]. \tag{M.13}$$

For these discussions, assume that patients are randomized to receive either a new intervention or to receive control group therapy. In this example, there is one primary endpoint that occurs with a cumulative event rate θ_c. In the intervention group the cumulative event rate for the primary endpoint is θ_t. The investigator does not know the value of θ_c, since he does not study every patient in the population. He therefore selects a sample from the population and uses that sample to compute p_c, which will serve as his estimate of θ_c. If the clinical trial has

---

[*] This is the total number of patients in the study (number of patients in the placebo group plus the number of patients in the control group).

been executed concordantly, then p_c is a good estimator of θ_c; this means that the investigator can expect that p_c will be close to the value of θ_c. Analogously p_t is the estimate from the investigator's sample of the cumulative incidence of the endpoint in the population θ_t.

Thus, if the trial was executed according to its protocol (and not subject to the destabilizing influences of random research), then $p_c - p_t$ can be expected to be an accurate estimate of $\theta_c - \theta_t$. If the null hypothesis is true, then $\theta_c - \theta_t$ will be zero and we would expect $p_c - p_t$ to be small. If the alternative hypothesis is correct, and the investigator's intuition that the therapy being tested in the clinical trial will reduce the cumulative event rate of the primary endpoint is right, then θ_c is much greater than θ_t, and $p_c - p_t$, the best estimate of $\theta_c - \theta_t$ will be large as well.

A key point in understanding the sample size formulation is the critical role played by the number of endpoint events produced by the sample. The research sample produces primary endpoints—the rate at which these endpoints are accumulated is directly linked to the cumulative event rate in the control group. This cumulative event rate therefore plays a central role in the sample size calculations. If the primary endpoint of a clinical trial is total mortality, then recruiting 1,000 patients into the study provides no useful information for the evaluation of the effect of therapy on total mortality if at the end of the study none of the 1,000 recruited patients have died.

Therefore, the more primary endpoint events that occur during the course of the trial, the greater the volume of germane data available to answer the scientific question of whether the occurrence of those endpoint events are influenced by the intervention being studied. It follows that the larger the cumulative control group event rate is, the greater the number of primary endpoint events that will be generated. The greater the rate at which primary endpoints are produced, the smaller the required sample size for the clinical trial will be, *ceteris paribus*.

A second measure that is critical in sample size considerations is the effectiveness of the therapy. This is often measured by the difference between the cumulative incidence rate of the primary endpoint in the population θ_c and the cumulative incidence of the primary event rate in the population if everyone in the population were to receive the treatment being studied in the clinical trial, θ_t. This difference is commonly referred to as "delta" or $\Delta = \theta_c - \theta_t$.[*] The greater the difference between θ_c and θ_t, then the fewer the number of patients required to obtain a reliable estimate of that difference.

To understand this principle, it may be helpful to think of the two primary sources of variability involved in the estimation of the treatment effect in a clinical trial. The test statistic used to test the statistical hypothesis that $\theta_c = \theta_t$ versus the alternative hypothesis that these events are not equal is

$$\frac{p_c - p_t}{\sqrt{Var\left[p_c - p_t\right]}}. \tag{M.14}$$

---

[*] Sometimes it is useful to refer to the percent reduction in events attributable to the therapy, otherwise known as the therapy's efficacy.

The first source of this variability is systematic; it is induced by the intervention being studied by the clinical trial and is an estimate of Δ, the difference between the treatment and control group event rates that are seen in the sample. This variability is estimated by $p_c - p_t$ and resides in the numerator of (M.14). This is the "signal." The denominator of (M.14) is the second source of variability or the "noise"; it is an expression of the fact that, since the research is sample-based, estimates of $p_c - p_t$ will vary from sample to sample. Since this sampling variability "noise" should not be confused with the systematic, intervention-induced "signal" measured by $p_c - p_t$, this noise must be removed from the estimate of the therapy's effect. Therefore using these characterizations, the greater the signal–to–noise ratio, the larger the expression in (M.14) will be.

The greater the signal–to–noise ratio as represented by (M.14), the easier it is to detect a genuine population effect of the intervention. If the magnitude of the difference $\theta_c - \theta_t$ is small in the population, then $p_c - p_t$ is also likely to be small. In this circumstance where the magnitude of the signal is small, the noise must be coincidently reduced to detect the weak signal with precision. One useful tool the investigator has to reduce the background noise is to increase N, the sample size of the clinical trial. Part of the genius of choosing the reliable estimate $p_c - p_t$ of $\theta_c - \theta_t$ is that this estimate's sampling variability decreases as the sample size increases.

It is useful to consider the sample size computation as a three phased calculation. For each demonstration, there will be three phases of the computation.

Phase 1:   under the null
Phase 2:   under the alternative
Phase 3:   consolidation

We will step through each of these phases as we compute the sample size for the clinical trial as outlined earlier in this appendix.

M.3.1 Phase 1: Under the Null Hypothesis
Note that the test statistic

$$\frac{p_c - p_t - (\theta_c - \theta_t)}{\sqrt{Var[p_c - p_t]}} \qquad (M.15)$$

follows a normal distribution. Under the null hypothesis that $\theta_c - \theta_t = 0$, the previous equation reduces to

$$\frac{p_c - p_t}{\sqrt{Var[p_c - p_t]}}. \qquad (M.16)$$

One useful way to think of this test statistic is as a normed effect size. Under the null hypothesis, we expect this normed effect size to have a mean of zero and a variance of one. It will follow the normal or bell-shaped distribution. Then, the null hypothesis will be rejected when[*]

$$\frac{p_c - p_t}{\sqrt{Var\left[p_c - p_t\right]}} > Z_{1-\alpha/2} \qquad (M.17)$$

or,

$$p_c - p_t > Z_{1-\alpha/2}\sqrt{Var\left[p_c - p_t\right]}. \qquad (M.18)$$

M.3.2 Phase 2: Under the Alternative Hypothesis

We now consider what should have if the alternative hypothesis was true. In this case, we start with the definition of statistical power.

Power = Probability [the null hypothesis is rejected | alternative hypothesis is true]

The null hypothesis is rejected when the test statistic falls in the critical region or when $p_c - p_t > Z_{1-\alpha/2}\sqrt{Var\left[p_c - p_t\right]}$. The alternative hypothesis is true if $\theta_c - \theta_t = \Delta \geq 0$. This allows us to write

$$Power = 1-\beta = P\left[p_c - p_t > Z_{1-\alpha/2}\sqrt{Var\left[p_c - p_t\right]} \mid \theta_c - \theta_t = \Delta\right]. \qquad (M.19)$$

We now standardize the argument in the probability statement of (M.19) so that the quantity on the left follows a standard normal distribution. This requires subtracting the population mean effect under the alternative hypothesis (i.e., Δ) and dividing by the square root of the variance of $p_c - p_t$. These operations must be carried out on both sides of the inequality in the probability expression in (M.19) as follows.

---

[*] This is not the only circumstance under which the null hypothesis will be rejected. It will also be rejected when harm is caused by the intervention or when $p_t - p_c$ is very much less than zero. However, in the sample size computation, attention is focused on the tail of the distribution in which the investigators are most interested.

$$1-\beta = P\left[\frac{p_c-p_t-\Delta}{\sqrt{Var[p_c-p_t]}} > \frac{Z_{1-\alpha/2}\sqrt{Var[p_c-p_t]}-\Delta}{\sqrt{Var[p_c-p_t]}}\right]$$

$$= P\left[\frac{p_c-p_t-\Delta}{\sqrt{Var[p_c-p_t]}} > Z_{1-\alpha/2} - \frac{\Delta}{\sqrt{Var[p_c-p_t]}}\right] \qquad \text{(M.20)}$$

$$= P\left[N(0,1) > Z_{1-\alpha/2} - \frac{\Delta}{\sqrt{Var[p_c-p_t]}}\right].$$

By the definition of a percentile value from a probability distribution, we can now write

$$Z_\beta = Z_{1-\alpha/2} - \frac{\Delta}{\sqrt{Var[p_c-p_t]}}. \qquad \text{(M.21)}$$

M.3.3 Phase 3: Consolidation

We are now ready to conclude this computation, by solving for N, the size of the trial. The sample size is embedded in the variance term in the denominator of expression (M.21).

$$Var[p_c-p_t] = \frac{p_c(1-p_c)}{n_c} + \frac{p_t(1-p_t)}{n_t}. \qquad \text{(M.22)}$$

where n_c is the number of patients to be recruited to the control group in the clinical trial and n_t is the number of patients to be recruited to the active group. The sample size or trial size is the total number of patients required for the experiment $= N = n_c + n_t$. If we assume that the number of patients in the control group will equal the number of patients in the treatment group, then $n_c = n_t = n$ and $N = 2n$. Then (M.21) can be rewritten as

$$Z_\beta = Z_{1-\alpha/2} - \frac{\Delta}{\sqrt{\dfrac{p_c(1-p_c)}{n} + \dfrac{p_t(1-p_t)}{n}}}. \qquad \text{(M.23)}$$

We only need solve this equation for n

$$n = \frac{\left[p_c(1-p_c)+p_t(1-p_t)\right]\left[Z_{1-\alpha/2}-Z_\beta\right]^2}{\Delta^2}. \qquad \text{(M.24)}$$

The trial size $N = 2n$ may be written as

$$N = \frac{2\left[p_c\left(1-p_c\right)+p_t\left(1-p_t\right)\right]\left[Z_{1-\alpha/2}-Z_\beta\right]^2}{\Delta^2}. \qquad (M.25)$$

To compute the power we only need to adapt the following equation from the last line of expression (M.20),

$$1-\beta = P\left[N(0,1) > Z_{1-\alpha/2} - \frac{\Delta}{\sqrt{Var\left[p_c-p_t\right]}}\right] \qquad (M.26)$$

and rewrite the Var $[p_c - p_t]$ to find

$$1-\beta = P\left[N(0,1) > Z_{1-\alpha/2} - \frac{\Delta}{\sqrt{\dfrac{p_c\left(1-p_c\right)}{N/2}+\dfrac{p_t\left(1-p_t\right)}{N/2}}}\right]. \qquad (M.27)$$

M.4 Example

If the experiment is designed for a two–sided α of 0.05, 90 % power ($\beta = 0.10$), $p_c = 0.20$, and $\Delta = 0.03$, then we compute that $p_t = 0.17$. This corresponds to a $\left(0.20-0.17\right)/0.20 = 0.15$ or 15% reduction in events attributable to the intervention). The trial size can be computed from

$$N = \frac{2\left[p_c\left(1-p_c\right)+p_t\left(1-p_t\right)\right]\left[Z_{1-\alpha/2}-Z_\beta\right]^2}{\left[p_c-p_t\right]^2}. \qquad (M.28)$$

Inserting the data from this example reveals

$$N = \frac{2\left[(0.20)(0.80)+(0.17)(0.83)\right]\left[1.96-(-1.28)\right]^2}{\left[0.20-0.17\right]^2} = 7024 \qquad (M.29)$$

or 3,512 subjects per group. If only 2,000 subjects per group can be identified, the power can be formulated from

$$Power = P\left[N(0,1) > Z_{1-\alpha/2} \; - \; \frac{\Delta}{\sqrt{\dfrac{p_c(1-p_c)}{N/2} + \dfrac{p_t(1-p_t)}{N/2}}} \right] \qquad (M.30)$$

and including the data from this example

$$Power = P\left[N(0,1) > 1.96 - \frac{0.03}{\sqrt{\dfrac{(0.20)(0.80)}{2000} + \dfrac{(0.17)(0.83)}{2000}}} \right] = 0.69.$$

M.5 Continuous Outcomes

Many clinical trials have outcome measures that are continuous. Consider a clinical experiment that is designed to test the effect of an intervention on the change in left ventricular end diastolic volume (EDV). Patients are recruited using a random-sampling plan and have their baseline EDV measured. They are then randomized to receive placebo care or the intervention, and followed for three months, at the end of which they have their EDV measured again. The investigator assumes that the EDVs will be normally distributed, and wishes to analyze the change in EDV over time across the two groups. He believes that there will be a large increase in EDV in the placebo group, reflecting the natural progression of the disease. It is his hope that the EDV change will be smaller in the treatment arm of the experiment.

Let $\mu_d(c)$ be the population mean change in the end diastolic volumes for the placebo group and $\mu_d(t)$ be the population mean change in the end diastolic volume in the active group. Let's begin with the null hypothesis,

$$H_0 : \mu_d(c) = \mu_d(t) \text{ versus } H_a : \mu_d(c) \neq \mu_d(t).$$

Clearly, the investigator does not believe the alternative hypothesis as stated, he believes that $\mu_d(c)$ the population mean change in EDV in the placebo group, will be greater than $\mu_d(t)$, the population mean change in EDV in the active group. However, since he recognizes that he does not know the effect of therapy, he states the alternative hypothesis as two-sided. However, his true belief in the ability of the treatment to affect the change in EDV will be reflected in phase 2.

M.5.1 Phase 1: The Null Hypothesis

The purpose of phase 1 is simply to construct the test statistic and identify its critical region. The distribution of the test statistic is the distribution under the null hypothesis, i.e., under the assumption that there is no treatment effect on the mean change in EDV. As was stated before, the investigator believes the difference in EDVs will follow a normal distribution. Let d_c be the sample mean change in the placebo group, and d_t is the sample mean change in the active group, and $Var[d_c - d_t]$ be the variance of the difference in chance of the EDVs We note that under the null hypothesis the quantity

$$\frac{d_c - d_t}{\sqrt{Var[d_c - d_t]}} \tag{M.31}$$

follows a normal distribution. Then the null hypothesis will be rejected when

$$\frac{d_c - d_t}{\sqrt{Var[d_c - d_t]}} > Z_{1-\alpha/2}, \tag{M.32}$$

where $Z_{1-\alpha/2}$ is the $1 - \alpha/2$ percentile value from the standard normal distribution with mean zero and variance one. We may rewrite equation (M.32) to see that we will reject the null hypothesis in favor of the alternative if

$$d_c - d_t > Z_{1-\alpha/2}\sqrt{Var[d_c - d_t]}. \tag{M.33}$$

This ends phase 1.

M.5.2 Phase 2: The Alternative Hypothesis
This next phase combines the result of phase 1 with the notion of power. Begin with the definition of power:

Power = Prob[The null hypothesis is rejected | the alternative hypothesis is true]

The null hypothesis is rejected when the test statistic falls in the critical region. The alternative hypothesis is true if $d_c - d_t = \Delta \geq 0$. This quantity Δ is the difference that the investigator hopes to see between the changes in the two groups. This consideration is not two-sided at this point, and is the opportunity for the investigator to state precisely state the magnitude of efficacy he believes this treatment will produce.

Using the result of Phase 1 we can write the power equation as

$$Power = P\left[d_c - d_t > Z_{1-\alpha/2}\sqrt{Var[d_c - d_t]} \mid \Delta\right]. \tag{M.34}$$

We now standardize this so that the quantity on the left follows a standard normal distribution. Under phase 2, the alternative hypothesis the mean of the treatment difference $d_c - d_t = \Delta \geq 0$. This leads to

$$Power = P\left[\frac{d_c - d_t - \Delta}{\sqrt{Var\left[d_c - d_t\right]}} > \frac{Z_{1-\alpha/2}\sqrt{Var\left[d_c - d_t\right]} - \Delta}{\sqrt{Var\left[d_c - d_t\right]}}\right], \qquad \text{(M.35)}$$

which can be simplified to

$$= P\left[\frac{d_c - d_t - \Delta}{\sqrt{Var\left[d_c - d_t\right]}} > Z_{1-\alpha/2} - \frac{\Delta}{\sqrt{Var\left[d_c - d_t\right]}}\right] \qquad \text{(M.36)}$$

$$= P\left[N(0,1) > Z_{1-\alpha/2} - \frac{\Delta}{\sqrt{Var\left[d_c - d_t\right]}}\right].$$

These steps are simply algebra. At this point, we can use the fact that
$P\left[N(0,1) \geq Z_\beta\right] = 1 - \beta$ to write

$$Z_\beta = Z_{1-\alpha/2} - \frac{\Delta}{\sqrt{Var\left[d_c - d_t\right]}}. \qquad \text{(M.37)}$$

This concludes Phase 2

M.5.3 Phase 3: Consolidation
Phase 2 concluded with an equation, that we must now solve for n. We assume that there were be an equal number of subjects in the treatment group and the intervention group. The sample size n is embedded in the variance term in the denominator of equation (M.37).

$$Var\left[d_c - d_t\right] = \frac{\sigma_D^2}{n} + \frac{\sigma_D^2}{n} = \frac{2\sigma_D^2}{n}, \qquad \text{(M.38)}$$

where σ_D^2 is the variance of an intrasubject difference. The trial size (i.e., the total number of subjects needed for the experiment) $= N = 2n$. Replacing the denominator of the expression on the right–hand side of equation (M.37) with the right-hand side of (M.38), we have

$$Z_\beta = Z_{1-\alpha/2} - \frac{\Delta}{\sqrt{Var\left[d_c - d_t\right]}}. \qquad \text{(M.39)}$$

We need only solve this equation for n

$$n = \frac{2\sigma_D^2\left[Z_{1-\alpha/2} - Z_\beta\right]^2}{\Delta^2}, \qquad \text{(M.40)}$$

and the trial size* N, is

$$N = \frac{4\sigma_D^2 \left[Z_{1-\alpha/2} - Z_\beta \right]^2}{\Delta^2}.$$ (M.41)

To compute the power one need only adapt the following equation from Phase 2,

$$1 - \beta = P \left[N(0,1) > Z_{1-\alpha/2} - \frac{\Delta}{\sqrt{Var\left[d_x - d_y \right]}} \right],$$ (M.42)

and rewrite the variance to find

$$1 - \beta = P \left[N(0,1) > Z_{1-\alpha/2} - \frac{\Delta}{\sqrt{\dfrac{2\sigma_D^2}{n}}} \right].$$ (M.43)

M.5.4 Example
If, for this experiment, the investigator chooses a two-sided alpha of 0.05, 90% power (beta = 0.10), delta = 10 and $\sigma_D = 18$, the trial size is

$$N = \frac{4\sigma_D^2 \left[Z_{1-\alpha/2} - Z_\beta \right]^2}{\left[\Delta \right]^2} = \frac{4(18)^2 \left[1.96 - (-1.28) \right]^2}{\left[10 \right]^2} = 136.$$ (M.44)

Or 68 subjects per group. If the delta of interest is 5 rather than 10, the power is

---

* The trial size is the total number of patients required for the experiment; here it is the number of patients randomized to the placebo group plus the number of patients randomized to the intervention group.

$$1 - \beta = P\left[N(0,1) > Z_{1-\alpha/2} - \frac{\Delta}{\sqrt{\dfrac{2\sigma^2}{n}}} \right]$$

(M.45)

$$= P\left[N(0,1) > 1.96 - \frac{5}{\sqrt{\dfrac{2(18)^2}{68}}} \right]$$

$$= P[N(0,1) > 0.34] = 0.37.$$

Appendix N

Predictive Power Comp tations

In Chapter Ten, we focused on the computation of conditional power for a test statistic in a study to test the effectiveness of therapy to prevent Alzheimer's disease. We began with the prior distribution $\pi(\theta)$ of the effect size θ, expressed as a relative risk.

$$\pi(\theta) = \frac{a}{\theta\sqrt{2\pi}} e^{-(a\ln\theta + b)^2/2}.$$

This is the log normal distribution (i.e., the log of θ follows a normal distribution). Investigators choose the values of the constants a and b consistent with the current medical knowledge. Our goal is to incorporate this prior distribution into the conditional power computation,

$$CP(H_0) = \gamma = P\left[TS(1) \geq Z_{1-\alpha/2} \mid TS(I) = s\right]. \tag{N.1}$$

where $TS(I)$ is the value of the test statistic at information time $0 \leq I \leq 1$.

In order to solve for s, we first convert expression (N.1) to a statement involving a Brownian motion event by multiplying each term on the right-hand side of expression (N.1) by $\sqrt{I}$.

$$\gamma = P\left[TS(1) \geq Z_{1-\alpha/2} \mid TS(I) = s\right]$$
$$= P\left[(\sqrt{I})TS(1) \geq (\sqrt{I})Z_{1-\alpha/2} \mid (\sqrt{I})TS(I) = \sqrt{I}\,s\right]$$
$$= P\left[B(1) \geq Z_{1-\alpha/2} \mid B(I) = \sqrt{I}\,s\right].$$

which we can write as

$$\gamma = P\left[B(1-I) \geq Z_{1-\alpha/2} - \sqrt{I}\,s\right]. \tag{N.2}$$

The traditional conditional power approach assumes that there is no efficacy for the unexpired duration of the study. In this case the normal distribution that $B(1 - I)$ follows would have mean 0 and variance $1 - I$. However, in the Bayesian setting, we assume that there is nonzero efficacy for the remainder of the study, expressed in terms of the relative risk θ. This will change the mean location of Brownian motion, but the mean is typically expressed in terms of a drift parameter μ, i.e., Brownian motion at time I with drift parameter μ follows a normal distribution with mean μ and variance I. Our plan is to therefore link the drift parameter μ to the relative risk θ.

Let the drift parameter be μ. Then $B(I - I)$ follows a normal distribution with mean $\mu(I - I)$ and variance $I - I$ we may transform expression (N.2) to

$$\gamma = P\left[N\left(\mu(1-I), 1-I\right) \geq Z_{1-\alpha/2} - \sqrt{I}\, s \right].$$ (N.3)

This probability can be evaluated conditional on the value of μ if we knew the value of μ. The relationship between the drift parameter and the relative risk θ can be written as

$$\mu = -\ln\theta\sqrt{\frac{E}{4}},$$ (N.4)

where E is the anticipated total number of primary endpoint events in the trial. To convert the prior probability distribution for θ, $\pi(\theta)$ to the probability distribution for μ, $\pi(\mu)$ using expression recall that

$$\pi(\theta) = \frac{a}{\theta\sqrt{2\pi}} e^{-(a\ln\theta + b)^2/2}.$$ (N.5)

Begin by writing $w = \ln(\theta)$. Then $\theta = e^w$, and $d\theta = e^w dw$. Then we may write

$$\pi(w) = \frac{a}{e^w\sqrt{2\pi}} e^{-(a\ln e^w + b)^2/2} e^w$$

$$= \frac{a}{\sqrt{2\pi}} e^{-(aw+b)^2/2}.$$

Letting $\mu = -\sqrt{\frac{E}{4}}\, w$, we may transform $\pi(w)$ to $\pi(\mu)$.

$$\pi(w) = \frac{a}{\sqrt{2\pi}} e^{-\left(a\sqrt{\frac{4}{E}}\mu + b\right)^2/2} \sqrt{\frac{4}{E}}$$

$$= \frac{1}{\sqrt{2\pi\frac{E}{4a^2}}} e^{\frac{-1}{2\frac{E}{4a^2}}\left(\mu - \sqrt{\frac{E}{4a^2}}b\right)^2}.$$

Thus, the prior distribution of μ, $\pi(\mu)$ is normal with mean $\sqrt{E/4a^2}\, b$ and variance $\sqrt{E/4a^2}$. It is this normal distribution result that motivated the use of the log normal distribution for $\pi(\theta)$.

Our goal is to now find the distribution of Brownian motion with mean $\mu(1-I)$ and variance $(1-I)$ where μ itself is a random variable following a normal distribution with mean $\sqrt{E/4a^2}\, b$ and variance $\sqrt{E/4a^2}$.

We will solve the problem in general. Let X be a variable that follows a normal distribution with mean $\mu(1-I)$ and variance σ^2. Let μ itself follow a normal distribution with mean ϕ and variance ω^2. We must identify the unconditional probability for X. From $f_X(x) = \int f_X(x \mid \mu)\pi(u)$, we may write

$$f_X(x) = \int f_X(x \mid \mu)\pi(u)$$

$$= \int_{-\infty}^{\infty} \frac{1}{\sqrt{2\pi\sigma^2}} e^{-\frac{(x-\mu(1-I))^2}{2\sigma^2}} dx \frac{1}{\sqrt{2\pi\omega^2}} e^{-\frac{(\mu-\phi)^2}{2\omega^2}} d\mu \qquad (N.6)$$

$$= \int_{-\infty}^{\infty} \frac{1}{\sqrt{2\pi\sigma^2\omega^2}} e^{-\left[\frac{(x-\mu(1-I))^2}{2\sigma^2} + \frac{(\mu-\phi)^2}{2\omega^2}\right]} dx\, d\mu$$

Our goal will be to complete the square in the exponential, adding the terms that will allow us to carry out the integration with respect to μ following the development in Appendix I. It will then remain for us to recognize the remaining terms which will be in terms of ϕ, σ^2, and ω^2. We proceed by defining the exponent in the last line of expression (N.6) as A and writing

$$A = -\left[\frac{(x-\mu(1-I))^2}{2\sigma^2} + \frac{(\mu-\phi)^2}{2\omega^2}\right] = -\frac{1}{2}\left[\frac{(x-\mu(1-I))^2}{\sigma^2} + \frac{(\mu-\phi)^2}{\omega^2}\right]$$

$$= -\frac{1}{2}\left[\frac{\omega^2(x-\mu(1-I))^2}{\sigma^2\omega^2} + \frac{\sigma^2(\mu-\phi)^2}{\sigma^2\omega^2}\right].$$

Continuing,

$$A = \frac{-1}{2\sigma^2\omega^2}\left[\omega^2(x-\mu(1-I))^2 + \sigma^2(\mu-\phi)^2\right]$$

$$= \frac{-1}{2\sigma^2\omega^2}\left[\omega^2(x-\mu(1-I))^2 + \sigma^2(\mu-\phi)^2\right]$$

$$= \frac{-1}{2\sigma^2\omega^2}\left[\left(\omega^2+(\sigma(1-I))^2\right)\mu^2 - 2\left(\omega^2\phi+\sigma^2(1-I)x\right)\mu + \omega^2\phi^2 + \sigma^2x^2\right].$$

Define ρ as

$$\rho = \frac{\sigma^2\omega^2}{\left(\omega^2+(\sigma(1-I))^2\right)}.$$

Continuing, with the goal of substituting the value one for the coefficient of μ^2, we find

$$A = \frac{-1}{2\rho}\left[\mu^2 - 2\frac{\left(\omega^2\phi+\sigma^2(1-I)x\right)}{\omega^2+(\sigma(1-I))^2}\mu + \frac{\omega^2\phi^2+\sigma^2x^2}{\omega^2+(\sigma(1-I))^2}\right],$$

which may be rewritten as

$$A = \frac{-1}{2\rho}\left[\mu^2 - 2\frac{\left(\omega^2\phi+\sigma^2(1-I)x\right)}{\omega^2+(\sigma(1-I))^2}\mu\right] - \frac{1}{2\rho}\left[\frac{\omega^2\phi^2+\sigma^2x^2}{\omega^2+(\sigma(1-I))^2}\right]. \quad \text{(N.7)}$$

Completing the square for the term

$$\mu^2 - 2\frac{\left(\omega^2\phi+\sigma^2(1-I)x\right)}{\omega^2+(\sigma(1-I))^2}\mu,$$

we find

$$\mu^2 - 2\frac{\left(\omega^2\phi + \sigma^2(1-I)x\right)}{\omega^2 + \left(\sigma(1-I)\right)^2}\mu$$

$$= \mu^2 - 2\frac{\left(\omega^2\phi + \sigma^2(1-I)x\right)}{\omega^2 + \left(\sigma(1-I)\right)^2}\mu + \frac{\left(\omega^2\phi + \sigma^2(1-I)x\right)}{\omega^2 + \left(\sigma(1-I)\right)^2} - \frac{\left(\omega^2\phi + \sigma^2(1-I)x\right)}{\omega^2 + \left(\sigma(1-I)\right)^2} \qquad \text{(N.8)}$$

$$= \left(\mu - \frac{\left(\omega^2\phi + \sigma^2(1-I)x\right)}{\omega^2 + \left(\sigma(1-I)\right)^2}\right)^2 - \frac{\left(\omega^2\phi + \sigma^2(1-I)x\right)}{\omega^2 + \left(\sigma(1-I)\right)^2}.$$

Substituting the last line of (N.8) for $\mu^2 - 2\dfrac{\left(\omega^2\phi + \sigma^2(1-I)x\right)}{\omega^2 + \left(\sigma(1-I)\right)^2}\mu$ in expression

(N.7), we may now write

$$A = \frac{-1}{2\rho}\left(\mu - \frac{\left(\omega^2\phi + \sigma^2(1-I)x\right)}{\omega^2 + \left(\sigma(1-I)\right)^2}\right)^2 - \frac{1}{2\rho}\left[\left[\frac{\left(\omega^2\phi + \sigma^2(1-I)x\right)}{\omega^2 + \left(\sigma(1-I)\right)^2}\right]^2 - \frac{\omega^2\phi^2 + \sigma^2 x^2}{\omega^2 + \left(\sigma(1-I)\right)^2}\right]$$

$$= \frac{-1}{2\rho}\left(\mu - \frac{\left(\omega^2\phi + \sigma^2(1-I)x\right)}{\omega^2 + \left(\sigma(1-I)\right)^2}\right)^2 + C(x).$$

Returning to expression (N.6) we may write

$$f_X(x) = \int_{-\infty}^{\infty}\frac{1}{\sqrt{2\pi\sigma^2\omega^2}}e^{-\left[\frac{(x-\mu(1-I))^2}{2\sigma^2} + \frac{(\mu-\phi)^2}{2\omega^2}\right]}dxd\mu$$

$$= \frac{1}{\sqrt{2\pi\left(\omega^2 + \left(\sigma(1-I)\right)^2\right)}}e^{C(x)}\int_{-\infty}^{\infty}\frac{1}{\sqrt{2\pi\frac{\sigma^2\omega^2}{\omega^2 + \left(\sigma(1-I)\right)^2}}}e^{\frac{-1}{2\frac{\sigma^2\omega^2}{\omega^2 + (\sigma(1-I))^2}}\left(\mu - \frac{\left(\omega^2\phi + \sigma^2(1-I)x\right)}{\omega^2 + (\sigma(1-I))^2}\right)^2}du$$

$$= \frac{1}{\sqrt{2\pi\left(\omega^2 + \left(\sigma(1-I)\right)^2\right)}}e^{C(x)}.$$

The last line of this equality follows from the observation that the integrand is the probability density function of a normally distributed random variable with mean

$$\frac{\left(\omega^2\phi+\sigma^2\left(1-I\right)x\right)}{\omega^2+\left(\sigma\left(1-I\right)\right)^2}$$

and variance $\dfrac{\sigma^2\omega^2}{\omega^2+\left(\sigma\left(1-I\right)\right)^2}$. It now remains to identify $C(x)$.

$$-2\rho C(x)=\left[\frac{\omega^2\phi^2+\sigma^2 x^2}{\omega^2+\left(\sigma\left(1-I\right)\right)^2}-\frac{\left(\omega^2\phi+\sigma^2\left(1-I\right)x\right)}{\omega^2+\left(\sigma\left(1-I\right)\right)^2}\right]^2$$

$$=\frac{\left(\omega^2\phi^2+\sigma^2 x^2\right)\left(\omega^2+\left(\sigma\left(1-I\right)\right)^2\right)}{\left[\omega^2+\left(\sigma\left(1-I\right)\right)^2\right]^2}-\frac{\left(\omega^2\phi+\sigma^2\left(1-I\right)x\right)^2}{\left[\omega^2+\left(\sigma\left(1-I\right)\right)^2\right]^2}.$$

Further simplification reveals

$$-2\rho C(x)=\frac{\left(\omega^4\phi^2+\sigma^2\omega^2 x^2+\omega^2\phi^2\left(\sigma\left(1-I\right)\right)^2+\sigma^2 x^2\left(\sigma\left(1-I\right)\right)^2\right)}{\left[\omega^2+\left(\sigma\left(1-I\right)\right)^2\right]^2}$$

$$-\frac{\left(\omega^4\phi^2+2\omega^2\phi\sigma^2\left(1-I\right)x+\left(\sigma^2\left(1-I\right)x\right)^2\right)}{\left[\omega^2+\left(\sigma\left(1-I\right)\right)^2\right]^2}.$$

Cancellation of terms produces

$$C(x)=\frac{-1}{2\left(\omega^2+\left(\sigma\left(1-I\right)\right)^2\right)}\left(x^2-2\phi(1-I)x+\phi^2\left(1-I\right)^2\right)$$

$$=\frac{-1}{2\left(\omega^2+\left(\sigma\left(1-I\right)\right)^2\right)}\left(x-\phi(1-I)\right)^2.$$

Thus, the probability function of X is

$$f_X(x) = \frac{1}{\sqrt{2\pi\left(\omega^2 + \left(\sigma(1-I)\right)^2\right)}} e^{\frac{-1}{2\left(\omega^2 + \left(\sigma(1-I)\right)^2\right)}\left(x - \phi(1-I)\right)^2}.$$

a function that we recognize as a normal distribution with mean $\phi(1-I)$ and variance $\omega^2 + \left(\sigma(1-I)\right)^2$. For the setting that was discussed and elaborated in Chapter Ten, $\phi = \sqrt{E/4a^2}\, b$, $\sigma = (1-I)$, $\omega^2 = \sqrt{E/4a^2}$.

Thus

$$f_X(x) = \frac{1}{\sqrt{2\pi\left(E/4a^2 + (1-I)^4\right)}} e^{\frac{-1}{2\left(E/4a^2 + (1-I)^4\right)}\left(x - \sqrt{E/4a^2}\, b(1-I)\right)^2}.$$

Since the setting of Chapter Ten requires a mixture of probability functions, we must evaluate this normal distribution for two settings. That is, since

$$\pi(\theta) = \left(\frac{1}{2}\right)\frac{10}{\theta\sqrt{2\pi}} e^{-(10\ln\theta + 5)^2/2} + \left(\frac{1}{2}\right)\frac{10}{\theta\sqrt{2\pi}} e^{-(10\ln\theta)^2/2}$$

Then the distribution of Brownian motion is a mixture

$$f_X(x) = \frac{1}{2\sqrt{2\pi\left(5.88 + (1-I)^4\right)}} e^{\frac{-1}{2\left(5.88 + (1-I)^4\right)}(x)^2} + \frac{1}{2\sqrt{2\pi\left(5.88 + (1-I)^4\right)}} e^{\frac{-1}{2\left(5.88 + (1-I)^4\right)}\left(x - 12.12(1-I)\right)^2}.$$

Predictive Power Computation

To compute the predictive power using this prior distribution $\pi(\theta)$ and $\pi(\mu)$ we recall that the investigators chose to compute the predictive power of stopping at information time I_1 based on the value of the test statistic $TS(I_1) = s_1$. They would compute

$$P\left[TS(1)\geq 1.96\mid TS(I_1)=s\right]$$
$$=P\left[B(1)\geq 1.96 \mid B(I_1)=\sqrt{I_1}s\right] = P\left[B(1-I_1) \geq 1.96-\sqrt{I_1}s\right]$$
$$=P\left[N\left(\mu(1-I_1),(1-I_1)\right)\geq 1.96-s\sqrt{I_1}\right].$$

The right-hand side of the previous expression is a computation that would be a function of the drift parameter μ. However, we know that μ has a prior distribution. The work from the previous section demonstrates that μ is normally distributed with mean $\sqrt{E/4a^2}\,b(1-I)$ and variance $E/4a^2+(1-I)^4$. Thus, we may complete the conditional power computation by writing

$$P\left[TS(1)\geq 1.96\mid TS(I_1)=s\right]$$
$$=P\left[N\left(\mu(1-I_1),(1-I_1)\right)\geq 1.96-s\sqrt{I_1}\right]$$
$$=P\left[N\left(\sqrt{\frac{E}{4a^2}}b(1-I),\frac{E}{4a^2}+(1-I)^4\right)\geq 1.96-s\sqrt{I_1}\right].$$

Continuing, we can write

$$=P\left[N(0,1)\geq\frac{1.96\ -\ s\sqrt{I_1}\ -\ \sqrt{\dfrac{E}{4a^2}}b(1-I_1)}{\sqrt{\dfrac{E}{4a^2}+(1-I_1)^4}}\right]$$

$$=1-F_Z\left[\frac{1.96\ -\ s\sqrt{I_1}\ -\ \sqrt{\dfrac{E}{4a^2}}b(1-I_1)}{\sqrt{\dfrac{E}{4a^2}+(1-I_1)^4}}\right].$$

And the predictive power is a function of the value of test statistic s at information time I_1, and values of the parameters a and b in the prior distribution $\pi(\theta)$.

Index

Printed and bound by CPI Group (UK) Ltd, Croydon, CR0 4YY

23/10/2024

01778262-0003